Clinical Methods in
RESPIRATORY MEDICINE

Clinical Methods in RESPIRATORY MEDICINE

Second Edition

Editors

Jyotirmoy Pal
MBBS MD(General Medicine) FRCP FICP FACP WHO Fellow
Professor
Department of Medicine
College of Medicine and
Sagore Dutta Hospital
Kolkata, West Bengal, India

Nandini Chatterjee
MD FRCP(London, Glasgow) FICP
Professor
Department of Medicine
Institute of Postgraduate Medical Education and
Research (IPGMER) and SSKM Hospital
Kolkata, West Bengal, India

Supriya Sarkar
MD(Respiratory Medicine) FICP FCCP
Professor and Head
Department of Respiratory Medicine
College of Medicine and
Sagore Dutta Hospital
Kolkata, West Bengal, India

Sekhar Chakraborty
MD(Medicine) MRCP FRCP(Glasgow) FRCP(Ireland) FACP FICP
Medical Director
Kins Diabetes Speciality Centre
Siliguri, West Bengal, India
Governing Body Member of API
Vice President of IMA Bengal State Branch and
IMA Siliguri Branch

Foreword
BB Thakur

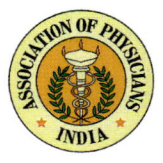 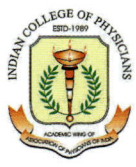

Association of Physicians of India
Indian College of Physicians

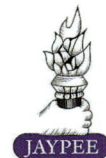

JAYPEE BROTHERS MEDICAL PUBLISHERS
The Health Sciences Publisher
New Delhi | London

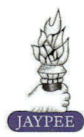

Jaypee Brothers Medical Publishers (P) Ltd

Headquarters
EMCA House
23/23-B, Ansari Road, Daryaganj
New Delhi 110 002, India
Landline: +91-11-23272143, +91-11-23272703
+91-11-23282021, +91-11-23245672
E-mail: jaypee@jaypeebrothers.com

Corporate Office
Jaypee Brothers Medical Publishers (P) Ltd.
4838/24, Ansari Road, Daryaganj
New Delhi 110 002, India
Phone: +91-11-43574357
Fax: +91-11-43574314
E-mail: jaypee@jaypeebrothers.com

Overseas Office
JP Medical Ltd.
83, Victoria Street, London
SW1H 0HW (UK)
Phone: +44-20 3170 8910
Fax: +44(0)20 3008 6180
E-mail: info@jpmedpub.com

Website: www.jaypeebrothers.com
Website: www.jaypeedigital.com

© 2025, Jaypee Brothers Medical Publishers

The views and opinions expressed in this book are solely those of the original contributor(s)/author(s) and do not necessarily represent those of editor(s) or publisher of the book.

All rights reserved. No part of this publication may be reproduced, stored or transmitted in any form or by any means, electronic, mechanical, photocopying, recording or otherwise, without the prior permission in writing of the publishers.

All brand names and product names used in this book are trade names, service marks, trademarks or registered trademarks of their respective owners. The publisher is not associated with any product or vendor mentioned in this book.

Medical knowledge and practice change constantly. This book is designed to provide accurate, authoritative information about the subject matter in question. However, readers are advised to check the most current information available on procedures included and check information from the manufacturer of each product to be administered, to verify the recommended dose, formula, method and duration of administration, adverse effects and contraindications. It is the responsibility of the practitioner to take all appropriate safety precautions. Neither the publisher nor the author(s)/editor(s) assume any liability for any injury and/or damage to persons or property arising from or related to use of material in this book.

This book is sold on the understanding that the publisher is not engaged in providing professional medical services. If such advice or services are required, the services of a competent medical professional should be sought.

Every effort has been made where necessary to contact holders of copyright to obtain permission to reproduce copyright material. If any have been inadvertently overlooked, the publisher will be pleased to make the necessary arrangements at the first opportunity.

Inquiries for bulk sales may be solicited at: jaypee@jaypeebrothers.com

Clinical Methods in Respiratory Medicine / Jyotirmoy Pal, Nandini Chatterjee, Supriya Sarkar, Sekhar Chakraborty

First Edition: 2018
Second Edition: **2025**
ISBN: 978-93-6616-445-8
Printed at: Samrat Offset Pvt. Ltd.

Dedicated To

(Late) Dr YP Munjal

Contributors

AG Ghoshal MD DNB
FCCP(Pulmonary Medicine)
Medical Director
National Allergy Asthma
Bronchitis Institute
Kolkata, West Bengal, India

Angira Das Gupta MD
DNB(Respiratory Diseases)
MRCP(UK)
Consultant Pulmonologist
Department of Respiratory
Diseases
BR Singh Hospital and Centre for
Medical Education and Research
Kolkata, West Bengal, India

Arunabha Datta Chaudhuri
MD(Pulmonary Medicine)
Professor
Department of Pulmonary
Medicine
RG Kar Medical College and
Hospital
Kolkata, West Bengal, India

Atin Dey MD(Pulmonary Medicine)
Professor
Department of Pulmonary
Medicine
RG Kar Medical College and
Hospital
Kolkata, West Bengal, India

Bhoomi Angirish MD DNB FRCR
Assistant Professor
Department of Radiology
GMERS Medical College
Himmatnagar, Gujarat, India

Biva Bhakat MD(General
Medicine) MBBS DM Neurology(PDT)
Resident
Department of Neurology
Medical College, Kolkata
Kolkata, West Bengal, India

Dhiman Ganguly MD(General
Medicine) MRCP(UK)
Consultant Pulmonologist
Calcutta Heart Clinic and
Hospital, Salt Lake
Kolkata, West Bengal, India

Indranil Halder DCH(Cal) MD(Cal)
FCCP(USA) FICP FICS European
Diploma in Adult Respiratory
Medicine FRCP(Glasgow)
Associate Professor
Department of Pulmonary
Medicine
College of Medicine and JNM
Hospital, Kalyani
Kolkata, West Bengal, India

Jaydip Deb MD(Pulmonary
Medicine)
Professor
Department of Pulmonary
Medicine
NRS Medical College and
Hospital
Kolkata, West Bengal, India

Jyotirmoy Pal MBBS MD(General
Medicine) FRCP FICP FACP WHO
Fellow
Professor
Department of Medicine
College of Medicine and
Sagore Dutta Hospital
Kolkata, West Bengal, India

Nandini Chatterjee MD
FRCP(London, Glasgow) FICP
Professor
Department of Medicine
Institute of Postgraduate
Medical Education and Research
(IPGMER) and SSKM Hospital
Kolkata, West Bengal, India

Pradip Kumar Chowdhury MD
RMO-Cum Clinical Tutor
Department of Pulmonary
Medicine, RG Kar Medical
College and Hospital
Kolkata, West Bengal, India

Raja Dhar MBBS MD(Chest
Medicine) FRCP(London, UK)
FCCP(USA) CCT(Respiratory and
General Medicine, UK) MSc(Evidence-
Based Medicine, UK)
Director and Head
Department of Pulmonology
Calcutta Medical Research
Institute
Kolkata, West Bengal, India

Sekhar Chakraborty
MD(Medicine) MRCP FRCP(Glasgow)
FRCP(Ireland) FACP FICP
Medical Director
Kins Diabetes Speciality Centre
Siliguri, West Bengal, India
Governing Body Member of API
Vice President of IMA Bengal
State Branch and
IMA Siliguri Branch

Shubham Sharma DNB Trainee
2nd Year
Department of Pulmonology
Fortis Hospital
Kolkata, West Bengal, India

Shyam Krishnan
DNB(Respiratory Medicine)
Senior Resident
Department of Pulmonology
Fortis Hospital
Kolkata, West Bengal, India

Contributors

Subhadeep Gupta MBBS
Junior Resident
Department of Medicine
RG Kar Medical College and Hospital
Kolkata, West Bengal, India

Subhadip Mukherjee
DNB(Internal Medicine)
Department of Medicine
BR Singh Hospital and Centre for Medical Education and Research
Kolkata, West Bengal, India

Subhasis Mukherjee
MD(Respiratory Medicine)
Associate Professor
Department of Respiratory Medicine
College of Medicine and Sagore Dutta Hospital
Kolkata, West Bengal, India

Subhra Mitra MD(Pulmonary Medicine) DTCD MRCP(UK)
Professor and Head
Department of Pulmonary Medicine
Calcutta National Medical College
Kolkata, West Bengal, India

Subir Kumar Dey MBBS DTMCH DTCD MD(TCD) FNCCP(I)
Ex-Head, Chest Medicine
NMC Kolkatta
Director, DE's Research Centre
Howrah
Kolkata, West Bengal, India

Sukanta Kumar Dey BDS MDS
Assistant Professor
Awadh Dental College and Hospital
Director, DE's Research Centre, Howrah
Kolkata, West Bengal, India

Sumit Roy Tapadar MD (Pulmonary Medicine)
Associate Professor
Department of Pulmonary Medicine
RG Kar Medical College and Hospital
Kolkata, West Bengal, India

Supriya Sarkar MD(Respiratory Medicine) FICP FCCP
Professor and Head
Department of Respiratory Medicine
College of Medicine and Sagore Dutta Hospital
Kolkata, West Bengal, India

Surya Kant MD(Gold Medalist) MNAMS FCCP(USA) FIMSA FNCCP FCAI FIAB FICS FUPDA FIAMS FIACM
Professor and Head
Department of Respiratory Medicine
King George's Medical University
Lucknow, Uttar Pradesh, India

Tanuka Mandal MD(General Medicine)
Consultant
Department of General Medicine
RG Kar Medical College and Hospital
Kolkata, West Bengal, India

Udas Chandra Ghosh MBBS MD(Medicine) DNB(Medicine) DNB(Respiratory Diseases) DTCD FICP FRCP(Glasgow)
Professor
Department of Medicine
Medical College, Kolkata
Kolkata, West Bengal, India

Uddalok Chakraborty
MD(Internal Medicine)
DM(Neurology)
Senior Resident
Department of Neurology
Bangur Institute of Neurosciences
IPGMER and SSKM Hospital
Kolkata, West Bengal, India

Foreword

It is indeed a great pleasure to write about the compendium on *"Clinical Methods in Respiratory Medicine"* edited jointly by professor Jyotirmoy Pal, professor Nandini Chatterjee, professor Supriya Sarkar, and Dr Sekhar Chakrabarty.

For hundreds of years, the history and physical examination have been the most powerful tools to understand the patient's clinical mysteries. During my career as a medical student, the science of medicine was in the primitive stage, and we had to depend on clinical workup for diagnosis and management of the patients, and in more than half of the patients, the history used to be the main determinant. Currently with a limited or no physical examination, a long list of laboratory and imaging tests to be done is handed over to the patients. However, even the proper choice of tests depends on a good differential diagnosis based on a good clinical examination. In addition to that a careful questioning and examination strengthens the doctor–patient relationship, builds the patient's confidence in the doctor, and makes them feel that the doctor cares.

As physical examination skills have declined, fewer physicians are confident enough in their skills to teach routinely at the bedside. Teaching rounds that used to be spent in the presence of the patient are now relegated to the hallway or conference room. Time spent with patients is also more fragmented and fraught with distractions due to the electronic health record, pages, phone calls, and texts.

Due to overall apathy toward the clinical medicine, the American Medical Association held a large funeral service for the physical examination on September 14, 2016. A moving tribute was planned in which multiple healthcare providers demonstrated aspects of the physical examination; however, no one could remember any maneuvers.

Against this backdrop of, the authors have done a commendable job of bringing out a book on *"Clinical Methods in Respiratory Medicine"*. The clinical examination, a forgotten art and science of medicine, has very diligently been described. It encompasses the basic sciences of pulmonology like the anatomy and physiology, the clinical signs and symptoms, the basic investigations along with pulmonary function test, the stepwise approach to arterial blood gas (ABG) analysis, CT thorax, etc. Molecular diagnosis of tuberculosis and newer guidelines of the National Tuberculosis Elimination Program (NTEP) have also been nicely covered.

I enjoyed going through the manuscript of this book, which has a wealth of updated informations on different facets of *"Clinical Methods in Respiratory Medicine"*.

To author such a book, strong desire, determination, and dedication are required along with tremendous commitment and concentration, which is the foundation stone of such book. They must have spent many sleepless nights in selecting the most erudite teachers in respiratory medicine for sharing their thoughts to bring out such informative book.

I am confident that the wealth of information embedded in this book is going to be a treasure for all clinicians and postgraduates for both teaching and clinical practice.

The clinicians can maximize the value of time spent with patients and renew the importance of the clinical examination in 21st century.

The authors need to be complimented and congratulated for their efforts.

BB Thakur
MD FRCP FICP FIAMS FIACM FACP FISPD
Consultant Physician
Past Dean, Indian College of Physicians
Past President, Hypertension Society of India
Past President, Association of Physicians of India
Professor and Head, Department of Medicine (Retired)
Sri Krishna Medical College and Hospital
Muzaffarpur, Bihar, India

Preface

In spite of advancement of technology, the art of history taking and clinical examination have immense importance in clinical diagnosis and management. Clinical evaluation can help us in judicious and cost-effective use of diagnostic tools. Respiratory manifestations and disorders are possibly the most common challenges encountered by practicing physicians on one hand and by students in their examination on the other.

From this point of view, we tried to highlight clinical anatomy and physiology useful to understand respiratory diseases. We have elaborated common symptoms of respiratory diseases such as cough, sputum, hemoptysis, chest pain, and dyspnea. General examination is described in details and in a useful manner. Short case depictions with accompanying FAQs have been explained.

Respiratory system examination and interpretation also have incorporated that will be useful to both undergraduate and postgraduate students. Attempts have been made to include important diagnostic tools, new treatment guidelines along with National Tuberculosis Elimination Program as well.

We sincerely hope that this book will clear doubts and act as a ready reckoner for daily practice.

We are thankful to our authors and our publisher M/s Jaypee Brothers Medical Publishers (P) Ltd, New Delhi, India for bringing out this edition before APICON 2025. Lastly, we express our deepest respect to our mentors Late Professor YP Munjal, Professor BB Thakur, Dr Manotosh Panja, and Dr Amal Banerjee without whose guidance this book would not have seen the light of day.

Jyotirmoy Pal
Nandini Chatterjee
Supriya Sarkar
Sekhar Chakraborty

Contents

CHAPTER 1 **Introduction: A Clinical Approach to Respiratory Medicine** 1
Supriya Sarkar
- Collection of Clinical Data *1*
- Analysis of Individual Manifestation *2*
- Grouping of Clinical Manifestations *2*
- Understanding the Clinical Course of Disease *2*
- Analysis of Positive and Negative Clues *3*
- Identification and Analysis of Clinical Pattern *3*
- Interposing Epidemiology Over Clinical Pattern *4*
- Application of Clinical Expertise *4*

CHAPTER 2 **Clinical Anatomy of Thorax** 5
Arunabha Datta Chaudhuri
- Basic Anatomy of Thorax *5*
- The Anatomy of Airways *7*
- Anatomy of Lung, Pleura, and Diaphragm *9*
- Surface Anatomy *17*

CHAPTER 3 **Basic Science in Pulmonology** 21
Dhiman Ganguly
- The Blood Gases *21*
- The Oxygen Cascade *23*
- The Carbon Dioxide Story *25*
- Regulation of Respiration *28*

CHAPTER 4 **Clinical Approach and Analysis of Respiratory Symptoms** 31
Angira Das Gupta, Subhadip Mukherjee, Nandini Chatterjee,
Supriya Sarkar, Surya Kant, Raja Dhar, Shubham Sharma, Biva Bhakat,
Subhasis Mukherjee

A. Clinical Approach to Cough and Expectoration 31
Angira Das Gupta, Subhadip Mukherjee, Nandini Chatterjee, Supriya Sarkar
- What are the Causes of Cough? *32*
- Case Vignette 1 *35*
- Case Vignette 2 *38*
- Case Vignette 3 *38*

B. Clinical Approach to Hemoptysis 42
Surya Kant, Nandini Chatterjee
- Etiology 42
- Approach to Patient 42
- Investigations 44
- Case Vignette 46

C. Clinical Approach to Chest pain 49
Raja Dhar, Shubham Sharma, Supriya Sarkar
- Etiology 49
- Cardiac Causes of Chest Pain 49
- Pulmonary Causes of Chest Pain 52
- Musculoskeletal Causes of Chest Pain 56
- Psychiatric Causes of Chest Pain 56
- Other Causes of Chest Pain 56
- Case Vignette 57

D. Clinical Approach to Dyspnea 61
Supriya Sarkar, Nandini Chatterjee, Biva Bhakat
- Definition of Dyspnea 61
- Etiology of Dyspnea 61
- Approach to Dyspnea 63
- Case Vignette 1 66
- Case Vignette 2 68

E. Clinical Approach to Cyanosis 70
Subhasis Mukherjee, Nandini Chatterjee
- Pathophysiology of Cyanosis 70
- Causes of Cyanosis 71
- Types of Cyanosis 72
- Clinical Approach to a Patient with Cyanosis 73
- Limitations 74
- Case Vignette 75

CHAPTER 5 General Examination 77
Jyotirmoy Pal, Pradip Kumar Choudhury, Subhodeep Gupta, Tanuka Mondal, Uddalok Chakraborty
- Introduction and First Impression 77
- Appropriate Setting for Examination 78
- Examination of Higher Function or Cognition 78
- Posture and Decubitus 83
- Pallor 84
- Cyanosis 86
- Clubbing 87
- Edema 90

- Jaundice *93*
- Blood Pressure *94*
- Pulse *99*
- Respiration *104*
- Fever *110*
- Jugular Venous Pressure *113*
- Oral Examination *117*
- Tongue *118*
- Gait *120*
- Skin Lesions *121*
- Pigmentation *123*
- Generalized Lymphadenopathy *124*
- Anthropometry *127*
- Nutrition *130*
- Different Type of Nails in Clinical Medicine *133*
- Examination of Eyes *136*
- Face Examination *140*
- Hand Examination *144*
- Hair *151*

CHAPTER 6 Evaluation of Respiratory System 153
Supriya Sarkar
- Upper Respiratory Tract *153*
- Examination of Lower Respiratory System *154*

CHAPTER 7 Basic Investigations: Indications and Interpretations 169
Subir Kumar Dey, Sukanta Kumar Dey, AG Ghoshal, Shyam Krishnan, Udas Chandra Ghosh, Sekhar Chakraborty, Indranil Halder, Subhra Mitra, Jaydip Deb, Sumit Roy Tapadar

A. Examination of Sputum 169
Subir Kumar Dey, Sukanta Kumar Dey
- Sputum Analysis *169*
- How to Obtain a Sputum Sample? *170*
- Microscopic Features of Sputum *170*
- Clinical Application of Sputum in the Diagnosis of Pulmonary Diseases *171*
- Sputum Examination in Revised National Tuberculosis Control Program *172*

B1. Interpreting the Chest X-ray 174
AG Ghoshal, Shyam Krishnan
- Technical Aspects *174*
- Technique for Radiograph Viewing *176*
- Common Radiological Signs *180*

B2. Role of Chest X-ray (Lateral View) in Respiratory System 183
Udas Chandra Ghosh
- Importance of Lateral View *184*
- Clinical Importance *185*

C. Arterial Blood Gas Analysis—A Step-wise Approach 189
Sekhar Chakraborty
- Applications of Arterial Blood Gas *189*
- Step-wise Approach to Analyze Arterial Blood Gas *189*
- Case Vignette 1 *194*
- Case Vignette 2 *195*
- Case Vignette 3 *195*
- Case Vignette 4 *196*
- Case Vignette 5 *197*
- Case Vignette 6 *197*

D. Interpretation of the Spirometry 198
Indranil Halder
- Selecting the Best Value for Clinical Use *198*
- Calculating the Reference *198*
- Reporting the Spirometry Results *199*
- Types of Ventilatory Defects *199*
- Severity Classification *201*
- Bronchodilator Response *202*
- Central and Upper Airway Obstruction *202*

E. Investigations for Pleural Diseases 204
Subhra Mitra
- Thoracentesis *204*
- Imaging Study *207*
- Pleural Biopsy *211*
- Undiagnosed Pleural Effusion *212*

F. Basic Approach to Computed Tomography of Thorax 214
Bhoomi Angirish
- Technique *214*
- Image Reconstruction Techniques *215*
- High-resolution CT Anatomy *216*
- Patterns on High-resolution CT *216*
- Spatial Distribution of Disease *226*
- Airways Disease *227*
- Mediastinum *228*
- Pleura *229*
- Chest Wall *230*

G. Molecular Diagnosis of Tuberculosis 232
Sumit Roy Tapadar
- Nucleic Acid Amplification Test *232*
- Cbnaat (Xpert MTB/RIF) *232*
- CBNAAT Report Interpretation—Some Examples *235*
- Line Probe Assay *236*

CHAPTER 8 National Tuberculosis Elimination Program 238
Supriya Sarkar, Surya Kant, Arunava Dutta Choudhury
- Revised National TB Control Program *238*
- National Tuberculosis Elimination Program *239*
- National TB Prevalence Survey 2019–2021 *239*
- Diagnosis of TB in National Tuberculosis Elimination Program *240*
- Management of TB in National Tuberculosis Elimination Programme *241*
- Follow-up of TB Patients *242*
- Management of Drug-resistant TB *242*
- Extrapulmonary TB *245*
- Notification of TB *245*
- TB Prevention Treatment *245*
- Active Case Finding *246*
- Certification of Elimination of TB *246*
- Training and Research Activities *246*
- Strategies for Private Sector *246*
- Future Suggested Changes in National Tuberculosis Elimination Program *247*

Index 249

CHAPTER 1

Introduction: A Clinical Approach to Respiratory Medicine

Supriya Sarkar

Junior doctors are often confused, whether they should select the shortcut of modern technology or they should take the age-old, long, tough, and difficult path of clinical medicine. The question may come, is clinical medicine relevant today? Even in today's era of modern technology, clinical medicine has not lost its relevance. In fact, clinical medicine is more relevant now. Today any delay or any advancement of investigation will be questioned by patients and their family members, and they may drag the matter to the court of law. As e.g., common possibilities in a patient having chronic cough are tuberculosis, asthma, chronic obstructive pulmonary disease (COPD), postnasal dripping, gastroesophageal reflux, or lung malignancy. Every condition needs specific investigation to establish the diagnosis. In our country, due to financial and other reasons, a battery of investigations is not possible. Failure to prescribe appropriate investigation will cause trouble to patients as well as to doctors.

The art of medicine is a combination of medical knowledge, intuition, experience, and judgment. Medical decision making is an important responsibility of physicians. It is important at each stage of diagnosis and therapeutic process. Clinical data analysis is a systemic effort to achieve a provisional diagnosis or to narrow differential diagnosis to least number of possible probabilities, and to plan least number of investigations. Clinical data analysis requires knowledge, experience, analytic skill, and most importantly time to spend with patient.

■ COLLECTION OF CLINICAL DATA

Collecting relevant clinical information, as much as possible, is essential before going to next step. Collection of clinical data from patients and patients' relatives (detail sleep event or daytime sleepiness) is the most essential and important step. It should be informative, complete, and perfect; otherwise next steps will be ineffective. It is important to remember that we are dealing with a human being who has sentiments, personality, ego, and self-respect.

During history taking, we may have to ask personal questions. It is important to make patient comfortable. An emphatic attitude is essential for extracting necessary information. A clear knowledge and understanding of diseases will help the process. Similarly, during examination, we must be careful and should not hurt patients' sentiment, privacy, and ego. While examining private areas, always explain him/her about what, how, and why this is done. For better elicitation of physical signs, it is essential that both patient and doctor are comfortable at the time of examination. As e.g., important abdominal findings may not be elicited if the patient makes his/her abdomen tough.

Chest X-ray is now considered a part of clinical examination of respiratory system. Many lung diseases, particularly in deep seated lung pathology surrounded by normal lung parenchyma, may not yield any clinical sign. In those situations, chest X-ray can give an initial idea about the disease that can suggest future investigation protocol.

It is important to remember that history (questionnaires) may have to be taken many times (at least thrice). Firstly, at the beginning, history is taken to have an idea about the disease. Secondly, after completion of physical examination. Thirdly, after completion of investigations, some questions or points need to be clarified. As e.g., high-resolution computed tomography (CT) scan thorax shows usual interstitial pneumonia (UIP) pattern then to confirm the diagnosis of idiopathic pulmonary fibrosis (IPF), and you have to exclude other causes by asking some questions such as drug history.

■ ANALYSIS OF INDIVIDUAL MANIFESTATION

After collecting information, next step is to critically analyze each symptom or sign. As e.g., a chest pain may arise from chest wall, pleura, mediastinum, pericardium, or myocardium. By a detailed review of chest pain, the probable origin of chest pain is to be determined. Every effort is to be made to differentiate them with some degree of reasonable certainty.

■ GROUPING OF CLINICAL MANIFESTATIONS

After analyzing each manifestation, the next step is to group few symptoms and signs into a meaningful combination that will reflect some pathology. As e.g., fever with chill, impaired percussion note without shift of mediastinum and bronchial breath sound with crepitations indicate consolidation. A combination of cough without expectoration, dyspnea without wheeze, and bilateral mainly basal end inspiratory crepitations suggest interstitial/alveolar involvement. The identification of such pathology will direct you to plan for further investigation and symptomatic treatment.

■ UNDERSTANDING THE CLINICAL COURSE OF DISEASE

Clinical course means onset, duration, progression, interval, and chronology of manifestation. Onset may be acute or chronic. Acute onset means when patient can definitely tell the starting of disease or symptoms like fever for 10 days, dyspnea for 1 week, etc. Insidious onset means when patient cannot tell when the manifestation started, as e.g., the patient is telling that he has fever for 2–3 months (as if 2 and 3 months are equal), and that may suggest chronic inflammation such as tuberculosis. Sudden onset is a subset of acute onset when patients can pinpoint the moment from where the disease has been started. Examples of sudden onset diseases are pneumothorax and any vascular event such as pulmonary thromboembolism. Duration-wise, clinical manifestations are classified into acute, subacute, and chronic. Cough with profuse purulent expectoration and local crepitations may indicate lung abscess if history is of short duration, but the same manifestations of longer duration will point toward bronchiectasis. Symptoms may be progressive without symptom-free intervals, and with or without episodes of exacerbations as in case of COPD, interstitial lung disease, cardiomyopathy, etc. On the other hand, disease may be episodic with symptom-free intervals as in case of asthma. Chronology of manifestations is also helpful as, e.g., a sudden onset of pleuritic chest pain followed by dyspnea and that event starts with a bout of cough is almost suggestive of pneumothorax.

■ ANALYSIS OF POSITIVE AND NEGATIVE CLUES

Proper identification and analysis of every positive or negative clue are an important step. The identification of overt and covert risk factors is a distinctive step. As e.g., for the diagnosis of COPD, it is essential to take history of smoking (overt clue) and biomass fuel exposure (covert clue). Similarly, in a tuberculosis patient with persistent hypotension, the finding of pigmentations in tongue or oral mucosa suggests Addition's disease due to bilateral adrenal gland involvement. Negative clues are equally important. As e.g., in a case of pleural effusion, the absence of pleuritic chest pain, a sign of pleural inflammation, may point against tuberculosis and may favor malignancy. The absence of crepitation including post-tussive crepitation practically rules out lung parenchymal fibrosis. Negative clues should be analyzed with caution as the absence of obliteration of Traube's space usually excludes left-sided pleural effusion, but that does not completely exclude encysted pleural effusion.

■ IDENTIFICATION AND ANALYSIS OF CLINICAL PATTERN

Clinicians identify a clinical pattern where each manifestation is important, but overall clinical picture is more important. Scoring systems for the diagnosis of certain disease, such as allergic bronchopulmonary aspergillosis, may be considered a scientifically grafted form of pattern identification. A male patient with positive diagnostic scoring for rheumatoid arthritis develops pleural effusion; we should consider rheumatoid pleural effusion along with other possibilities. But similar clinical picture in a female patient less likely indicates rheumatoid effusion as pleural involvement in rheumatoid arthritis is less common in female. Pattern identification needs knowledge as well as experience. Experience may be acquired directly by observing cases or may be acquired from reading books or case reports.

It is not sufficient to identify a clinical pattern, but we should interpose the pattern on the background of clinical setting. As e.g., a 60-year-old smoker with superior vena caval obstruction, we should suspect lung malignancy. On the other hand, a 30-year-old nonsmoker with superior vena caval obstruction with cervical lymphadenopathy points to lymphoma.

■ INTERPOSING EPIDEMIOLOGY OVER CLINICAL PATTERN

Epidemiology is not a paraclinical subject, but all physicians are using it as an assisting tool in clinical medicine, probably not appreciating its influence. Viral infections are often identified by their epidemiological pattern such as influenza, swine flu, and hepatitis. A right upper lobe fibrocavitary disease may suggest tuberculosis in India, melioidosis in Vietnam, or histoplasmosis in Northern America.

■ APPLICATION OF CLINICAL EXPERTISE

Clinical expertise is the most complicated thing to explain. Clinical expertise is a combination of scientific knowledge, experience, prudence, analytic, and problem-solving capability. Clinical expertise requires not only cognitive proficiency, integration of verbal and visual information but also complex fine motor skills necessary for invasive and noninvasive procedures. Clinical expertise can be acquired through experience.

We know that during clinical examination, some incidental finding may be uncovered that is completely unrelated to the clinical problem at hand. Clinical reasoning is the skill for deciding whether a clinical clue is worth pursuing or should be diminished in totality.

Clinical judgment is a process that will help in selecting investigation or treatment protocol. Whether bronchoscopy will be helpful in a particular hypoxic patient? Whether patient can tolerate lung biopsy? Whether patient can tolerate chemotherapy? Risk-benefit and cost-effective analysis are parts of clinical judgment. It is an essential skill that every clinician must possess and apply.

■ CONCLUSION

Clinical medicine is an art of possibilities and probabilities. It is an interesting and challenging job. Clinical medicine is a journey where surprise is waiting for you at every bend. Please enjoy the challenge and learn it throughout your life as there is no end of this journey. When you can combine clinical medicine with modern technologies, you will be a good clinician.

SUGGESTED READINGS

1. Kasper DL, Hauser SL, Jameson JL, Gauci AS, Longo DL, Loscalzo J. Harrison's Principles of Internal Medicine. 19th edition. McGraw-Hill Education, New York, 2017. pp. 18-25, 95-102, 123-6, 243-6, 1661-2.
2. Munro JF, Campbell IW. Macleod's Clinical Examination. 7th edition. ELBS. Reprinted 1987. pp. 1-16, 54-96.

CHAPTER 2

Clinical Anatomy of Thorax

Arunabha Datta Chaudhuri

■ INTRODUCTION

The clinical anatomy of the thorax is a vital area of study that focuses on the structures within the chest cavity, which includes the heart, lungs, major blood vessels, and the components of the respiratory and cardiovascular systems. Understanding the thoracic anatomy is crucial for medical professionals, particularly in diagnosing and treating conditions related to the heart, lungs, and other thoracic organs.

The thoracic cavity is bordered by the ribs, sternum, and vertebral column, forming a protective structure for the vital organs. The lungs, responsible for gas exchange, occupy most of the cavity, while the heart lies centrally within the mediastinum. Other key structures include the trachea, esophagus, diaphragm, and major blood vessels such as the aorta, superior vena cava, and pulmonary arteries and veins.

Clinical knowledge of thoracic anatomy is essential for a wide range of medical procedures, including chest tube insertion, mechanical ventilation, cardiac surgery, and diagnosing conditions such as pneumonia, pleurisy, pulmonary embolism, and heart failure. By comprehending the anatomical relationships within the thorax, healthcare professionals can accurately assess symptoms, interpret diagnostic imaging, and perform interventions to improve patient outcomes. This understanding is foundational for both medical education and clinical practice.

■ BASIC ANATOMY OF THORAX

The thorax is a region of the body between neck and abdomen. The frame of work of the walls of the thorax (thoracic cage) is formed by the vertebral column behind the ribs and intercostal spaces on either side and the sternum and the costal cartilages in front. The cavity of the thorax can be divided into median partitions called the mediastinum and the laterally placed pleura and the lungs.

The thoracic cage communicates above through the "thoracic inlet" with the root of the neck; and below, it is separated from the abdominal cavity by the diaphragm.

The thoracic cavity communicates with the route of the neck through an opening called thoracic inlet, which is bounded posteriorly by the first thoracic vertebra, laterally by the medial borders of the first ribs and their costal cartilage and anteriorly by the superior border of the manubrium sterni. Esophagus, trachea, major vessels, and nerves pass through thoracic inlet. The apices of the lung and the pleura projects upward into the neck because of the obliquity of the opening.

The thoracic cavity communicated with the abdomen through a large opening, covered by the diaphragm, which is bounded posteriorly by the 12th thoracic vertebra, laterally by the costal margin and anteriorly by the xiphisternal joint. The esophagus, descending aorta, and inferior vena cava pass though separate openings and small vessels and nerves pierce through the diaphragm.

The Intercostal Spaces

There are slight variations between the different intercostal spaces, but typically each space contains three muscles, comparable to those of the abdominal wall, and an associated neurovascular bundle. The muscles are: (1) External intercostal muscles; (2) internal intercostal muscles, and (3) innermost intercostal muscles, those are incompletely separated from internal intercostal muscle by the neurovascular bundles.

Like their counterpart in abdomen, the nerves and vessels of the thoracic wall lie between the middle and innermost layers of muscles. This neurovascular bundle consists of vein, artery, and nerve from above downward. Intercostal veins lie in grooves on the undersurface of the corresponding ribs.

Important Surface Markings

- Superior angle of the scapula (T2)
- Upper border of the manubrium sterni, the suprasternal notch (T2/3)
- Spine of the scapula (T3)
- Sternal angle (of Louis)—the transverse ridge at the manubriosternal junction (T4/5)
- Inferior angle of scapula (T8)
- Xiphisternal joint (T9)

Since the first and 12th ribs are difficult to feel, the ribs should be counted from the second costal cartilage, which articulates with the sternum at the angle of Louis. The spinous processes of all the thoracic vertebrae can be palpated in the midline posteriorly, but it should be remembered that the first spinous process that can be felt is that of C7 vertebra prominence. The *trachea* is palpable in the suprasternal notch midway between the heads of the two clavicles.

Clinical Importance

- *Thoracic outlet syndrome*: The brachial plexus of nerves (C5–C8, and T1) and the subclavian artery and vein are closely related to the upper surface of the first ribs and the clavicle. The nerves or the blood vessels may be compressed here between bones. Most of the symptoms are caused by pressure on the lower trunk of the plexus, producing pain on the medial side

of the forearm, and the hand and wasting of the small muscles of the hand and pressure on the blood vessel may compromise the circulation of the upper limb.
- Local irritation of the intercostal nerves by conditions such as Pott's disease of the thoracic vertebrae (tuberculosis) may give rise to pain, which is referred to the front of the chest or abdomen in the region of the peripheral termination of the nerves.
- Local anesthesia of an intercostal space is easily produced by infiltration around the intercostal nerve trunk and its collateral branch—a procedure known as *intercostal nerve block*. During intercostal nerve block, the needle is directed toward the rib near the lower border, and the tip comes to the rest near the subcostal groove, where the local anesthetics are infiltrated around the nerve.
- Pus from the region of the vertebral column tends to track around the thorax along the course of the neurovascular bundle and to three "point" of exit (lateral to erector spinae, in the midaxillary line and just lateral to the sternum) of the cutaneous branches of the intercostal nerves.
- Fractures of the ribs are common in chest injuries. The ribs prone to fracture as they are relatively fixed. Fifth to tenth ribs are commonly fractured. The first four ribs are protected by the clavicle and pectoral muscles anteriorly and by the scapula and its associated muscles posteriorly. The 11th and 12th ribs are floating ribs, and they move with the force of impact. During the impact, the jagged end of a fractured rib may penetrate into the lungs and may produce pneumothorax. Flail chest is an emergency condition that occurs due to severe crush injuries commonly by road traffic accidents. Multiple ribs may be fractured near the rib angles posteriorly and near the costochondral junctions anteriorly. Flail chest is characterized by multiple rib fractures at two ends as a result that part is disconnected to the rest of the thoracic wall. The stability of the chest wall is lost, and the flail segments are sucked in during inspiration and driven out during expiration, producing paradoxical and ineffective respiratory movements.

■ THE ANATOMY OF AIRWAYS

Airway anatomy can be further subdivided into the following two segments: (1) Extrathoracic airway including the supraglottic region, glottis, and infraglottic region of larynx and upper part of trachea, and (2) intrathoracic airways including lower part of trachea, right and left main bronchi, lobar, segmental and subsequent generations of bronchi, and bronchioles up to terminal bronchioles. Bronchioles can be differentiated from bronchus by the absence of cartilages and mucosal glands. Air passages distal to terminal bronchioles are included in lung parenchyma as in respiratory bronchioles, alveolar ducts, and alveolar sac the diffusion process takes place.

The Trachea

The trachea is about 4.5 inches (11.5 cm) in length and nearly 1 inch (2.5 cm) in diameter. It commences at the lower border of the cricoid cartilage (C6) and terminates by bifurcating at the level of the sternal angle of Louis (T4/5) to form the right and left main bronchi (Carina). In the living subject, the level of bifurcation varies slightly with the phase of respiration; in deep inspiration it descends to T6, and in expiration it rises to T4. The patency of the trachea is maintained by a series of 15–20 "U"-shaped cartilages. Posteriorly, where the cartilage is deficient, the trachea is flattened and its wall completed by fibrous tissue and a sheet of smooth muscles (the trachealis). Mucous membrane of trachea is lined by a ciliated columnar epithelium with many goblet cells.

Clinical Importance

- In the neck, a unilateral or bilateral enlargement of thyroid gland can cause gross displacement or compression of the trachea.
- The intimate relationship between the arch of the aorta and the trachea and left bronchus is responsible for the physical sign known as "tracheal-tug", characteristic of aneurysms of the aortic arch. With each cardiac systole, the pulsating aneurysm may tug at the trachea and left bronchus, a clinical sign that can be felt by palpating the trachea in the suprasternal notch.

The Bronchi

The *right main bronchus* is wider, shorter, and more vertical than the left. It is about 1 inch (2.5 cm) long and passes directly to the root of the lung at T5. Before joining the lung, it gives off its *upper lobe branch* and then passes below the pulmonary artery to enter the hilum of the lung. On entering the hilum, it divides into a middle and inferior lobar bronchus. It has two important relations: (1) The azygos vein, which arches over it from behind to reach the superior vena cava (SVC); and (2) the pulmonary artery, which lies first below and then anterior to it. The *left main bronchus* is nearly 2 inches (5 cm) long and passes downward and outward below the arch of the aorta, in front of the esophagus and descending aorta. Unlike the right, it gives off no branches until it enters the hilum of the lung. The pulmonary artery spirals over the bronchus, lying first anteriorly and then above it. On entering the hilum of left lung, it divides into a superior and inferior lobar bronchus.

Clinical Importance

- The greater width and more vertical course of the right bronchus accounts for the greater tendency for foreign bodies and aspirated material to pass into the right bronchus and then especially into lower lobes of the right lung rather than into the left.
- Widening and distortion of the angle between the bronchi (carina) as seen at bronchoscopy are a serious prognostic sign, since it usually indicates carcinomatous involvement of the tracheobronchial lymph nodes around the bifurcation of the trachea or by a dilated atrium. The former may be subjected to transtracheal needle biopsy or aspiration at this point.
- All the intrinsic muscles of the larynx except the cricothyroids are supplied by the recurrent laryngeal nerves. Injury to these nerves therefore prevents abduction or adduction of the vocal cords lying into neutral position. Bilateral paralysis, which may occur as a result of thyroid carcinoma or following thyroidectomy, causes fixation of both cords and therefore seriously compromised airways. More usually, unilateral paralysis occurs as a result of tumor or occasionally fibrosis or surgery, and one cord becomes fixed. The most common paralytic lesions seen are due to damage to the left recurrent laryngeal nerve, which leaves the vagus at the level of aortic arch, hooks round the aorta and ligamentum arteriosum and runs up. In the mediastinum, the nerve passes between trachea and esophagus. This long

intrathoracic course makes the left recurrent laryngeal nerve vulnerable to involvement by pulmonary and other neoplasms around the aortic arch as well as by the aortic aneurysm. The involvement of the nerve in fibrosis, tuberculosis, or radiotherapy may occasionally cause paralysis. Right recurrent nerve has a shorter course, as it hooks round right subclavian artery. The nerve may be affected by tumor or lymph nodes in the cervical or thoracic inlet, e.g., thyroid carcinoma, aneurysm, or surgery on the thyroid gland.
- The primary ciliary dyskinesia—the primary disorder associated with ciliary dysfunction is responsible for 5–10% cases of bronchiectasis. In this condition, ultrastructural defect in the cilia of the bronchial mucosa causes asynchronous movement of cilia. The cilia become dyskinetic within coordinated movement results in ineffective mucociliary escalator system. There is impaired bacterial clearance that results in recurrent upper and lower respiratory tract infection such as sinusitis, otitis media, and bronchiectasis. Approximately half of the patients with primary ciliary dyskinesia fall into the subgroup of Kartagener's syndrome characterized by situs inversus, sinusitis, and bronchiectasis.

■ ANATOMY OF LUNG, PLEURA, AND DIAPHRAGM

The Lungs

Each lung is conical in shape, having a blunt apex which reaches above the sternal end of the first rib, projects upward into the neck about 1 inch above the clavicle, a concave base overlying the diaphragm, an extensive costovertebral surface molded into the form of the chest wall and a mediastinal surface which is concave to accommodate the pericardium and other mediastinal structures. The right lung is slightly larger than the left and is divided into three lobes—upper, middle, and lower, by the oblique and horizontal fissures. The left lung has only an oblique fissure and hence has only two lobes. For physical examination, upper lobes are to be examined from the front of the chest and the lower lobes from the back.

Blood Supply

The peculiarity of pulmonary circulation is that here arteries carry deoxygenated blood to pulmonary capillaries where it gets oxygenated. Blood returns to the left atrium through pulmonary veins. Pulmonary arteries follow the airways and their division, whereas the pulmonary veins pass through connective tissues in the septal walls. Another noteworthy matter in pulmonary circulation is its enormous reserve and its ability to maintain low pressure even it accommodates the same amount of blood as systemic circulation. Airways are supplied by bronchial arteries derived from descending aorta, having the pressure of systemic circulation.

Lymphatic Drainage

The lymphatics of the lung drain centripetally from the pleura toward the hilum. From the *bronchopulmonary lymph nodes* in the hilum, efferent lymph channels pass to the *tracheobronchial nodes* at the bifurcation of the trachea, then to the *paratracheal nodes,* and the mediastinal lymph trunks to drain usually directly into the brachiocephalic veins or, rarely, indirectly via the thoracic or right lymphatic duct.

Nerve Supply

At the root of each lung is a pulmonary plexus composed of efferent and afferent autonomic nerve fibers. It is formed from branches of the sympathetic trunk and receives parasympathetic fibers from the vagus nerve. The sympathetic efferent fiber produces bronchodilatation and vasoconstriction. The parasympathetic efferent fiber produces bronchoconstriction, vasodilatation, and increased glandular secretion. Afferent impulses derived from bronchial mucous membrane and from stretch receptor in the alveolar walls pass to the central nervous system in both sympathetic and parasympathetic nerves.

The Surface Marking of the Lungs and Fissures

The surface projection of the lung is somewhat less extensive than that of the parietal pleura, and in addition it varies quite considerably with the phase of respiration. The *apex* of the lung closely follows the line of the cervical pleura, and the surface marking of the *anterior border of the right lung* corresponds to that of the right mediastinal pleura. On the left side, however, the *anterior border* has a distinct notch (the *cardiac notch*), which passes behind the fifth and sixth costal cartilages. The *lower border* of the lung has an excursion of as much as 2–3 inches (5–8 cm) in the extremes of respiration, but in the neutral position (midway between inspiration and expiration) it lies along a line which crosses the sixth rib in the midclavicular line, the eighth rib in the midaxillary line, and reaches the tenth rib adjacent to the vertebral column posteriorly. The *oblique fissure*, which divides the lung into upper and lower lobes, is indicated on the surface by a line drawn obliquely downward and outward from 1 inch (2.5 cm) lateral to the spine of the second thoracic vertebra to the sixth costal cartilage about 1.5 inches (4 cm) from the midline. This can be represented approximately by abducting the shoulder to its full extent; the line of the oblique fissure then corresponds to the position of the medial border of the scapula. The surface marking of the *transverse fissure* (separating the middle and upper lobes of the right lung) is a line drawn horizontally along the fourth costal cartilage and meeting the oblique fissure where the latter crosses the fifth rib.

Clinical Importance

- Malignancy of the lung apex may compress subclavian artery resulting in diminished pulses in the arm, the pressure on the lower trunk of brachial plexus leads to radiating pain in the arm with muscle wasting (Pancoast syndrome), the involvement of SVC leads to SVC syndrome, and the involvement of cervical sympathetic chain leads to Horner syndrome.
- Lung tissue and the visceral pleura are devoid of pain sensitive nerve endings. Chest pain occurs only when the disease involves surrounding structures. Once lung disease crosses the visceral pleura and the pleural cavity to involve the parietal pleura, pain becomes prominent. Similarly, the pleurisy of the central part of diaphragmatic pleura, which receives sensory innervations from the phrenic nerve (C3–C5), can lead to referred pain over the shoulders.
- A sequestrated segment is a part of the lung that has become isolated during development. Its bronchi do not connect bronchial tree, and its blood supply is derived from the aorta. It is most common in lower lobe, especially on the left. It creates a problem only when it is infected.

CHAPTER 2: Clinical Anatomy of Thorax

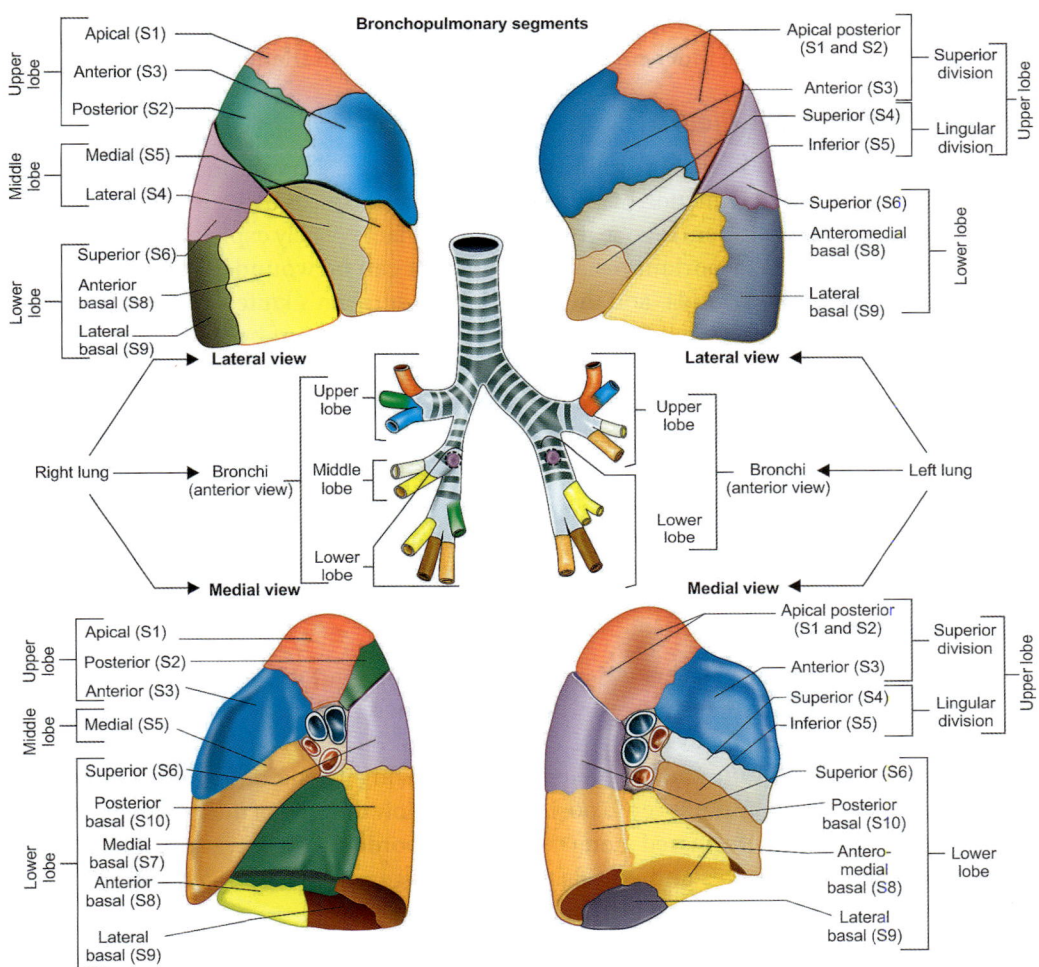

FIG. 2.1: Lobar and segmental distribution of lungs.

Lung anatomy includes the lung parenchyma, which is further subdivided into lobes and segments **(Fig. 2.1)**.

The Pleurae

The two pleural cavities are totally separate from each other. Each *pleura* consists of two layers: (1) A *visceral layer* intimately related to the outer surface of the lung and extends into the depth of interlobar fissures and (2) a *parietal layer* lining the inner aspect of the chest wall, the upper surface of the diaphragm, and the sides of the pericardium and mediastinum. The two layers are continuous in front and behind the root of the lung, but below this the pleura hangs down in a loose fold, the *pulmonary ligament*, which forms a "dead space" for distension of the pulmonary veins. The lungs do not occupy all the available space in the pleural cavity even in forced inspiration. The parietal and visceral layers of pleura are separated from one another by a slit-like space, the pleural cavity. This pleural cavity normally contains a small amount of tissue fluid (5-10 mL)—the pleural fluid which covers the surfaces of the pleura as a thin film and permits the two layers to move on each other with minimum friction.

Surface Marking of the Pleura

The *cervical pleura* can be marked out on the surface by a curved line drawn from the sternoclavicular joint to the junction of the medial and middle thirds of the clavicle; the apex of the pleura is about 1 inch (2.5 cm) above the clavicle. This fact is easily explained by the oblique slope of the first rib. It is important because the pleura can be wounded (with consequent pneumothorax) by a stab wound—and this includes the surgeon's knife and the anesthetist's needle—above the clavicle. The lines of pleural reflexion pass from behind the sternoclavicular joint on each side to meet in the midline at the second costal cartilage (the angle of Louis). The right pleural edge then passes vertically downward to the sixth costal cartilage. Lower border of pleura crosses the eighth rib in the midclavicular line, the 10th rib in the midaxillary line and the 12th rib at the lateral border of the erector spinae. On the left side, the pleural edge arches laterally at the fourth costal cartilage and descends lateral to the border of the sternum, due, of course, to its lateral displacement by the heart. Apart from that deviation, the left pleural borders are the same as that of right side.

Clinical Importance

- Normally the two pleural layers are in close apposition, and the space between them is only a potential one. It may, however, fill with air (pneumothorax), blood (hemothorax), or pus (empyema).
- Fluid can be drained from the pleural cavity by inserting a wide bore needle through an intercostal space usually the seventh posteriorly or below the area of maximum dullness on percussion. The needle is passed along the superior border of the lower rib, thus avoiding injury to intercostal nerves and vessels. There is danger of penetrating the diaphragm if needle passes in the lower intercostal space.
- Since the parietal pleura is segmentally innervated by the intercostal nerves, inflammation of the pleura results in pain referred to the cutaneous distribution of these nerves (i.e., to the thoracic wall or in the case of the lower nerves to the anterior abdominal wall, which may mimic an acute abdominal emergency).
- The formation of this pleural fluid results from hydrostatic and osmotic pressure. Since the hydrostatic pressures are greater in capillaries of parietal pleura than in the capillaries of the visceral pleura (pulmonary circulation), the pleural fluid is normally absorbed into the capillaries of the visceral pleura. Any condition which increases the production of the fluid (e.g., inflammation, malignancy, etc.) or impairs the drainage of fluid results in abnormal accumulations of fluid, called pleural effusion. The presence of 300 mL of pleural fluid in the costodiaphragmatic recess in an adult is sufficient to enable clinician to detect effusion.
- Inflammation of the pleura (pleuritis or pleurisy), secondary of the inflammation of the lungs, results in the pleural surfaces coated with inflammatory exudates, causing the surfacing to be roughened, which produces friction, and a pleural rub can be heard with stethoscope on inspiration and expiration. Often the exudate is invaded by fibroblasts, which lay down the collagen and bind the visceral pleura to the parietal pleura formed pleural adhesion in the form of pleural fibrosis.

The Diaphragm

The diaphragm is the dome-shaped septum dividing the thoracic from the abdominal cavity. It comprises two portions: a peripheral muscular part which arises from the margins of the thoracic outlet and a centrally placed aponeurosis.

The muscular fibers are arranged in three parts:
1. A *vertebral part* from the crura and from the arcuate ligaments.
2. A *costal part* is attached to the inner aspect of the lower six ribs and costal cartilages.
3. A *sternal portion* consists of two small slips from the deep surface of the xiphisternum. The central tendon, into which the muscular fibers are inserted, is trefoil in shape and is partially fused with the undersurface of the pericardium.

Opening of the Diaphragm

- The aortic opening lies anterior to the body of the 12th thoracic vertebra between the crura, and it transmits the aorta, the thoracic duct, and the azygos vein.
- The esophageal opening lies at the level of 10th thoracic vertebra, and it transmits the esophagus, the right and left vagus nerves, branches of left gastric vessels, and lymphatics.
- The caval opening lies at the level of eighth thoracic vertebra, and it transmits inferior vena cava and terminal branches of phrenic nerve.
- Other openings transmit splanchnic nerves, sympathetic trunk, superior epigastric vessels, left phrenic nerve, and the neurovascular bundles of seventh to 11th intercostal space.

The diaphragm receives its entire motor supply from the phrenic nerve (C3–C5) whose long course from the neck follows the embryological migration of the muscle of the diaphragm from the cervical region. Injury or operative division of this nerve results in paralysis and elevation of the corresponding half of the diaphragm.

Radiographically, the paralysis of the diaphragm is recognized by its elevation and paradoxical movement, instead of descending on inspiration it is forced upward by pressure from the abdominal viscera. The sensory nerve fibers from the central part of the diaphragm also run in the phrenic nerve, hence irritation of the diaphragmatic pleura (in pleurisy) or of the peritoneum on the undersurface of the diaphragm by subphrenic collections of pus or blood produces referred pain in the corresponding cutaneous area, the shoulder tip. The peripheral part of the diaphragm, including the crura, receives sensory fibers from the lower intercostal nerves.

Clinical Importance

- A number of defects may occur in the diaphragm, giving rise to a variety of:
  - Congenital herniae through the diaphragm. These may be:
    - Through the foramen of Morgagni, anteriorly between the xiphoid and costal origins
    - Through the foramen of Bochdalek—the pleuroperitoneal canal—lying posteriorly
    - Through a deficiency of the whole central tendon (occasionally such a hernia may be traumatic in origin)
    - Through a congenitally large esophageal hiatus

- Far more common are the acquired hiatus herniae (subdivided into sliding and rolling herniae). These are found in patients usually of middle age where weakening and widening of the esophageal hiatus have occurred. In the *sliding hernia,* the upper stomach and lower esophagus slide upward into the chest through the lax hiatus when the patient lies down or bends over; the competence of the cardia is often disturbed and peptic juice can therefore regurgitate into the gullet. This may be followed by esophagitis with consequent heartburn, bleeding, and, eventually, stricture formation. In the *rolling hernia* (which is far less common), the cardia remains in its normal position and the cardioesophageal junction is intact, but the fundus of the stomach rolls up through the hiatus in front of the esophagus, hence, the alternative term of paraesophageal hernia. In such a case, there may be epigastric discomfort, flatulence, and even dysphagia, but *no* regurgitation because the cardiac mechanism is undisturbed.
- *Paralysis of the diaphragm*: A single dome of diaphragm may be paralyzed by crushing or sectioning of phrenic in the neck or may be due to phrenic nerve palsy due to malignancy. In some cases, it may be due to neurological cause (e.g., cervical myelitis, encephalitis, etc.), mechanical cause (e.g., retrosternal goiter, aortic aneurysm, etc.), infection (tuberculosis, etc.), pulmonary infarction, etc.
- *Eventration of diaphragm*: It is a condition in which all or part of the diaphragm is largely composed by fibrous tissue with only a few or no interspersed muscle fibers. It is usually congenital but may be acquired. It may be complete which invariably occurs in the left side, or it may be incomplete which occurs virtually exclusively on the right side.

The Mediastinum

The mediastinum is thoracic cavity which lies between the lungs. It is bound laterally by the parietal pleurae, anteriorly by the sternum, posteriorly by the vertebral column and paravertebral gutter, superiorly by the thoracic outlet, and inferiorly by the diaphragm. Contents of the mediastinal compartment have been described in **Table 2.1**.

Clinical Importance

- *Pneumomediastinum*: Free air in the mediastinum detected on a chest X-ray or computed tomography (CT) scan is pneumomediastinum. It is spontaneous when occurring without surgical or medical procedures, chest trauma or mechanical ventilation, and in the absence of underlying lung disease. Secondary pneumomediastinum is far more common in recent times with mechanical ventilation patients. Anatomical continuity may lead to extensive subcutaneous emphysema over the head and neck area, pneumoperitoneum or

Table 2.1: Contents of the mediastinal compartment.		
Anterior	Middle	Posterior
Pericardial fat, thymus gland, substernal extension of thyroid and parathyroid glands, lymph node, and connective tissues	Heart and pericardium, trachea, main bronchus, innominate vein and superior vena cava, aortic arch and great vessels, phrenic nerves, vagus nerves, lymph node, and connective tissues	Azygos and hemiazygos veins, esophagus, descending aorta, sympathetic trunk, intercostal nerves, thoracic duct, and connective tissues

air may dissect the pleural layers or the pericardium, leading to associated pneumothorax or pneumopericardium.
- *Mediastinitis*: Inflammation of the mediastinal structures is defined as mediastinitis. Based on the duration and severity of symptoms, it may be broadly classified to acute and chronic. Clinical presentation is dramatic and often life threatening in acute mediastinitis, whereas chronic inflammation leads to present as mediastinal mass.
- *Anterior mediastinal mass*:
  - *Thymoma*: It accounts for 20% anterior mediastinal neoplasm in adults.
  - *Mediastinal germ cell tumors (GCTs)*: Primitive germ cell that fails to migrate completely during early embryonic development is the currently accepted theory regarding the origin of GCTs. This is classified into three groups based on cell type—benign teratomas, seminomas, and embryonal tumors or malignant teratomas or nonseminomatous GCTs.
  - Mediastinal goiters
  - Mediastinal lymphomas
- *Tumor of the middle mediastinum*:
  - Mediastinal cysts
  - Bronchogenic cysts
  - Enterogenous cysts
  - Pericardial cysts
  - Lymphangiomas
- *Tumor of the posterior mediastinum*:
  - Neuroenteric cysts
  - *Neurogenic tumors*: It arises from various neural elements such as peripheral nerve routes (e.g., neurofibroma), from the sympathetic ganglia (e.g., ganglioneuroma), etc.
  - Nerve sheath tumors
  - *Tumor of the autonomic nervous system*: It arises from neural cells rather than from the nerve sheath. It constitutes about half to two-thirds of neural tumor of posterior mediastinum and is benign.
- *Superior vena cava syndrome* (*SVCS*): It is a common complication of lung cancer and non-Hodgkin lymphoma, and it constitutes 90% of the cases of SVCS. Benign cases (5–10%) are usually due to tuberculosis, fungal diseases, and thrombosis due to iatrogenic procedures.

Bronchopulmonary Segments

These are the anatomic, functional, and surgical units of the lungs. Each lobar bronchus which passes to the lobe of the lung gives off branches called segmental (tertiary) bronchi **(Fig. 2.2)**. Each segmental bronchus passes to a structurally and functionally independent unit of a lung lobe called bronchopulmonary segment, which is surrounded by connected tissue. The segmental bronchus is accompanied by a branch pulmonary artery, but the tributaries of the pulmonary vein run in the connected tissue between adjacent bronchopulmonary segments. Each segment has its own lymphatic and nerve supply. On entering a bronchopulmonary segment, each segmental bronchus divides repeatedly. The smallest bronchia divides and gives rise to bronchioles, which are less than 1 mm diameter, no cartilage in their walls, and lined by columnar ciliated epithelium. The bronchioles then divide and give rise to terminal

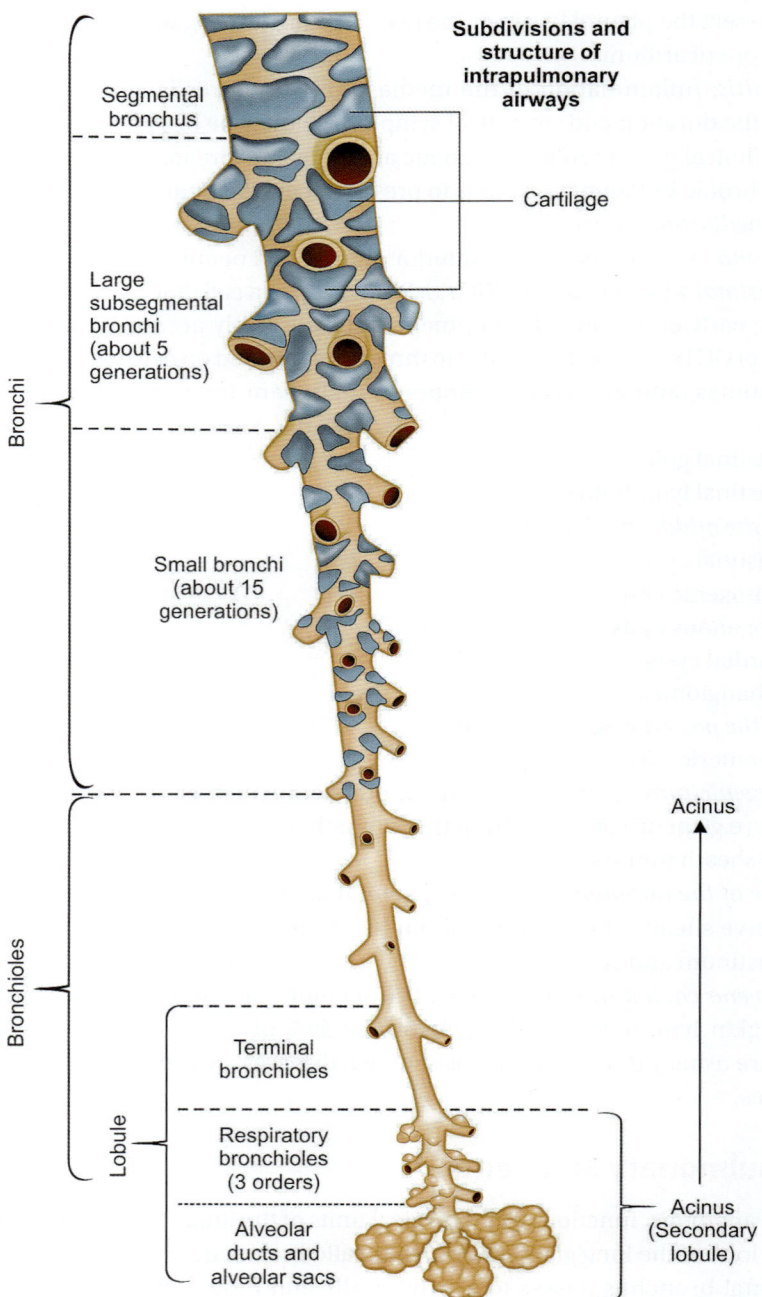

FIG. 2.2: Subdivision of airways.

bronchioles, which show delicate outpouchings from their walls, which is called respiratory bronchioles, where gaseous exchange between blood and air take place, and diameter of it is about 0.5 mm. The respiratory bronchioles end by branching into alveolar ducts, which lead into tubular passage with numerous thin-walled alveolar sacs. The alveolar sacs consist of several alveoli opening into a single chamber **(Fig. 2.3)**.

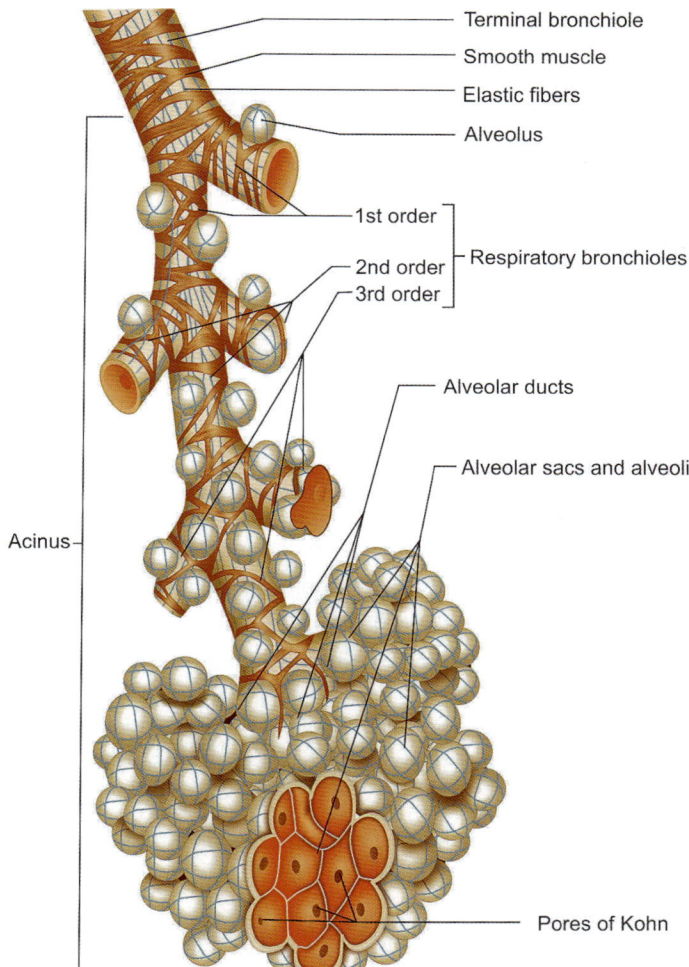

FIG. 2.3: Subdivisions and structure of intrapulmonary airways.

Clinical Importance

Excessive accumulation of bronchial secretions in a lobe or segment interferes with airflow and prone to subsequent infection. To aid in the normal drainage of a bronchial segment, a physiotherapist often alters the position of the patient so that gravity assists in the process of drainage. Further disease processes localized to a particular segment, or a lobe can be approached surgically.

■ SURFACE ANATOMY

Important surface markings of thorax have been described in **Tables 2.2 to 2.5**. **Table 2.2** describes important thoracic landmarks used as references. **Table 2.3** describes important lines used in clinical examination. **Tables 2.4 and 2.5** describe surface markings of pleura, lungs, fissures, and Traube's space.

Table 2.2: Important thoracic cage landmarks.

The sternocostal angle	It corresponds with the second costal cartilage, and it is used as a starting-point from which ribs are counted. It also corresponds with the fifth thoracic vertebra
The junction between the body and xiphoid process of the sternum	It corresponds with the fibrocartilage between the ninth and tenth thoracic vertebrae
The lower border of the pectoralis major	It corresponds with the fifth rib
The inferior angle of the scapula, while the arms are at the sides	It corresponds with the sternum between the fourth and fifth ribs, the fifth rib in the nipple line, and the ninth rib posteriorly
The uppermost visible digitation of serratus anterior muscle	It corresponds with the sixth rib

Table 2.3: Important lines used for clinical examination of thorax.

Midclavicular line/mammary line	A line drawn vertically downward from a point midway between the center of the jugular notch and the tip of the acromion
Midsternal line	A line drawn vertically downward from the middle line of the sternum
Lateral sternal line	A line drawn vertically downward along the sternal margin
Parasternal line	A line drawn vertically downward midway between the lateral sternal and the midclavicular line
Anterior axillary line	A line drawn vertically downward from the anterior axillary folds
Posterior axillary lines	A line drawn vertically downward from posterior axillary fold
Midaxillary line	A line drawn vertically downward from the apex of the axilla
Scapular line	A line drawn vertically downward through the inferior angle of the scapula

Table 2.4: Surface marking of pleura.

Right pleura	Anterior border	The line begins at the sternoclavicular articulation, then runs downward and medially to the midpoint at the junction between the manubrium and body of the sternum, then follows the midsternal line to the lower end of the body of the sternum or xiphoid process
	Lower border	The line starts at midline of xiphoid process, then turns laterally and downward across the seventh sternocostal junction, then crosses the eighth costochondral junction in the midclavicular line, the 10th rib in the midaxillary line, and then ends at spinous process of the 12th thoracic vertebra
Left pleura	Anterior border	The line runs similar to that of right side up to the level of the fourth costal cartilage in midline, then diverges laterally, continues downward slightly lateral to the sternal border and ends at the sixth costal cartilage
	Lower border	The line starts at the sixth costal cartilage, then runs downward and laterally, crosses the seventh costal cartilage, and then follows that of right side, but at a slightly lower level

Table 2.5: Surface markings of lungs and fissures.	
Apex of the lung	Apex of lung is situated in the neck above the medial third of the clavicle. The height is generally about 2.5 cm above the clavicle but may varies (± 2.5 cm)
Anterior borders of the right lung	Line starts at apex point—2.5 cm above the clavicle and nearer to anterior border of sternocleidomastoid; then runs downward and medially across the sternoclavicular joint and manubrium sterni until it meets almost midline at the junction between the manubrium and body of the sternum; then runs downwards vertically near the midsternal line up to the level of the sixth costal cartilage at sixth or seventh chondrosternal junction
Anterior border of left lung	Line runs similarly as far as the level of the fourth costal cartilages; then curves laterally and downward across the fourth sternocostal joint to reach the parasternal line at the fifth costal cartilage; and then turns medially and downward to the sixth sternocostal joint
Lower border of the lungs (in expiration)	Lines run slightly curved with convexity downward; start from the sixth or seventh chondrosternal junction; run downward and laterally to the eighth rib in the mid-axillary line; then run slightly upward to cut the 10th rib in scalpula line; and continue medially to about 1.75 cm lateral to the spinous process of 10th thoracic vertebrae
Posterior borders of lungs	Lines start from the level of the spinous process of the seventh cervical vertebra and run vertically downwards on either side of the vertebral column up to the level of the spinous process of the 10th thoracic vertebra
Oblique fissures	Lines run from the spinous process of the second thoracic vertebra around the side of the thorax, then cross the midclavicular line across sixth ribs; then lines correspond roughly with the vertebral border of the scapula when the hand is placed on the top of the head; and continues along contour of the sixth rib
Horizontal fissure	Line starts from the midpoint of the oblique fissure or from the point where it cuts the midaxillary line and ends in the midsternal line at the level of the fourth costal cartilage or Line starts from the costal cartilage of the fourth rib and crosses fifth rib at the midaxillary line to join the oblique fissure
Traube's space is a crescent-shaped space bounded by left lung, anterior border of the spleen, and left lobe of the liver	The space is bounded by the left sixth rib superiorly, the left midaxillary line laterally, and the left costal margin inferiorly

The Movements of Respiration

During inspiration, the movements of the chest wall and diaphragm result in an increase in all diameters of the thorax. This, in turn, brings about an increase in the negative intrapleural pressure and an expansion of the lung tissue. Conversely, in expiration, the relaxation of the respiratory muscles and the elastic recoil of the lung reduce the thoracic capacity and force air out of the lungs. In quiet *inspiration,* the first rib remains relatively fixed, but the contraction of the external intercostals elevates and everts the succeeding ribs. In the case of the second to seventh ribs, this principally increases the anteroposterior diameter of the thorax (by the forward thrust of the sternum), like a pump handle. The corresponding movement of the lower ribs raises the costal margin and leads mainly to an increase in the transverse diameter of the thorax, like a bucket handle. The depth of the thorax is increased by the contraction of the diaphragm, which draws down its central tendon. Normal quiet *expiration* is aided by the tone of the abdominal musculature, which, acting through the contained viscera, forces the diaphragm upward. In deep and forced inspiration, additional muscles are called into play (e.g., scalenus anterior, sternocleidomastoid, serratus anterior, and pectoralis major) to increase further the capacity of the thorax. Similarly, in deep expiration, forced contraction of the abdominal muscles aids the normal expulsive factors.

■ CONCLUSION

The thorax plays a crucial role in housing and protecting vital organs while supporting respiration and circulation. This chapter comprehensively outlines the anatomy of the thorax, including the thoracic cage, airways, lungs, pleura, diaphragm, and mediastinum. It highlights the functional significance and intricate relationships between these structures.

The thoracic cage offers a dynamic yet robust framework that accommodates vital respiratory and circulatory processes. Detailed descriptions of airways and lung structures emphasize their specialization for efficient gas exchange. The pleura ensures seamless lung movement during respiration, while the diaphragm functions as the principal muscle for breathing. The mediastinum, containing vital structures such as the heart, esophagus, and major vessels, underscores the thorax's complex anatomical organization.

Clinically, this chapter emphasizes conditions like rib fractures, thoracic outlet syndrome, and pneumothorax, demonstrating the thorax's vulnerability and its impact on systemic health. Insights into pleural effusions, lung malignancies, and mediastinal disorders enrich its relevance for medical practice.

Overall, the chapter provides a foundational understanding of thoracic anatomy and its applied clinical significance, equipping readers with knowledge critical for diagnosing and managing thoracic diseases effectively.

SUGGESTED READINGS

1. Ellis H (Ed). Clinical Anatomy: A Revision and Applied Anatomy for Clinical Students, 10th illustrated edition. Blackwell Science; 2002.
2. Seaton A, Seaton D, Litch GA (Eds). Crofton and Douglas's Respiratory Diseases, 5th edition. John Wiley & Sons; 2008.
3. SK Jindal (Ed). Handbook of Pulmonary and Critical Care Medicine, 1st edition. New Delhi: Jaypee Brothers Medical Publisher Pvt. Ltd.; 2012.

CHAPTER 3

Basic Science in Pulmonology

Dhiman Ganguly

■ INTRODUCTION

Practice of pulmonology is essentially learning to assess two major presenting symptoms, namely—breathlessness and cough, by clinical means, interpretation of laboratory results, and then deciding upon the site of pathology—which could be the airways, or the lung parenchyma or both, and coming up to a diagnostic label. At times, disease elsewhere can produce a clinical manifestation in respiratory system (i.e., breathing in metabolic acidosis), but those are not common and can usually be diagnosed quite easily. Therapy has to be decided next, but if the initial steps are not right, treatment invariably remains suboptimal.

To be able to do this, it is important to understand the physiological disturbance involved in the disease process. In vast majority of respiratory diseases, this is a ventilation perfusion mismatch. Hypoventilation can result from neuromuscular diseases—but most of the time complicates long-standing ventilation/perfusion (V/Q) mismatch due to respiratory muscle fatigue.

As respiration is all about a regular supply of oxygen and removal of carbon dioxide, to understand the disturbed physiology, we need clear concepts on properties of gases in general, and how these are involved in a biological system, we need to understand mechanics of breathing (as movement of air follows laws of mechanics) and how that gets altered in diseases of airways and lung parenchyma, and lastly, how do we manage to maintain and control the respiratory function under changing circumstances of daily life.

■ THE BLOOD GASES

Respiratory system remains in close contact and interacts with the ambient air all our life. This is because we breathe to collect oxygen from and release carbon dioxide into the atmosphere, through the respiratory system. Hence, to understand the physiology of respiration, it is mandatory for us to have a clear picture about the atmosphere that we live in. The atmosphere is a gaseous envelope of the earth that spreads for a few hundred kilometers above its surface. This gaseous envelope is actually a mixture of gases—for the purpose of our understanding, the composition of air may be taken as 79% of nitrogen and 21% of oxygen. For the present, we are ignoring traces of carbon dioxide, carbon monoxide, and other gases in our calculation.

Gases differ in physical properties from solids and liquids in the sense that these do not have either a definite shape or a volume. Because the mutual attraction between gas molecules is almost nonexistent, the molecules are in ceaseless, high velocity, and random motion. If the molecules in a gas are in motion, it is only natural that these will bang against each other and against the surface of the earth continuously. The pressure (force per unit area) that a gas exerts is the summation of the impacts of its myriad rapidly moving elastic molecules on the surface of the earth or the walls of the container of the gas (partial pressure). The magnitude of pressure depends on the average kinetic energy and the concentration of the gas molecules (number of molecules per unit volume). The molecules rebound from the collisions without loss of energy, and this is why these are regarded as perfectly elastic. The rapidly moving gas molecules in a mixture of gases make sure that the composition of the mixture remains the same through the space occupied by the mixtures of gases. At sea level, air pressure will support a column of mercury 760 mm high; this is called the barometric pressure (Pb). As the pressure depends on the number of molecules per unit volume and as the concentration of gas molecules is higher nearer to surface of earth (because of gravitational pull), the pressure drops as one goes to higher altitudes, although the composition of the atmosphere, as explained earlier remains the same. This means air at the top of Mount Everest contains 21% oxygen, as on the sea surface, but the pressure exerted on the mountain top is much lower compared to sea level. Gases also exert pressure, when dissolved in a liquid. The gas pressure in a liquid is at times called tension; in this context partial pressure and tension are interchangeable terms. Pressure exerted by a gas in solution is directly proportional to the concentration of the gas and inversely proportional to its solubility coefficient. The solubility coefficient of CO_2 is about 20 times higher than oxygen—this is why 0.03 mL of oxygen dissolved in 100 mL of blood produces a pressure of 100 mm Hg, whereas 2.5 mL of dissolved CO_2 in the same volume of arterial blood results in a partial pressure of 40 mm Hg.

There are two other facts of gas physics that are essential as background information in respiratory physiology—firstly, water vapor is water in gas phase, and it exerts a pressure of 47 mm Hg when it fully saturates a sample of air at 37°C, and secondly, Dalton's law states that the pressure of a gas mixture is the arithmetic sum of the partial pressures of individual constituent gas pressures in the mixture. In other words, the barometric pressure of 760 mm Hg is the sum of partial pressure of oxygen (PO_2) and nitrogen as 160 mm (159.2) and 600 mm (593.44), respectively. The partial pressure of a gas remains the same irrespective of the presence or absence of other gases, in the same volume.

The composition of our atmosphere has changed to a great extent since the earth was formed 4.5 billion years ago. However, the rate of change has been exceedingly slow, until recently. Certain pollutants are now regularly present in the atmosphere, especially around areas of human habitations. Within a short space of several generations, we are going to convert all the carbon in fossil fuels, which accumulated through half a billion years, into carbon dioxide.

THE OXYGEN CASCADE

Let us now consider how exactly the oxygen from the source, i.e., the ambient air, reaches the place where it is utilized, i.e., the mitochondria.

The first step is to visualize the changes in the composition of inhaled air as it travels down the bronchial tree. The water in the mucous membrane gets vaporized and becomes a third constituent of the air, until a state of equilibrium is reached, i.e., the volume of water getting vaporized and the volume of vapor getting condensed to water are equal. When saturated, the water vapor constitutes approximately 6.2% of nitrogen, oxygen, and water vapor mixture and exerts a partial pressure of 47 mm Hg. Consequently, the partial pressure of nitrogen and oxygen drops by about 37 mm Hg and 10 mm Hg, respectively by the time the air reaches the alveoli. It means the PO_2 in inspired air will drop from 160 mm Hg to 150 mm [partial pressure of inspired O_2 (PiO_2)] on reaching the gas exchanging surface. Once the inhaled gas reaches the gas-exchanging surface, further changes take place. Oxygen gets taken up from the air and carbon dioxide gets added to it—keeping the total pressure at 760 mm Hg. It might appear under the circumstances that the PO_2 of the air, as it enters the gas exchanging surface (i.e., 150 mm), should be the sum of PO_2 and partial pressure of carbon dioxide (PCO_2) in the alveolar air, but this is not exactly true, because ordinarily we do not produce a molecule of CO_2 against utilization of a molecule of O_2. On a mixed diet, our respiratory exchange ratio is 0.8—a healthy adult at rest uses 250 mL of oxygen and produces 200 mL of carbon dioxide every minute. The other important fact to keep in mind is that the ventilation is controlled in such a way—that the PCO_2 in alveoli is maintained at 40 mm Hg. In fact, hanging onto the right volume of CO_2 is a priority to the homeostasis of *milieu interior*. For example, if someone is hyperventilating—he or she will soon start feeling dizzy and if the individual does not stop—there will be a syncopal attack due to cerebral vasoconstriction—thereby stopping the hyperventilation. This means our physiology would rather let the brain suffer from lack of oxygen—then let go the carbon dioxide. Because of the respiratory exchange ratio of 0.8 the PO_2 in alveolar air can be calculated as follows—$PiO_2 - PaCO_2/R = PAO_2$ or $150 - 40/0.8 = 100$ mm Hg. This is known as alveolar air equation. Calculations have been made assuming that the person has normal minute ventilation—keeping the $PaCO_2$ at 40 mm Hg. Some of the modern blood gas analyzers give the figures in kilopascal (kPa). It is easy to convert these figures—760 mm Hg is 100 kPa—this means kPa figures are to be multiplied by 7.6 to get mm Hg figures.

The difference between the PAO_2 so calculated and the PaO_2 in arterial blood (as measured) is called alveolar arterial oxygen tension gradient $P(A-a)O_2$, this is a measure for ventilation perfusion mismatch. Even for normal, healthy people, there is usually a small mismatch of (2–5) mm Hg, and this usually increases with advancing age. A normal $P(A-a)O_2$ means there is nothing wrong with the lung or pulmonary circulation.

Respiratory dysfunction of any kind, be it in the airways, in lung parenchyma, or pulmonary vasculature invariably results in a V/Q mismatch.

The next sequence in oxygen story is the passage of the oxygen molecules across the alveolar capillary wall to get on to the oxygen transport system. The driving force that pushes the gas molecules is provided by the PO_2 inside the alveoli as this is much higher than the PO_2 of mixed venous blood present in the capillaries which is only about 40 mm Hg under ordinary circumstances. To make things a little complicated, the relation between the "push" of partial pressure of the volume of oxygen actually getting on to the transport system (and saturating hemoglobin) is not linear. Oxygen is transported by and large as oxyhemoglobin with red blood cells (RBCs). Each gram of hemoglobin has the capacity of carrying a maximum of 1.34 mL of oxygen when the hemoglobin is fully saturated oxygen is relatively insoluble in blood at 37°C only 0.03 mL of oxygen can dissolve in 100 mL of blood. Therefore, this virtually has no role in oxygen carriage.

Despite large number of layers, the overall thickness of the respiratory membrane is as little as 0.2 µm in some areas—it averages about 0.6 µm except where there are cell nuclei. The total surface area of respiratory membrane is 70 m^2 in normal adults. This is equivalent to the floor area of a 25 × 30 feet room. The total quantity of blood in capillaries of lung at any given point of time is about 60–140 mL. One can easily imagine how thin the "sheet" of blood is, and this explains the rapidity of gas exchange. Under normal conditions, the arterial blood gets fully saturated within one-third of the time it takes to traverse from venous end of the capillary to the arterial end (0.25 seconds and 0.75 seconds). This is why, patients with interstitial lung disease (ILD), until very late in the course of illness, maintain a normal oxygen saturation while at rest, but exercise or febrile illness (because of tachycardia reducing the transit time) rapidly desaturates arterial blood **(Table 3.1)**.

Normal human erythrocytes are biconcave disk with a diameter of about 7.6 mm. Hemoglobin is the vital protein that transports oxygen from lungs to the tissues and facilitates transport of carbon dioxide from tissues to the lungs. The hemoglobin molecule consists of a protein moiety called goblin and four ferrous—protoporphyrin complexes. The molecular weight is about 67,000 Daltons. It has already been made clear that under normal circumstance, dissolved oxygen of 0.03 mL per 100 mL of blood is of no practical significance and with 15 g of hemoglobin in 100 mL of blood, the bulk of oxygen (i.e., 20 mL) is actually carried as oxyhemoglobin. Unlike dissolved oxygen the volume of O_2 combined with hemoglobin is not linearly related to PO_2 but is described by an "S"-shaped curve **(Fig. 3.1)** that slopes steeply between 10 and 50 mm Hg. The unique shape of oxyhemoglobin dissociation curve is an important example of physiologic adaptation. The relatively flat portion above 70 mm Hg ensures saturation of most hemoglobin despite wide variations of alveolar PO_2, and the steep fall below 50 mm Hg ensures rapid extraction of oxygen from arterial blood in the tissues. When the arterial blood reaches the tissue capillaries, O_2 diffuses to the mitochondria where the PO_2 is much lower. The tissue PO_2 differs considerably throughout the body, normal intracellular PO_2 ranges from as low as 5 mm Hg to as high as 40 mm Hg averaging (by direct measurement in animal experiments) 23 mm Hg. Because only 1–3 mm Hg oxygen pressure

Table 3.1: Partial pressures of oxygen and carbon-dioxide values at different levels.		
Levels	PO$_2$ in mm Hg	PCO$_2$ in mm Hg
Atmosphere	160	0.3
Inspired air	150	0.3
Alveolus	104	40
Artery	95	40
Vein	40	46
Tissue level	Less than 40 (Average 23)	46
Expired air	120	27

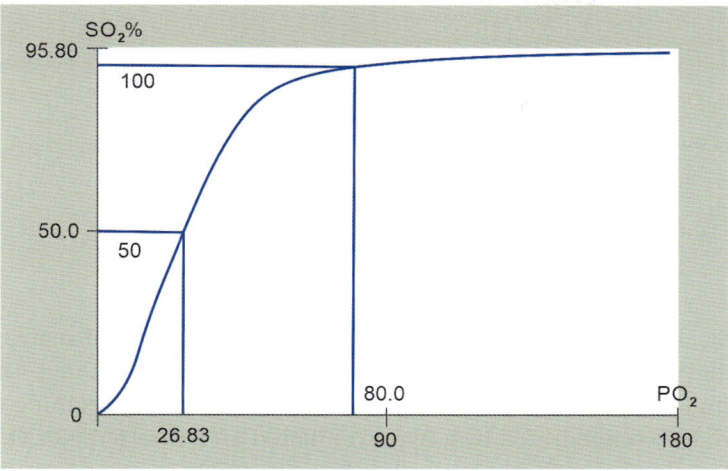

FIG. 3.1: Oxyhemoglobin dissociation curve.

is normally required for full support of chemical processes that use oxygen in the cell, one can see that even this low PO_2 of 23 mm Hg is more than adequate and provides a large safety margin.

P_{50} is the oxygen tension of blood at 50% saturation. It is an index that characterizes the oxygen affinity for hemoglobin and, as such, affects the shape and position of oxyhemoglobin dissociation curve. Alterations to the standard dissociation curve are reflected as a decreased P_{50} (left shift) or increased P_{50} (right shift). Normal P_{50} at pH 7.4 is approximately 27 mm Hg.

■ THE CARBON DIOXIDE STORY

Utilization of oxygen in the cells produces carbon dioxide and therefore increases intracellular PCO_2—which is about 46 mm Hg. The PCO_2 of arterial blood is 40 mm Hg. This small difference in partial pressure is good enough for diffusion of carbon dioxide because this gas is 20 times more diffusible compared to oxygen. Transport of CO_2 in blood is a little more complicated affair compared to transport of oxygen **(Table 3.2)**.

The dissolved carbon dioxide in the blood reacts with water to form carbonic acid inside the RBCs. This reaction would occur much too slowly to be of importance, were it not for the fact that inside the red blood cells is an enzyme called carbonic anhydrase. Almost instantaneously, the carbonic acid dissociates into hydrogen and bicarbonate ions. Most of the hydrogen ions then combine with hemoglobin in the red blood cells, because this protein is a powerful acid base buffer. Many of the bicarbonate ions diffuse out into the plasma, while chloride ions diffuse into the red cells to take their place. This has been termed chloride shift. The presence of reduced (deoxygenated) hemoglobin in tissue capillaries helps with loading of CO_2 while the oxygenation that occurs in the pulmonary capillaries assists in unloading. The fact that deoxygenated blood increases its ability to carry CO_2 is known as *Haldane effect*.

The reverse process occurs at pulmonary capillaries. The rather small pressure gradient of 5–6 mm Hg of CO_2 proves to be enough to unload about 4 mL of CO_2 from each 100 mL of blood.

Table 3.2: Forms of carbon dioxide in blood.		
	Arterial	Mixed venous
Pressure (mm Hg)	40	46
Content (mL/100 mL of blood)	48.5	52.5
Solution	2.5 mL	2.8
HCO_3	43	46
Carbamino	3	3.7

Hypercapnia almost never results from ventilation or perfusion mismatching, as long as the overall minute ventilation (VE) remains normal. This is because, although a hypoventilated area of lung can result in increased PCO_2 in the pulmonary vein draining the area—this is almost invariably compensated by a hyperventilated area where the PCO_2 is lower than normal. In fact, patients usually hyperventilate bringing PCO_2 down and causing a degree of respiratory alkalosis. Hypoxemia cannot be compensated by hyperventilated areas, as oxygen is nearly 100% saturated at 100 mm Hg tension, and hemoglobin can never be made to carry more oxygen, however, raised the PO_2 may be. $PaCO_2$ reflects ventilation in a linear manner, if the ventilation is halved, PCO_2 will double and vice versa.

Mechanics of Breathing

The alveolar air gets partly replaced with each cycle of respiration by fresh air from atmosphere. The volume and frequency of such replenishment are determined by the ventilatory drive, which in turn is normally determined by the metabolic requirements of a given instant. This replenishment of alveolar air is a purely mechanical process, accomplished by the respiratory bellows. Air moves only when there is a difference in pressure and during inspiration a negative pressure (3 cm in tidal breath) is created by diaphragm (alveolar pressure-0.5 to -1 cmH_2O) and air rushes in; during expiration the diaphragm relaxes and the elastic recoil of lung (and partly of the chest wall) in healthy individuals proves to be enough to drive the tidal breath out—without spending any energy.

Functional residual capacity (FRC) denotes the end of a tidal expiration; this is a remarkably reproducible measurement of lung mechanics. This capacity is dependent on a balance between inward recoil of lung and outward recoil of chest wall. Hence, this is larger in patients with emphysema (loss of recoil) and smaller in patients with interstitial fibrosis (increased recoil).

The statement that "air moves only when there is a difference of pressure" is somewhat incomplete when it comes to breathing mechanics, it must be added that the "difference in pressure must be good enough to overcome the resistance offered to passage of air". The first seat of resistance to the flow of air up to the gas exchanging surface of the lung is at two levels. The airways are a series of branching tubes that are divided into conducting airways and gas exchanging areas. The frictional resistance of a gas passing through a pipe is directly proportional to the length of the tube and inversely proportional to the fourth power of its radius. In other words, the longer the tube the larger the resistance, and doubling the radius of a tube reduces resistance to one-sixteenth of its previous value. Human airways are designed to take advantage of both these physical laws. After each division, the daughter bronchi are almost as big as the dividing bronchus. Therefore, cross-section is nearly doubled after each division, and the bronchi divide after only a small length. This is why the smaller airways (i.e., airways of 2–3 mm diameter or less) offer only about 10% of total airway resistance. The flow in larger airways is turbulent, hence dependent on the density of the gas that is flowing, whereas the flow in small airways is linear, hence independent of the density of the gas. This is the basis of using helium-oxygen mixture in treating diseases of airway obstruction and measurement of volume of isoflow. Airway resistance (Raw) is expressed as the difference of pressure needed to generate airflow of 1 L/s. This is normally about 2 cmH$_2$O. To generate the same rate of flow through a smoker's pipe, one would need a difference of pressure of at least 500 cmH$_2$O.

The second seat of resistance is provided partly by the elastic recoil of lung tissue and mostly by the surface tension of the liquid lining the alveoli. Elasticity is defined as the force that brings back the original shape and size of an object after the deforming force has been removed. By this definition, a steel plate is more elastic than a rubber band. The elasticity of the lung parenchyma depends on the interaction of collagen and elastin fibers. The slope of the pressure volume curve of lungs, or the volume change per unit pressure change, is known as the compliance. In the normal working range (intrapleural pressure of about −5 to −10 cmH$_2$O), the lung is remarkably distensible or very compliant. The compliance of both lungs taken together is about 200 mL/cmH$_2$O. To distend the lungs by 500 mL, usually about 3 cmH$_2$O pressure is enough. However, at higher volumes, the lungs become stiffer (less compliant) as seen by the flatter slope of the curve. Lung compliance drops in ILD, acute lung injury/acute respiratory distress syndrome (ARDS), and pulmonary edema (making it difficult to inflate), and reverse occurs in emphysema (making it difficult to deflate).

Surface tension has been defined as a force that is active on a gas liquid interface trying to reduce the interface to a minimum area. This is why a drop of water on the floor or a bubble is always circular (smallest surface area for a given volume). A certain pressure generated inside a bubble or a drop according to Laplace's law is directly proportional to the surface tension of the liquid and inversely proportional to the radius. If we apply this physical principle on human lung, one can easily see the probable disaster. The alveoli are not of uniform size; therefore, the alveolar lining fluid in a small alveolus will produce a higher pressure inside compared to that inside a larger alveolus, resulting in a situation where the smaller alveoli will empty their air content to a larger ones, and some of the smallest alveoli will never open at all. This will result in a situation where a lot of right ventricular output will get shunted to pulmonary veins—passing through atelectatic alveoli. In clinical practice, we see this happening in patients with ARDS. The only way to prevent this sequence of events in normal lung is to reduce the surface tension in smaller alveoli.

In normal lungs, this ventilation perfusion mismatching does not occur because of the presence of a chemical called surfactant that adjusts the surface tension in such a way that larger and smaller alveoli, both during inspiration and expiration, maintain an uniform pressure in the alveoli so that ventilation gets evenly distributed.

Surfactant molecules are synthesized by type II alveolar epithelial cells that lower the surface tension of alveolar lining fluid. Surface tension of water is 72 dynes/cm and that of alveolar lining fluid varies between 5 and 30 dynes/cm. Most important constituent of surfactant is dipalmitoylphosphatidylcholine (DPPC). Surfactant is formed relatively late in fetal life, and babies born prematurely may develop respiratory distress syndrome shortly after birth. Apart from DPPC, surfactants have protein (SP) molecules at both ends. These are called SP-A, B, C, and D. SP-A and D are water soluble (hydrophilic) and B and C are water insoluble—this results in the surfactant molecules orienting themselves perpendicular to the alveolar lining, one end pointing toward air, the other in the liquid. If the surface area is small, the concentration of surfactant molecules goes up and reduces the surface tension, thereby offsetting the effect of Laplace's law.

The important character of airways that one needs to keep in mind is that the caliber of airways (and consequently, the resistance offered) cyclically changes during inspiration and expiration. This is not difficult to understand, but the other important point to visualize is that extrathoracic and intrathoracic airways behave in exactly opposite way during the two phases of respiration. The upper extrathoracic airway tends to narrow down during inspiration—as the pressure inside is negative, but the negative intrapleural pressure makes the lung expand, thereby dilating all the intrathoracic airways. This is why airways obstruction in upper extrathoracic airway is more evident (at least initially) during inspiration (snoring and stridor) and that in intrathoracic airway is more evident during expiration (wheezing).

■ REGULATION OF RESPIRATION

At rest a normal healthy adult consumes about 250 mL (VO_2—5 mL/kg/min) of oxygen and produces about 200 mL of carbon dioxide every minute. Normal minute ventilation of about 5–10 L is usually enough to maintain life—under normal circumstances. But all these change during a stress (e.g., high fever or exercise). Obviously, the oxygen requirement goes up and so does the carbon dioxide output. The capability of utilizing oxygen while exercising has been taken as a measure of physical fitness. Of course, this depends not only on the respiratory system, and the ability of the cardiovascular system to transport oxygen to the tissues is equally important. In fact for normal individuals, the limiting factor for exercise capacity is cardiovascular, rather than respiratory. A fit athlete can push up the minute ventilation up to 120–150 L/min, and the cardiac output in contrast shown as modest rises from 5 L/min to about 25–30 L/min. Be that as it may, how does the respiratory control respond to oxygen demand and carbon dioxide excess in the system?

The Respiratory Center

This is composed of several groups of neurons located bilaterally in medulla oblongata and pons. These are divided into three groups: (1) Dorsal respiratory group, (2) ventral respiratory group, and (3) pneumotaxic center. The first one, dorsal respiratory group, plays the most fundamental role in control of respiration.

A fourth "apneustic center" has been described, the function of which is not clear; it presumably operates in association with the pneumotaxic center to control the depth of inspiration.

Control of Respiration Center Activity

The demands of ventilation will vary according to level of activity of the individual. We will now look at the mechanisms by which this is achieved.

Chemical Control of Ventilation

Excess of carbon dioxide and hydrogen ions stimulate the respiratory center directly.

Lack of oxygen, on the other hand, does not have a significant direct effort on respiratory center; instead, it acts almost entirely on peripheral chemoreceptors located in the carotid and the aortic bodies.

An additional chemosensitive area, separate from the three neuronal groups located in the medulla is sensitive to changes in either blood PCO_2 or hydrogen ion concentration, and in turn excites the other portions of respiratory center. Hydrogen ions do not easily cross the blood–brain barrier or the blood-cerebrospinal fluid barrier, for this reason changes in H^+ ion concentration in the blood have considerably less effect in stimulating the chemoreceptive neurons than do changes in CO_2. When $PaCO_2$ increases so does the PCO_2 of interstitial fluid and CSF. In both these fluids, CO_2 reacts with water to form hydrogen ions. Carbon dioxide losses it stimulatory defect within a few days as kidneys start retaining bicarbonate—which slowly diffuses to CSF—to combine with hydrogen ions. Changes in oxygen tension have virtually no direct effect on the respiratory center itself. Body has a special mechanism for respiratory control, located in peripheral chemoreceptors. These are located in several areas outside the brain and are especially important for detecting lack of oxygen in blood, in addition to responding to CO and H^+ ion concentrations. These receptors in turn transmit signals to the respiratory center in the brain, to help regulate respiratory activity. By far the largest number of chemoreceptors are located in the carotid bodies; however, a sizable number is in the aortic bodies too, a few are located elsewhere in association with thoracic and abdominal arteries. Each of these chemoreceptors receives a special blood supply through a minute artery directly from the adjacent arterial trunk—the blood flow through these bodies is 20 times the weight of the bodies themselves, each minute. This makes sure that the chemoreceptors are exposed to arterial blood all the time as removal of oxygen from the flowing blood is virtually nonexistent. Chemoreceptors are also sensitive to an increase in PCO_2 and hydrogen ion concentration. However, the direct effect of both these factors on respiratory center itself is much more powerful, the indirect effect through chemoreceptors is of no practical significance, with one exception; the reaction through chemoreceptors occurs as much as five times as rapidly as central stimulation; therefore, chemoreceptors increase the rapidity of response to carbon dioxide, as at the onset of exercise.

Lung Receptors

Pulmonary stretch receptors discharge in response to distension of lung, and the impulses travel to the brain in the vagus nerve. The result is that they inhibit further distension of lung and consequently slow down respiratory frequency, a phenomenon known as *Hering-Breuer* reflex. This was one of the first pulmonary reflexes described, but whether it is important in humans is unclear.

Irritant receptors are located in airways, when irritated (smokes or fumes) the reflex affects bronchoconstriction, and increased ventilation.

Juxtacapillary or J receptors are located in alveolar walls close to capillaries. Impulses from J receptors travel up vagus nerves and may be important in the rapid shallow breathing and dyspnea seen in ILD and pulmonary edema.

Irritant receptors exist in the nose, nasopharynx, larynx and trachea, and stimulation of these causes sneezing, coughing, bronchoconstriction, and laryngeal spasm.

■ CONCLUSION

Adequate supply of oxygen and removal of carbon dioxide in changing circumstances (healthy state at rest/during exercise/diseased states) essentially depends on adequately functioning respiratory system. Unless physicians understand the intricacies of normal mechanism of the system it is difficult to interpret the functional consequences of a diseased state and more importantly to assist/control the system in the critically ill with respiratory or multi organ failure. Training of elite athletes in different sports activities is another area, outside clinical medicine, where basic science of respiratory function is essential to develop training program for them.

SUGGESTED READINGS

1. Slonim NB, Hamilton LH. Respiratory Physiology, 5th edition. The CV Mosby Company; 1987.
2. Campbell EJ, Dickinson CJ, Slater JDH. Clinical Physiology, 4th edition. The English Language Book Society: Blackwell Scientific Publications; 1977.
3. Morgan Campbell EJ, Dickinson CJ, JDH Slater. Clinical Physiology, 4th edition. The English Language Book Society and Blackwell Scientific Publications; 1977.
4. West JB. Pulmonary Physiology and Pathophysiology, 1st edition. Lippincott Williams & Wilkins; 2001.
5. West JB Luks AM. West's Respiratory Physiology: The Essentials. South Asian Edition. Wolters Kluwer (India) Pvt Ltd. 2021.

CHAPTER 4

Clinical Approach and Analysis of Respiratory Symptoms

Angira Das Gupta, Subhadip Mukherjee, Nandini Chatterjee, Supriya Sarkar,
Surya Kant, Raja Dhar, Shubham Sharma, Biva Bhakat, Subhasis Mukherjee

A. CLINICAL APPROACH TO COUGH AND EXPECTORATION

Angira Das Gupta, Subhadip Mukherjee, Nandini Chatterjee, Supriya Sarkar

■ INTRODUCTION

Globally, cough is the most common reason for patients seeking medical attention. It is also one of the mechanisms by which infections can spread as droplets and most importantly it is one of many defense mechanisms that help clear excessive secretions and foreign material from the airways. Excessive cough is often a manifestation of various pulmonary and nonpulmonary diseases.

Estimates of prevalence of cough are scanty in our country. A population-based survey in rural India reports a prevalence of 3% among patients seeking medical care. Questionnaire-based estimates from the United States and Europe are between 9 and 33%. Cough, when chronic, can have serious impacts on various aspects of the patient's life. There can be problems with sleep, voice quality, musculoskeletal pain, and even rib fractures. Chronic cough can result in social problems such as relationship difficulties, decreased social interaction, and work-related problems, affecting physical, mental, and social health and even avoidance of public areas. Some patients, especially elderly women, also experience cough-related urinary incontinence with a dramatic impact on quality of life (QoL).

Cough is a reflex, and understanding its mechanism is of paramount importance in planning management and in future research. This chapter will discuss the main causes and outline a simple clinical approach to chronic cough.

WHAT ARE THE CAUSES OF COUGH?

Cough is commonly classified according to its duration as acute, subacute (lasting 3–5 weeks), and chronic (lasting more than 8 weeks). Such a classification is useful in framing the differential diagnoses and planning further management **(Table 4A.1)**.

The main concern in the management of acute cough is early recognition of life-threatening conditions which may be present such as pneumonia, severe exacerbations of preexisting lung diseases such as asthma and chronic obstructive pulmonary disease (COPD), pulmonary edema, and pulmonary embolism.

In cases of subacute onset cough, the most important task is to recognize the etiology as being infectious. When due to a noninfectious etiology, the approach is similar to chronic cough.

Chronic cough is a challenge to clinicians. Often cough is the only symptom in the absence of other clinical pointers to a specific disease.

In nonsmoker patients with chronic cough, normal chest radiology who are not in therapy with an angiotensin-converting enzyme (ACE) inhibitor, the most common causes are upper airway cough syndrome (UACS) (formerly called a postnasal drip syndrome), cough

Table 4A.1: Common causes of cough according to duration.	
Common causes	**Less common causes**
Acute cough (<3 weeks)	
Upper respiratory infections (sinusitis)	Acute exacerbations of underlying pulmonary diseases (COPD, ILD, asthma, and bronchiectasis)
Allergic rhinitis	Heart failure
Pneumonia	Acute exposure to noxious gases (occupational or environmental)
Subacute cough (3–8 weeks)	
Upper respiratory infections	Chronic heart failure
Acute exacerbations of underlying pulmonary diseases (COPD, ILD, asthma, and bronchiectasis)	Postviral infection
Chronic cough (>8 weeks)	
Upper airway cough syndrome	Connective tissue diseases (rheumatoid arthritis, scleroderma, SLE, Wegener's granulomatosis, and Sjögren's syndrome)
Obstructive airway diseases (asthma, COPD, bronchiectasis, cystic fibrosis, ILD, and bronchiectasis)	Inflammatory bowel disease
Gastroesophageal reflux	Tracheobronchomegaly
Nonasthmatic eosinophilic bronchitis	Foreign bodies (includes airway stents)
Lung cancer	Broncholithiasis
Sarcoidosis	Tracheoesophageal fistula
Indolent infections (tuberculosis and endemic fungi)	Psychogenic or habit cough

(COPD: chronic obstructive pulmonary disease; ILD: interstitial lung diseases; SLE: systemic lupus erythematosus)

variant asthma, nonasthmatic eosinophilic bronchitis (NAEB), or gastroesophageal reflux disease (GERD), alone or in combination. In fact, chronic cough may be simultaneously caused by more than one condition (19–62% of cases). However, despite comprehensive evaluation and treatment, up to 20% of patients with cough continue to remain symptomatic.

History and Clinical Examination

The current diagnostic protocols for chronic cough are based on the work of Irwin and colleagues first reported over 20 years ago. The first step is gathering a detailed medical history.

The importance of medical history in chronic cough is limited to seeking information on ACE inhibitor intake, smoking (past or current), having pets or birds at home or work, resident of a geographic area where tuberculosis or certain fungal diseases are endemic, previous history of cancer, tuberculosis, or acquired immunodeficiency syndrome (AIDS), or any current symptoms of fever, sweats, or weight loss.

Other important symptoms that may be useful in narrowing down the differential diagnoses are history of episodic wheezes, chest tightness, and shortness of breath suggestive of airway diseases or UACS.

Surprisingly, medical history in cough evaluation has been held to be of little value as regards the patient's description of his or her cough (i.e., character, timing, and aggravating factors), or the presence or absence of sputum production. None of these characteristics are of diagnostic value in terms of a specific etiology. Even when significant bronchorrhea is present, a nonsmoker patient with cough who is not on ACE inhibitors and has a normal chest roentgenogram will usually have UACS, asthma, GERD, or some combination of these diagnoses. In fact, clinical practice guidelines for patients with chronic cough suggest that neither the patient's description of his or her cough in terms of its character or timing, nor the presence or absence of sputum production, should be used to rule in or rule out a diagnosis or to determine the clinical approach. However, the presence of hemoptysis is a red flag sign for urgent evaluation.

Clinical examination is nonspecific for any specific etiology of cough. However, ear, nose, and throat (ENT) examination for ruling in a diagnosis of sinusitis or UACS must not be forgotten. The presence of wheeze on chest auscultation directs further diagnostic tests and empiric treatment. Most commonly, however, clinical examination is entirely normal.

Investigations

Radiology: A chest radiograph is the most important investigation for chronic cough patients. If abnormal and consistent with an etiology capable of causing cough, further tests are directed at diagnosing the specific etiology. But more than often chronic cough patients have normal chest X-rays.

There is no role for high-resolution CT (HRCT) scan in routine investigation of chronic cough. Its only role is to identify parenchymal or interstitial lung diseases, which are not apparent on simple chest roentgen. When used routinely, bronchiectasis can be identified in nearly a quarter of cases. Targeted use of HRCT in patients with chest radiographic abnormalities and/or clinical findings on chest examination has a diagnostic yield of only 17%.

The exact role and timing of sinus imaging in patients with chronic cough have yet to be established. Intuitively, it should follow ear, nose, and throat inspection to confirm or identify abnormalities not appreciated on examination. Plain sinus radiographs are considered to be of little value in the evaluation of chronic cough. This stems from the results of a prospective study where abnormalities of the plain sinus radiograph were identified in only 29% of patients, while in another prospective evaluation routine CT sinus imaging was no better than a good clinical examination. Thus, sinus CT scanning should be reserved for refractory cases, which may require surgical intervention.

Spirometry, bronchoprovocation test, and peak expiratory flow (PEF) measurements: Asthma is one such cause of chronic cough which can easily be diagnosed by spirometry even in busy clinics. When available, it should be performed with reversibility testing in all patients with chronic cough. Baseline spirometry results are likely to be normal in patients with cough variant asthma. This is when a bronchoprovocation test is required to demonstrate variable airflow obstruction.

Bronchoprovocation tests or bronchial challenge tests can provide useful information in patients with chronic cough. This test can be done either with agents working directly on airway musculature (histamine and methacholine) or by indirect methods (hypertonic saline, exercise, mannitol, and adenosine), where bronchoconstriction is stimulated by mediators released from inflammatory cells.

Bronchial hyperreactivity or a positive bronchoprovocation test in a patient with cough and normal spirometry helps in the diagnosis of asthma (cough variant asthma) by demonstrating variable airflow obstruction. Airway hyperreactivity may develop during or following an acute viral respiratory illness and may persist for some months afterward. A positive challenge test in such circumstances may be diagnostically misleading. A negative bronchial challenge test effectively excludes the diagnosis of asthma but does not eliminate a cough that may respond to steroid treatment. In fact, a negative bronchial challenge should prompt the clinician to look for evidence of underlying uncontrolled airway inflammation.

Sometimes, PEF measurement in patients with persistent cough presenting helps in diagnosing airflow obstruction, especially if spirometry is not available. Otherwise, the use of PEF measurements to assess bronchodilator response appears to have limitations compared to conventional methods. The value of serial PEF measurements for determining diurnal variability has not been properly assessed and is infrequently requested by specialist cough clinics.

Measuring airway inflammation: The major role of measuring airway inflammation (bronchitis) in chronic cough is to demonstrate the presence and nature of bronchitis in patients without functional or radiologic abnormalities, especially bronchial hyperreactivity associated with asthma. If the underlying inflammation is eosinophilic, the clinical condition is that of eosinophilic bronchitis without asthma. This forms almost 15% of cases of chronic cough in referral clinics and is possibly an underestimate due to nonavailability of tools for measuring airway inflammation in most centers.

The most well-described method for measuring airway inflammation is by sputum quantitative assay. The test entails selection of a small quantity of sputum from either a spontaneous or induced sample, treatment with a sputolysin (dithiothreitol) or subsequent filtering to obtain a homogeneous suspension of cells. The total cell count and viability are determined in a hemocytometer, while differential counts are obtained from Wright stained cytospins. According to the cellular nature, inflammation can be of four main types namely: (1) Eosinophilic, (2) neutrophilic, (3) combined eosinophilic and neutrophilic, and (4) paucigranulocytic.

Exhaled breath nitric oxide (FeNO) may be a simpler and operator friendly alternative to sputum quantitative assay, but currently it is not recommended routinely in the management of chronic cough. Its disadvantages are that it cannot distinguish between eosinophilic and noneosinophilic inflammation and has a wide normal range. However, a normal FeNO level can reliably rule out uncontrolled airway inflammation. The measurement of different inflammatory substances (e.g., hydrogen peroxide) in breath condensate, although currently a research procedure, may have a place in the diagnosis of chronic cough in the future.

Fiberoptic bronchoscopy: Despite a low diagnostic yield in the routine evaluation of chronic cough, bronchoscopy has significant diagnostic potential in patients where the more common causes have been rigorously excluded. In patients with refractory cough, bronchoscopic diagnoses included broncholithiasis, tracheobronchopathia, and laryngeal dyskinesia. Aspirated foreign bodies may go unrecognized for prolonged periods of time. Fiberoptic bronchoscopy may also sometimes be used for airway sampling either by mucosal biopsy or bronchial lavage in situations where the cause of cough remains undetected despite all noninvasive work-ups.

Gastrointestinal investigations: Since the association between gastroesophageal reflux and chronic cough has long been established, an empirical trial of antireflux therapy may be the best first-line approach for patients with cough with or without symptoms of heartburn. If a therapeutic trial fails, laboratory investigations such as 24-hour esophageal pH monitoring may be required. In fact, 24-hour esophageal pH monitoring is currently the best single test to help characterize any link between gastroesophageal reflux and cough. With the availability of dual probe technology, it is now possible to detect reflux to the hypopharynx and beyond (laryngopharyngeal reflux), which, though uncommon, occurs in some patients and may be the reason for their cough.

Another important concept that has evolved when evaluating patients who continue to cough despite complete acid suppression is that of nonacid refluxate. It is estimated that up to one-third of reflux episodes in patients with GERD are nonacid, and a recent development has been the simultaneous intraesophageal impedance and pH measurement of acid and nonacid reflux events. These patients with nonacid reflux might benefit from antireflux surgery.

Psychological assessment: A diagnosis of psychogenic cough (habit cough) in adults or children ("cough tic") warrants careful exclusion of organic causes. A psychological assessment is usually reserved as a last resort and, psychotherapy has shown favorable outcomes in such situations.

■ CASE VIGNETTE 1

A 73-year-old smoker developed high fever for 5 days associated with cough with blood stained purulent expectorant and pain in right lower chest aggravated with cough.

CHAPTER 4: Clinical Approach and Analysis of Respiratory Symptoms

a. What are the types of pneumonia?

Ans. Community-acquired pneumonia (CAP) and hospital-acquired pneumonia (HAP). Ventilator-associated pneumonia is a part of HAP. Recently added type is healthcare-associated pneumonia (HCAP).

b. What are the likely organisms in CAP?

Ans. Common organisms causing CAP are *Streptococcus pneumoniae, Haemophilus influenzae, Klebsiella pneumoniae, Chlamydia pneumoniae, Mycoplasma pneumoniae, Pseudomonas aeruginosa, Legionella* species. *Staphylococcus* is not a usual cause of CAP. Anaerobic infection occurs in setting of aspiration.

c. What are the CURB-65 criteria?

Ans. C for level of consciousness, U means blood urea nitrogen (more than 7 mmol/L), R means respiratory rate (≥30 breaths/min), B means blood pressure (systolic ≤ 90 mm Hg and/or diastolic ≤60 mm Hg), and 65 means age ≥ 65 years. Score 0 can be treated at home, score 1 and 2 should be admitted to a hospital and score ≥ 3 needs admission to intensive care unit (ICU).

d. What are the markers of severe pneumonia?

Ans. CURB-65 score 3 or more are indicators of severe pneumonia and need treatment at ICU. Multilobar involvement, hypoxemia [oxygen saturation (SpO_2) < 90%], acidosis (pH < 7.3), confusion, respiratory rate > 30 breaths/minute, neutropenia, thrombocytopenia, hypoalbuminemia, hyponatremia, and hypoglycemia are markers of severe pneumonia.

Other markers of severe pneumonia include complications of pneumonia such as parapneumonic effusion, empyema, septicemia, multiorgan failure, associated diseases such as diabetes, renal failure, and neurological diseases.

Another scoring system is pneumonia severity index (PSI) that includes 20 variables with age, coexisting illness, and abnormal physical and laboratory findings.

e. What are the antibiotic choices for CAP?

Ans. Beta-lactam antibiotics such as amoxycillin 1 g three times a day (TID), coamoxyclav 2 g two times a day (BID), cefuroxime 500 mg BID, cepodoxim 200 mg BID, and ceftriaxone 1–2 g intravenously (IV) BID.

Macrolide such as azithromycin 500 mg daily and clarithromycin 500 mg BID. Doxycycline 100 mg BID, levofloxacin 750 mg daily (fluoroquinolone should be avoided in CAP treatment).

Usual duration of treatment is 7 days.

Q1. What is your diagnosis?

Ans. Community-acquired pneumonia.

Q2. What are the points in favor?

Ans. Points in favor are high fever, cough, purulent/rusty expectoration, pleuritic chest pain along with findings of consolidation (high temperature, use of accessory muscles, diminished movement over the particular lobe, impaired to dull percussion notes, bronchial breath

CHAPTER 4: Clinical Approach and Analysis of Respiratory Symptoms

sound, increased vocal resonance, egophony and whispering pectoriloquy, and absence of mediastinal shift.

Q3. What are the physical signs of pneumonia?

Ans. High temperature, use of accessory muscles, diminished movement over the particular lobe, impaired to dull percussion note, bronchial breath sound, increased vocal resonance, egophony and whispering pectoriloquy, and absence of mediastinal shift.

Q4. What are the radiological signs of consolidation?

Ans. Homogenous opacity usually confined to a lobe with peripheral alveolar filling pattern and the presence of air bronchogram.

Q5. Is it possible to have mediastinal shift to the same side of pneumonia?

Ans. Usually, there is no mediastinum shift. Mediastinum may be shifted toward diseased side in case of associated lung volume loss due to fibrosis or collapse. Fibrosis may occur due to delayed resolution of pneumonia. Collapse may be due to postobstructive pneumonia or collapse-consolidation (middle lobe syndrome).

Q6. What are the indications for hospitalization in pneumonia?

Ans. CURB-65 score 1 or more.

Q7. What are the complications of pneumonia?

Ans. Parapneumonic effusion, empyema, delayed resolution of pneumonia, superinfection, septicemia, and septic embolism.

Q8. How will you investigate pneumonia?

Ans. Routine peripheral blood examination, blood sugar, urea, creatinine, liver function test (LFT), chest X-ray, sputum gram-stain, sputum culture and sensitivity (C/S), sputum for acid-fast bacilli (AFB)/cartridge-based nucleic acid amplification test (CBNAAT), blood C/S; computed tomography (CT) of thorax and bronchoscopy in selected case (hemoptysis, delayed resolution, and mediastinum shifted to disease side), examination of pleural fluid; and urine antigen analysis for *Legionella* infection. Other tests such as polymerase chain reaction (PCR) and serology may be required.

Q9. How to suspect development of effusion with pneumonia?

Ans. Mediastinum shift toward opposite side, dullness/stony dullness/diminished or absent breath sound, and vocal resonance.

Q10. How will you investigate pneumonia?

Ans. Already given.

Q11. What is the line of management of pneumonia?

Ans. Appropriate antibiotic and supportive treatment with paracetamol for fever/chest pain, oxygen for hypoxemia, aspiration, and examination of pleural fluid. Hospitalized patients should be treated with intravenous antibiotics. Some cases may require invasive ventilation.

CASE VIGNETTE 2

A 65-year-old man presents with insidious onset of cough with mucoid to mucopurulent expectoration and sometimes hemoptysis for many years along with a past history of tuberculosis (TB) 15 years ago.

The outline of findings in this case:
Insidious onset of cough with mucoid to mucopurulent expectoration and occasional hemoptysis for more than 5 years; flattening of left hemithorax, scoliosis with concavity toward left, dropping left shoulder, winging of left scapula, diminished movement of left hemithorax, trachea shifted toward left, apical impulse at left anterior axillary line, rib crowding in left hemithorax, and crackles scattered over left hemithorax.

Q1. What is the diagnosis?
Ans. Left lung fibrosis.

Q2. What are the types of fibrosis of the lung?
Ans. Lung parenchymal fibrosis, pleural fibrosis, pleuropulmonary fibrosis, and interstitial fibrosis.

Q3. What is "diffuse fibrosis" of the lung?
Ans. This is interstitial fibrosis usually bilateral involving mainly lower parts of the lungs. That may be idiopathic interstitial disease (ILD), also called diffuse parenchymal lung disease (DPLD), or secondary to diseases such as collagen vascular disease, occupational and drug induced.

Q4. What are the classical features of fibrosing alveolitis at the bedside?
Ans. Progressive dyspnea, dry cough, bilateral disease, diminished movement of thorax, end inspiratory crackles predominantly at lung bases.

CASE VIGNETTE 3

A 65-year-old man presents with acute onset of cough, dyspnea, and two episodes of hemoptysis in the last 1 month.
  He had been a heavy smoker for the last 30 years. On examination, there was shifting of the trachea to left side, the left side of chest is flattened, drooping of the shoulder present on the left, percussion note is impaired, the breath sound is diminished and impaired resonance on left hemithorax present.

Q1. What is the diagnosis?
Ans. It is a left-sided collapse of lung.

Q2. How do you classify collapse of the lung?
Ans. Absorption collapse (due to absorption of air distal to airway obstruction such as lung cancer and foreign body); relaxation collapse (due to release of negative pleural pressure

such as pneumothorax and pleural effusion); cicatricial collapse (due to stiffening of lung due to fibrosis); microatelectasis [adhesive atelectasis due to loss of surfactant found in acute respiratory distress syndrome (ARDS)].

Q3. What are the common causes of absorption collapse in relation to age?

Ans. In children—foreign body inhalation, and in elderly persons—bronchogenic carcinoma are the most important causes. Other causes include extraluminal obstruction as a result of compression by lymph nodes usually occurs in children; intraluminal disease such as malignant and benign diseases arising from the bronchus such as carcinoma (CA) or adenoma; and intraluminal obstruction due to foreign-body, blood clot, mucus clot, etc.

Q4. What is "middle lobe syndrome"?

Ans. Collapse consolidation of middle lobe without intraluminal obstruction.

Q5. What are the clinical features of bronchiectasis?

Ans. Cough with profuse mucoid/mucopurulent expectoration that will be separated into three layers while kept in a test tube and hemoptysis. There may be weight loss or failure to thrive, clubbing, and course/lathery biphasic crackles.

Q6. What are the clinical features of pulmonary tuberculosis (postprimary)?

Ans. Cough for more than 2 weeks, unexplained fever for more than 2 weeks, significant weight loss or no weight gain in children, hemoptysis, and abnormal chest X-ray. Signs are usually nonspecific or due to complications. Sign may be absent.

Q7. What are the clinical stigmata of evidence of past or present tuberculous infections?

Ans. The word stigmata should not be used with TB as this can lead to serious socioeconomic consequences and as a result increase the delay in contacting healthcare professional.

Q8. What are the effects of asbestos exposure in respiratory system?

Ans. Pleural plaque, benign pleural effusion, malignant pleural effusion, interstitial lung disease, bronchogenic carcinoma, and mesothelioma.

Q9. What is "pack year"?

Ans. The number of cigarette packets (20/pack) multiplied by years of smoking. If a patient smokes 10 cigarettes/day for 10 years then pack year will be $10/20 \times 10 = 5$.

Q10. What is the position of mediastinum in collapse of the lung?

Ans. Mediastinum will be shifted toward diseased side in whole lung collapse; trachea will be shifted in upper lobe collapse; whereas, heart will be shifted in lower lobe collapse.

Q11. What are the bronchopulmonary segments in the lung?

Ans. Collapse of bronchopulmonary segment is unlikely as there are communications among segments. There are 18–20 bronchopulmonary segments. In right side, upper lobe—apical, posterior and anterior; middle lobe—medial and lateral; lower lobe—apical and medial, anterior, lateral, posterior basal segments. In left side, upper lobe—apical and posterior (or apicoposterior segment), anterior, superior, and inferior lingular; lower lobe—medial segment may be absent.

Q12. What investigations would you like to perform (fibrosis or collapse)?

Ans. Chest X-ray, HRCT thorax in fibrosis/contrast-enhanced computed tomography (CECT) in collapse; sputum for AFB, CBNAAT, and malignant cell; fiberoptic bronchoscopy (FOB) in selected cases; apart from routine blood examination and blood biochemistry.

SUGGESTED READINGS

1. Irwin R, Boulet LP, Cloutier MM, Fuller R, Gold PM, Hoffstein V, et al. Managing cough as a defense mechanism and as a symptom: a consensus panel report of the American College of Chest Physicians. Chest. 1998;114(suppl 2):133S-81S.
2. Fochsen G, Deshpande K, Diwan V, Mishra A, Diwan VK, Thorson A, et al. Health care seeking among individuals with cough and tuberculosis: a population-based study from rural India. Int J Tuberc Lung Dis. 2006;10(9):995-1000.
3. Morice AH. Chronic cough: epidemiology. Chron Respir Dis. 2008;5(1):43-7.
4. Chung KF, Pavord ID. Prevalence, pathogenesis and causes of chronic cough. Lancet. 2008;371(9621):1364-74.
5. Morice AH, Fontana GA, Belvisi MG, Birring SS, Chung KF, Dicpinigaitis PV, et al. ERS guidelines on the assessment of cough. Eur Respir J. 2007;29:1256-76.
6. Swigris JJ, Stewart AL, Gould MK, Wilson SR. Patients' perspectives on how idiopathic pulmonary fibrosis affects the quality of their lives. Health Qual Life Outcomes. 2005;3:61.
7. Birring SS, Prudon B, Carr AJ, Singh SJ, Morgan MD, Pavord I, et al. Development of a symptom specific health status measure for patients with chronic cough: Leicester Cough Questionnaire (LCQ). Thorax. 2003;58:339-43.
8. Bradaia F, Lazor R, Khouatra C, Poissonnier L, Cottin V, Cordier JF. Incontinence urinaire a la toux au cours des pneumopathies interstitielles diffuses [Urinary incontinence due to chronic cough in interstitial lung disease]. Rev Mal Respir. 2009;26:499-504.
9. Lee K, Birring S. Cough. Medicine. 2012;40:173-6.
10. Pacheco A. Chronic cough: from a complex dysfunction of the neurological circuit to the production of persistent cough. Thorax. 2014;69:881-3.
11. Morice AH, Millqvist E, Belvisi MG, Bieksiene K, Birring SS, Chung KF, et al. Expert opinion on the cough hypersensitivity syndrome in respiratory medicine. Eur Respir J. 2014;44:1132-48.
12. Polverino M, Polverino F, Fasolino M, Andò F, Alfieri A, De Blasio F. Anatomy and neuro-pathophysiology of the cough reflex arc. Multidiscip Respir Med. 2012;7(1):5.
13. Banner KH, Igney F, Poll C. TRP channels: emerging targets for respiratory disease. Pharmacol Ther. 2011;130:371-84.
14. Jones RM, Hilldrup S, Hope-Gill BD, Eccles R, Harrison NK. Mechanical induction of cough in idiopathic pulmonary fibrosis. Cough. 2011;7:2.
15. Harrison NK, Pynn MC. Nerves, cough, and idiopathic pulmonary fibrosis. EMJ Respir. 2015;3:38-45.
16. Lieu TM, Myers AC, Meeker S, Undem BJ. TRPV1 induction in airway vagal low-threshold mechanosensory neurons by allergen challenge and neurotrophic factors. Am J Physiol Lung Cell Mol Physiol. 2012;302:L941-8.
17. Comroe JH. Special acts involving breathing. In: Cugell DW (Ed). Physiology of Respiration: An Introductory Text, 2nd edition. Chicago, IL: Year Book Medical Publishers Inc.; 1974. pp. 230-1.
18. Irwin RS, Corrao WM, Pratter MR. Chronic persistent cough in the adult: the spectrum and frequency of cases and successful outcome of specific therapy. Am Rev Respir Dis. 1981;123:414-7.
19. Irwin RS, Baumann MH, Bolser DC, Boulet LP, Braman SS, Brightling CE, et al. Diagnosis and Management of Cough Executive Summary: ACCP Evidence-Based Clinical Practice Guidelines. Chest. 2006;129:1S-23S.
20. McGarvey LPA, Heaney LG, Lawson JT, Johnston BT, Scally CM, Ennis M, et al. Evaluation and outcome of patients with chronic non-productive cough using a comprehensive diagnostic protocol. Thorax. 1998;53:738-43.
21. Palombini BC, Villanova CA, Araujo E, Gastal OL, Alt DC, Stolz DP, et al. A pathogenic triad in chronic cough: asthma, postnasal drip syndrome and gastro-oesophageal reflux disease. Chest. 1999;116:279-84.
22. Poe HR, Harder RV, Israel RH. Chronic persistent cough: experience in diagnosis and outcome using an anatomic diagnostic protocol. Chest. 1989;95:723-7.

23. Mello CJ, Irwin RS, Curley FJ. Predictive values of the character, timing, and complications of chronic cough in diagnosing its cause. Arch Intern Med. 1996;156:997-1003.
24. Smyrnios NA, Irwin RS, Curley FJ. Chronic cough with a history of excessive sputum production: the spectrum and frequency of causes, key components of the diagnostic evaluation, and outcome of specific therapy. Chest. 1995;108:991-9.
25. Ojoo J, Kastelik JA, Mulrennan S, et al. Selective use of thoracic tomographs in patients with chronic cough (abstract). Eur Respir J. 2002;20(Suppl 38):449s.
26. Pratter MR, Bartter T, Lotano R. The role of sinus imaging in the treatment of chronic cough in adults. Chest. 1999;116:1287-91.
27. Cockroft DW, Ruffin RE, Dolovich J, Hargreave FE. Allergen-induced increase in non-allergic bronchial reactivity. Clin Allergy. 1977;7(6):503-13.
28. de Kluijver J, Grünberg K, Sont JK, Hoogeveen M, van Schadewijk WA, de Klerk EP, et al. Rhinovirus infection in nonasthmatic subjects: effects on intrapulmonary airways. Eur Respir J. 2002;20:274-9.
29. Gibson PG, Dolovich J, Denberg J, Ramsdale EH, Hargreave FE. Chronic cough: eosinophilic bronchitis without asthma. Lancet. 1989:1346-8.
30. Thiadens HA, De Bock GH, Van Houwelingen JC, Dekker FW, De Waal MW, Springer MP, et al. Can peak expiratory flow measurements reliably identify the presence of obstruction and bronchodilator response as assessed by FEV1 in primary care patients presenting with a persistent cough? Thorax. 1999;54:1055-60.
31. Gibson PG, Hargreave FE, Girgis-Gabardo A, Morris M, Denburg JA, Dolovich J. Chronic cough with eosinophilic bronchitis: examination for variable airflow obstruction and response to corticosteroid. Clin Exp Allergy. 1995;25:127-32.
32. Brightling C, Ward R, Goh KL, Wardlaw AJ, Pavord ID. Eosinophilic bronchitis is an important cause of chronic cough. Am J Respir Crit Care Med. 1999;160:406-10.
33. Pizzichini E, Pizzichini MM, Efthimiadis A, Hargreave FE, Dolovich J. Measurement of inflammatory indices in induced sputum: effects of selection of sputum to minimize salivary contamination. Eur Respir J. 1996;9:1174-80.
34. Sen RP, Walsh TE. Fibreoptic bronchoscopy for refractory cough. Chest. 1991;99:33-5.
35. Irwin RS, French CL, Curley FJ, Zawacki JK, Bennett FM. Chronic cough due to gastroesophageal reflux. Clinical, diagnostic, and pathogenetic aspects. Chest. 1993;104:1511-7.
36. Sifrim D, Holloway R, Silny J, Xin Z, Tack J, Lerut A, et al. Acid, nonacid, and gas reflux in patients with gastroesophageal reflux disease during ambulatory 24-hour pH impedance recordings. Gastroenterology. 2001;120:1588-98.
37. Ojoo JC, Kastelik JA, Morice AH. A boy with a disabling cough. Lancet. 2003;361:674.
38. Mastrovich JD, Greenberger PA. Psychogenic cough in adults: a report of two cases and review of the literature. Allergy Asthma Proc. 2002;23:27-33.

B. CLINICAL APPROACH TO HEMOPTYSIS

Surya Kant, Nandini Chatterjee

■ INTRODUCTION

Hemoptysis is the expectoration of blood that originates from the lower respiratory tract. Bleeding from the upper airways is excluded from this definition.

Pseudohemoptysis occurs due to infections with *Serratia marcescens*, which produces a red pigment. So, there is red expectoration, but there are no red blood cells (RBCs) in the sputum.

False hemoptysis/spurious hemoptysis is bleeding from the upper aerodigestive tract (gums, nose, or pharynx).

Hemoptysis is usually a self-limiting event, but in fewer than 5% of cases, it may be massive. Hemoptysis is mainly classified by the amount of blood expectorated into mild, moderate, and massive. Massive hemoptysis is either more than and equal to 500 mL of expectorated blood over a 24-hour period or bleeding at a rate more than and equal to 100 mL/h. A large volume of expectorated blood alone should not define massive hemoptysis, rather an amount of blood sufficient to threaten the patient's life can be a more correct and functional definition of severe hemoptysis. Massive hemoptysis is usually a life-threatening condition with mortality rate of more than 50%. Flooding of the airways with blood leads to asphyxiation, and this is usually the cause of death rather than exsanguination.

■ ETIOLOGY

Two arterial vascular systems supply blood to the lungs: (1) The pulmonary arteries and (2) the bronchial arteries. The pulmonary arteries provide 99% of the arterial blood to the lungs and are involved in gas exchange. The bronchial arteries supply nourishment to the extra- and intrapulmonary airways. The bronchial arteries are direct branches of the aorta; hence, blood flow is at systemic pressure, while pulmonary arteries have one-third systemic pressure. In cases of severe hemoptysis, the source of bleeding usually originates from bronchial vessels (in 90% cases) and pulmonary arteries in 5% cases.

Table 4B.1 shows the differentiation of hemoptysis from hematemesis. **Box 4B.1** shows the common causes that are to be searched for in a case of hemoptysis.

■ APPROACH TO PATIENT

History

The history should be directed toward the cause that is relevant to the setting as treatment is mainly treating the primary cause. The color, amount of blood, and associated symptoms should be asked to determine the cause of hemoptysis and to differentiate from upper gastrointestinal (GI) bleed or bleeding from nasal tract. Old age and smoking should warrant search for malignancy. Constitutional symptoms such as fever, fatigue, malaise,

Table 4B.1: Differentiation of hemoptysis from hematemesis.

Hemoptysis	Hematemesis
There is usually a tingling sensation in the throat prior to the episode	Patient will usually complain of nausea and an upset stomach
The blood is frothy and bright red	Blood is dark red, brown, and nonfrothy
Blood is associated with sputum	Blood is associated with food particles
pH will be neutral to alkaline	Blood will give an acidic pH
Stool examination for occult blood is usually negative	Stool is almost always positive for occult blood
There is a history of lung disease	There is a history of gastrointestinal or liver disease
Not associated with malena	Associated with malena

BOX 4B.1 Etiology of hemoptysis.

Infections:
- Pulmonary tuberculosis
- Posttuberculosis Rasmussen's aneurysm
- Pneumonia
- Lung abscess
- Bronchiectasis
- Fungal infections

Neoplasms:
- Bronchogenic carcinoma
- Metastatic nodules
- Carcinoid tumor
- Bronchial adenoma
- Hamartoma

Cardiovascular disorders:
- Mitral stenosis
- Pulmonary infarction from thromboembolism

Trauma:
- Penetrating lung injury
- Lung contusion

Hematologic disorders:
- Blood dyscrasia

Autoimmune disorders:
- Goodpasture's syndrome
- Wegener's granulomatosis
- Small and medium vessel vasculitis

Metabolic disorders:
- Uremia
- Liver cirrhosis

Vascular disorders:
- Pulmonary arteriovenous malformation (PAVM)
- Osler–Weber–Rendu syndrome

Drug-induced:
- Antiplatelet drugs
- Anticoagulant drugs
- Nonsteroidal anti-inflammatory drugs (NSAIDs)
- D-penicillamine

and expectoration are usually seen in infectious causes. Recurrent childhood infections, recurrent sinusitis, and infertility can be associated with bronchiectasis or cystic fibrosis. Foul smelling copious expectoration with postural variation is usually seen in lung abscess. Joint pains, skin lesions, epistaxis, hematuria, and a family history might be a clue to autoimmune disorders. Bronchogenic carcinoma might be associated with hoarseness of voice, superior vena cava (SVC) obstruction, loss of weight, and appetite. Sudden onset chest pain and dyspnea can be a feature of pulmonary thromboembolism.

Examination

Physical Examination

Severity of anemia has to be assessed. Clubbing may be a feature of bronchiectasis, cystic fibrosis, lung abscess, and pulmonary arteriovenous malformation (PAVM). Oral and nasal cavity should be examined to find alternate sources of bleeding. Pedal edema might give a clue toward cardiovascular cause. The patient might have tachypnea, tachycardia, the use of accessory muscles, cyanosis, fatigue, and diaphoresis, indicating any respiratory or cardiac cause. Features of SVC obstruction are seen in malignancy, and nasal septal deformity is associated with Wegener's granulomatosis.

Respiratory System

Auscultation of lungs plays an important role in localizing lesions. Findings that should be kept in mind are focal wheeze and crepitations.

Other System Examination

Auscultation of heart will be helpful in finding murmur of mitral stenosis or mitral regurgitation which is an important cause of hemoptysis. The examination of skin helps in identifying bruising potentially suggestive of coagulopathy, telangiectasia of Osler–Weber–Rendu, palpable purpura, or other rash suggestive of vasculitis.

■ INVESTIGATIONS

Pathological and Biochemical Tests

Hemoglobin and Blood Counts

Hemoglobin levels can be low due to hemoptysis, which should be corrected either orally or parenterally depending on the degree of anemia. Leukocyte count is an important indicator of infection in conditions such as pneumonia, lung abscess, and bronchiectasis.

Renal Function Tests

Deranged urea and creatinine levels indicate conditions such as Goodpasture's syndrome, Wegener's granulomatosis, and uremia. Urine microscopic examination might give clues to diagnose occult bleeding in the urinary tract and renal conditions such as vasculitis that may be a primary cause of hemoptysis.

Bleeding Profile

Prothrombin time/international normalized ratio (PT/INR), bleeding time, and clotting time should be done to detect intrinsic clotting defects. Deranged coagulation profile due to any cause can lead to hemoptysis. They include immune thrombocytopenic purpura (ITP), disseminated intravascular coagulation (DIC), and drug use such as antiplatelets and warfarin.

Bacteriologic

Sputum examination for acid fast bacilli, Gram-stain, and fungal elements, along with culture should be done in suspected infective cases.

Imaging

Chest X-ray

It is considered the initial imaging modality for evaluating patients with hemoptysis. It is quick, inexpensive, and readily available. Chest X-ray (CXR) can assist in lateralizing bleeding and reveal a focal or diffuse lung involvement. CXR may detect underlying parenchymal and pleural abnormalities such as mass, pneumonia, chronic lung disease, atelectasis, cavitary lesion, and alveolar opacities due to alveolar hemorrhage.

Contrast-enhanced Computed Tomography Thorax

Since the sensitivity of CXR is not very high and all causes of hemoptysis cannot be delineated by CXR, it is essential to get a contrast-enhanced computed tomography (CECT) thorax in a certain subgroup of patients. It represents a noninvasive and highly useful imaging tool in the clinical context of hemoptysis and allows a comprehensive evaluation of the lung parenchyma, airways, and thoracic vessels by using contrast material. Computed tomography (CT) may identify the bleeding site in 63–100% of patients with hemoptysis and has the ability to uncover the potential underlying causes of bleeding, such as bronchiectasis, pulmonary infections, and lung cancer.

Computed Tomography Pulmonary Angiography

Computed tomography pulmonary angiography is important to identify origin and course of arteries, causing the bleeding. Pulmonary hemorrhage usually appears as focal or diffuse hazy consolidation or ground-glass opacity, even though thickened interlobular septa superimposed on a background of ground-glass attenuation ("crazy-paving" pattern) have also been described.

Bronchoscopy

For many years, bronchoscopy has been considered the primary method for diagnosing and localizing hemoptysis, especially if massive. Bronchoscopy, performed with either a rigid or flexible endoscope, is helpful in identifying active bleeding and for assessment of the airways in patients with massive hemoptysis. Bronchoscopy yields additional information about endobronchial lesions, a mucosal abnormality, and site for biopsy, and allows samples for tissue diagnosis, microbial cultures, bronchoalveolar lavage (BAL) fluid for cell counts, cultures, and brush smears. Moreover, with bronchoscopy, cold saline solution can be instilled directly into the airways at the level of the bleeding source, if identified, and balloon inflation or laser coagulation may be used to control hemorrhage.

Other Investigations

Perinuclear antineutrophilic cytoplasmic antibody (p-ANCA), cytoplasmic antineutrophilic cytoplasmic antibody (c-ANCA), rheumatoid factor (RF), and anticyclic citrullinated peptide (anti-CCP) are important indicators for immune-mediated diseases such as vasculitis and rheumatologic disorders.

Flowchart 4B.1 shows the approach for evaluation and management of hemoptysis.

CHAPTER 4: Clinical Approach and Analysis of Respiratory Symptoms

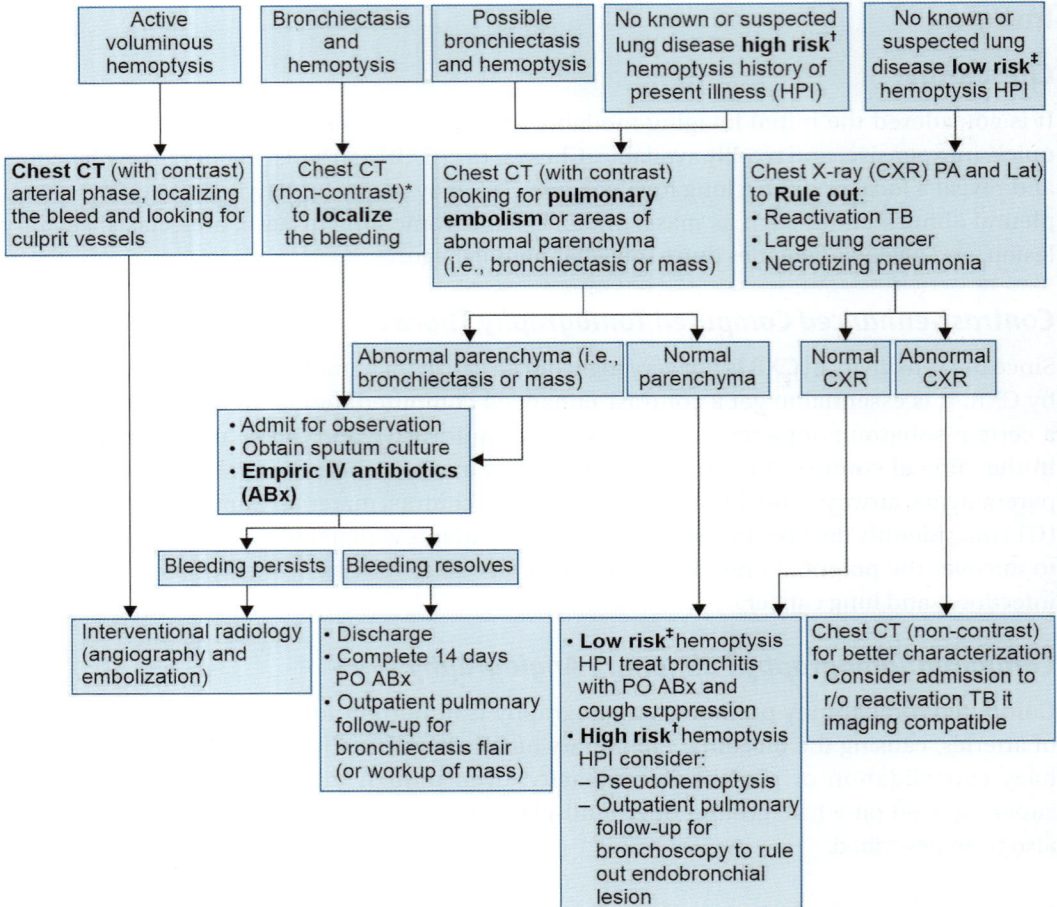

* Contrast (arterial phase) may be used if embolization is likely (i.e., **high risk** hemoptysis HPI) but is unnecessary with a **low risk** hemoptysis HPI.
† **High risk** hemoptysis HPI: No cough, phlegm, or respiratory illness.
‡ **Low risk** hemoptysis HPI: Productive cough, blood tinged sputum, respiratory illness.

FLOWCHART 4B.1: Schematic algorithm for approach to a patient with hemoptysis.
Courtesy: Jude W Landsberg. Manual for Pulmonary and Critical Care Medicine. pp. 569–70.

■ CASE VIGNETTE

A 24-year-old man presented with a history of low-grade fever for 1 month, weight loss, and night sweats. He came to emergency room (ER) with coughing out blood this morning. On examination, pallor was positive, pulse rate 90 beats/min, and temperature 99°F. Chest—few coarse crepitations present in infraclavicular area, bronchial breath sound in that area.

Q1. What is the differential diagnosis?
Ans. Pulmonary TB, post-TB sequela, bronchiectasis, lung abscess, bronchogenic carcinoma, bronchial adenoma, mitral heart disease, arteriovenous (AV) malformation, etc.

Q2. What are the investigations?
Ans. Chest X-ray, HRCT of thorax, ear, nose, and throat (ENT) examination, sputum examination for acid-fast bacillus (AFB), cartridge-based nucleic acid amplification test (CBNNAT), Gram-stain and culture and sensitivity (C/S), bronchoscopy, echocardiography, CT angiography, etc.

Q3. How to confirm the diagnosis?
Ans. Bronchiectasis can be confirmed by HRCT thorax though bronchography is the gold standard. TB can be confirmed by sputum/representative sample for AFB and CBNAAT.

Q4. What are causes of hemoptysis?
Ans. Pulmonary TB, post-TB sequelae, bronchiectasis, lung abscess, bronchogenic carcinoma, bronchial adenoma, mitral heart disease, AV malformation, etc.

Q5. How to differentiate from hematemesis?
Ans. Hemoptysis is coughing out of blood where blood is usually mixed with sputum, blood mixed expectoration or blood streak sputum, fresh red colored expectoration, associated with manifestations of primary lung disease. Whereas hematemesis is vomiting out of blood, blood is coffee colored, may be mixed with food particles, associated with acidity or heart burn, there may be manifestations of primary gastrointestinal or liver disease.

Q6. What are the causes of massive hemoptysis?
Ans. Bronchiectasis, rupture of AV malformation, rupture of aneurysm in tubercular cavity, or post-TB bronchiectasis. Usually in TB or lung cancer, hemoptysis is not massive.

Q7. What is massive hemoptysis?
Ans. Coughing out of blood more than 500 mL in a day or any amount of bleeding that causes hemodynamic instability.

Q8. What is a bronchial breath sound?
Ans. Bronchial breath sound is blowing in character with expiratory phase as long as inspiratory phase, and there is no gap between inspiration and expiration.

Q9. What are the findings in a cavity with patent bronchus?
Ans. Low-pitched bronchial (cavernous) breath sound, coarse crepitation, and rarely posttussive suction and crack pot resonance.

Q10. Sputum reveals AFB and CBNAAT are positive.
Ans. It is diagnostic of microbiologically confirmed pulmonary TB.

Q11. What are CBNAAT and line probe assay?
Ans. They are molecular tests to detect genome specific for *Mycobacterium tuberculosis* complex, drug-specific genes, and drug mutation gene.

Q12. What are the uses of CBNAAT?
Ans. The CBNAAT is used to confirm the presence of *Mycobacterium tuberculosis* complex and to detect rifampicin sensitivity/resistance.

Q13. How to treat the case?

Ans. Hemoptysis should be treated with rest, sedative, cough suppressants, coagulating agents along with management of the primary disease. Intravenous fluid and blood transfusion may be required in massive hemoptysis. Lung resection in localized disease or bronchial artery embolization is an option in some cases where medical treatment fails.

Q14. What are the complications of antitubercular therapy (ATT)?

Ans. Usual complications include nausea, vomiting, anorexia, liver toxicity (rise of liver enzymes to jaundice), peripheral neuropathy, optic neuritis, hyperuricemia, psychosis, etc.

Q15. What is ATT-induced hepatitis?

Ans. Hepatitis includes rise of liver enzymes to jaundice, sometimes with nausea, vomiting or anorexia, those are occurring following treatment with ATD.

Q16. What drugs to give in ATD-induced hepatitis?

Ans. Liver enzyme rise is usual with ATD therapy. If enzyme rise is >5 times or there is jaundice then stopping of ATD is indicated, except serious disease such as miliary TB, meningeal TB, or tubercular septicemia, etc., followed by restarting ATD from less to more hepatotoxic drugs after liver functions become normal. Surprisingly and fortunately, reintroduction of ATD is usually well tolerated. Treatment usually depends on seriousness of disease, degree of liver toxicity, and phase of treatment. Depending on those factors, several regimes may be prescribed with (1) no hepatotoxic drug with staphylococcal enterotoxin-like toxin X (SELX), (2) one hepatotoxic drug (2SHE/10), (3) two hepatotoxic drugs with H and R/Z.

■ CONCLUSION

Hemoptysis is a life-threatening condition, which can be the presenting complaint in a large number of respiratory as well as systemic disorders. If the cause of hemoptysis is diagnosed in time and aggressively managed, the patient's life can be saved.

SUGGESTED READINGS

1. Jeudy J, Khan AR, Mohammed T-L, Amorosa JK, Brown K, Dyer Debra S, et al. ACR Appropriateness Criteria Hemoptysis. J Thorac Imaging. 2010;25(3):W67-9.
2. Lordan JL, Gascoigne A, Corris PA. The pulmonary physician in critical care * Illustrative case 7: Assessment and management of massive haemoptysis. Thorax. 2003;58(9):814-9.
3. Ibrahim WH. Massive haemoptysis: the definition should be revised. Eur Respir J. 2008;32(4):1131-2.
4. Bruzzi JF, Remy-Jardin M, Delhaye D, Teisseire A, Khalil C, Rémy J. Multi-detector row CT of hemoptysis. Radiographics. 2006;26(1):3-22.
5. Chamilos G, Kontoylannis DP. Aspergillus, Candida and opportunistic mold infections of the lung. Fishman's Pulmonary Diseases and Disorders, 4th edition. New York, NY: Mc Graw-Hill; 2008. pp. 2291-304.
6. Hsiao EI, Kirsch CM, Kagawa FT, Wehner JH, Jensen WA, Baxter RB. Utility of fiberoptic bronchoscopy before bronchial artery embolization for massive hemoptysis. AJR Am J Roentgenol. 2001;177:861-7.
7. Kant S. Clinical approach to hemoptysis. Clinical Methods in Respiratory Medicine. New Delhi: Jaypee Brothers Medical Publishers Pvt. Ltd: 2018. pp. 45-53.
8. Kant S, Mehra S. An interesting case of haemoptysis. Int J Pulmon Med. 2007;9(1).
9. Kant S, Verma S. Fungal ball presenting as Haemoptysis. Int J Pulmon Med. 2008;10(1):1-4.
10. Kant S, Singhal S, Verma SK. Allergic bronchopulmonary aspergillosis presenting as haemoptysis: a case report. J Inter Med India. 2006;9(2):62-4.

C. CLINICAL APPROACH TO CHEST PAIN

Raja Dhar, Shubham Sharma, Supriya Sarkar

■ INTRODUCTION

- Chest pain is one of the most common chief complaints of patients presenting to emergency departments (EDs) annually.
- Etiologies of chest pain range from life-threatening conditions to those that are relatively benign.
- Most common causes of chest pain in outpatients are musculoskeletal and gastrointestinal conditions while stable angina constitutes 10%, 5% respiratory conditions, and approximately 2–4% acute myocardial ischemia (including myocardial infarction). Similarly, conditions presenting with chest pain that pose an immediate threat to life include acute coronary syndrome, aortic dissection, pulmonary embolism, tension pneumothorax, pericardial tamponade, and mediastinitis (e.g., esophageal rupture).
- The initial goal in the emergency room should be to identify these life threats.

■ ETIOLOGY

Different etiologies of chest pain may be grouped according to nature of onset of the chest pain as follows:
- *Instantaneous onset (within minutes)*:
  - Acute myocardial infarction
  - Acute pulmonary thromboembolism
  - Acute aortic dissection
  - Tension pneumothorax
  - Esophageal rupture
- *Acute onset (minutes to hours)*:
  - Pneumothorax
  - Stable and unstable angina pectoris
  - Myocardial ischemia
- *Gradual or insidious onset (hours to days)*:
  - Pleuritic chest pain (pleural effusion, pneumonia)
  - Pericarditis
  - Musculoskeletal chest pain

■ CARDIAC CAUSES OF CHEST PAIN

Myocardial Ischemia

- Angina pectoris is described as chest pain attributable to ischemia of the myocardium.
- Stable angina presents as pressure, heaviness, tightness, or constriction in the center or left side of the chest that is precipitated on exertion and is relieved at rest.

- Associated symptoms include pain in the chest precipitating with emotional stress or cold that radiates to the neck, jaw, and shoulder; dyspnea, nausea and vomiting, diaphoresis, presyncope, and palpitations.

Aortic Dissection (Table 4C.1)

- A rare condition but may be a surgical emergency as it could be life threatening, if left undiagnosed and untreated.
- Patients typically present with sudden onset chest and back pain that is severe, sharp, and "tearing" in quality.
- Pain can radiate anywhere in the chest or into the abdomen.
- Aortic dissection can be complicated by cerebrovascular accident, syncope, myocardial infarction, which is typically and usually due to involvement of the right coronary artery (RCA) territory, and heart failure.
- *Predisposing factors*:
  - Aortic aneurysm
  - Hypertension (HTN)
  - Vasculitis
  - Marfan's syndrome or other collagen diseases
  - Coronary artery bypass grafting (CABG)/cardiac catheterization
  - Drugs (crack cocaine)
  - Trauma

Diagnosis of Aortic Dissection

- History and physical examination may raise suspicion.
- Variations in pulse or blood pressure (>20 mm Hg difference between right and left arm)
- *Electrocardiography (ECG)*: Usually inconclusive, unless other cardiac complications associated with the dissection

Table 4C.1: Classifications of aortic dissection.	
Class	**Description**
Stanford classification	• Type A: Dissection involving the ascending aorta, regardless of the site of the primary tear • Type B: Dissection of the descending aorta
DeBakey classification	• Type 1: Dissection of the ascending and descending thoracic aorta • Type 2: Dissection of the ascending aorta • Type 3: Dissection of the descending aorta
Classification of different variants of aortic dissection	• Class 1: Classic dissection with separation of intima/media; intimal flap between dual lumens (true and false dissection) • Class 2: Medial disruption with intramural hematoma separation of intima/media; no intraluminal tear or flap imaged • Class 3: Discrete/subtle dissection; intimal tear without hematoma (limited dissection) and eccentric bulge at tear site • Class 4: Atherosclerotic penetrating ulcer; ulcer usually penetrating to adventitia with localized hematoma • Class 5: Iatrogenic/traumatic dissection

- *Imaging* (**Figs. 4C.1A to C**):
    - Chest radiograph: It may show mediastinal widening.
    - Computed tomography (CT) scan of the thorax.
    - Transesophageal echocardiography (TEE).
    - Magnetic resonance imaging (MRI).
    - Transthoracic echocardiography (TTE).

    Computed tomography scan of the thorax, TEE, and MRI are superior to TTE in terms of diagnostic accuracy.

Management of Aortic Dissection

- *In acute setting*:
    - Intensive care unit (ICU) admission
    - Pain control: Morphine

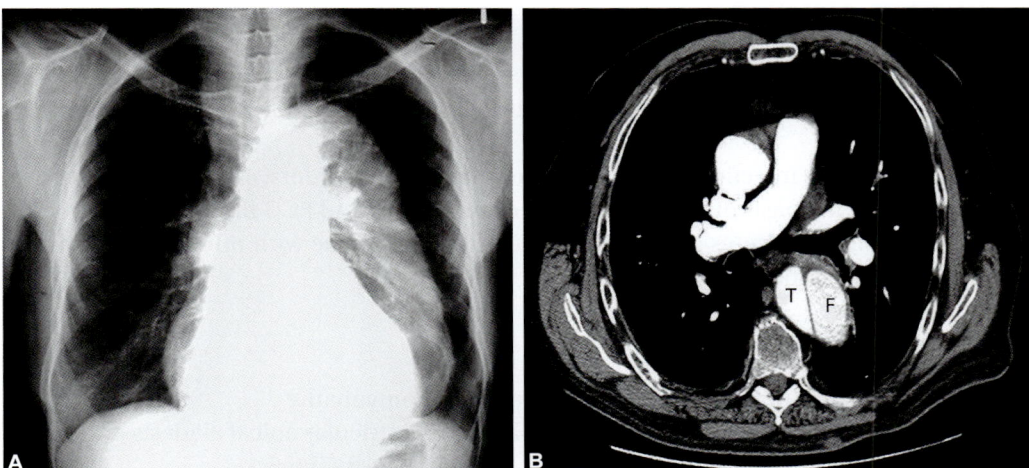
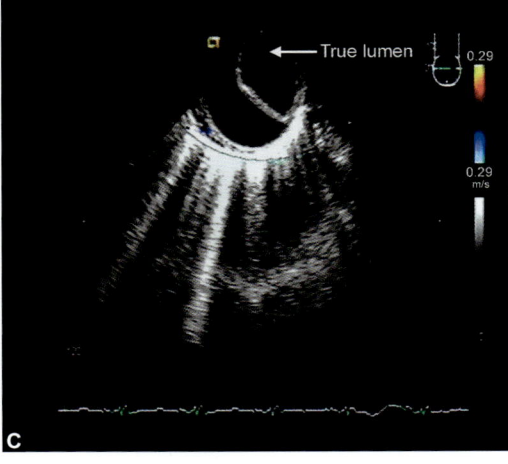

FIGS. 4C.1A TO C: Aortic dissection.

- Reduction of systolic blood pressure (SBP) with an aim of 100–120 mm Hg or lowest tolerated; heart rate (HR) aim should be <60 beats/min
- Intubate if unstable
- First-line treatment includes parenteral β-blockers (labetalol, propranolol, and esmolol).
- If HR < 60 beats/min and SBP >100 mm Hg with good mentation and renal function, nitroprusside can be given.
- If patient is hemodynamically unstable, look for blood loss, tamponade, or heart failure prior to volume replacement.

Heart Failure

- Heart failure may also present with chest pain.
- Acute decompensated heart failure may present with chest discomfort along with progressive dyspnea, cough, fatigue, and peripheral edema.

Pericarditis/Myopericarditis

- Pericarditis is the inflammation of the pericardial sac.
- Pleuritic chest pain that is improved by sitting up and leaning forward is characteristic of pericarditis.
- Etiologies include infection, medications, autoimmune disorders, and malignancy.
- Diagnosed on the basis of history, physical examination, and ECG findings
- Myopericarditis indicates a primarily pericarditis syndrome with minor involvement of the underlying myocardium.

Stress Cardiomyopathy

- Stress cardiomyopathy is also called takotsubo cardiomyopathy.
- It is a transient cardiac syndrome that involves left ventricular apical akinesis and mimics acute coronary syndrome.
- It often occurs in the setting of physical or emotional stress or critical illness.
- There is the presence of new ECG abnormalities such as ST segment elevation and/or T-inversion with mild elevation in cardiac enzymes. However, there is no significant coronary artery stenosis in coronary angiography.
- Left ventricular apical ballooning is present.

Mitral Valve Disease

- Mitral stenosis can infrequently cause chest pain.
- It is often a result of pulmonary HTN and right ventricular hypertrophy.

■ PULMONARY CAUSES OF CHEST PAIN

Life-threatening pulmonary etiologies of chest pain include pulmonary embolism and tension pneumothorax. Patients with pulmonary etiologies for chest pain generally also have respiratory symptoms and may be hypoxemic **(Table 4C.2)**.

CHAPTER 4: Clinical Approach and Analysis of Respiratory Symptoms

Table 4C.2: Various causes of chest pain due to pulmonary etiology and associated clinical features.

Pulmonary condition	Other associated clinical features
Pneumonia	Pleuritic chest pain; Fever and productive cough
Malignancy	Chest pain is typically on the same side as primary tumor; cough, dyspnea, and hemoptysis
Asthma and COPD	Feeling of chest tightness; dyspnea
Pleuritis	Pain due to inflammation of the lung pleura. Causes include autoimmune disease (e.g., SLE) and drugs (e.g., procainamide, hydralazine, and isoniazid); associated signs and symptoms of autoimmune disease such as fever, rash, arthralgias, and constitutional symptoms
Sarcoidosis	Cough and dyspnea: Cardiac sarcoidosis can cause arrhythmias and sudden death, which may be heralded by chest pain, palpitations, syncope, or dizziness
Acute chest syndrome	In patients with sickle cell anemia: Fever, hypoxia, tachypnea, and cough
Pulmonary hypertension	Exertional chest pain; exertional dyspnea and syncope

(COPD: chronic obstructive pulmonary disease; SLE: systemic lupus erythematosus)

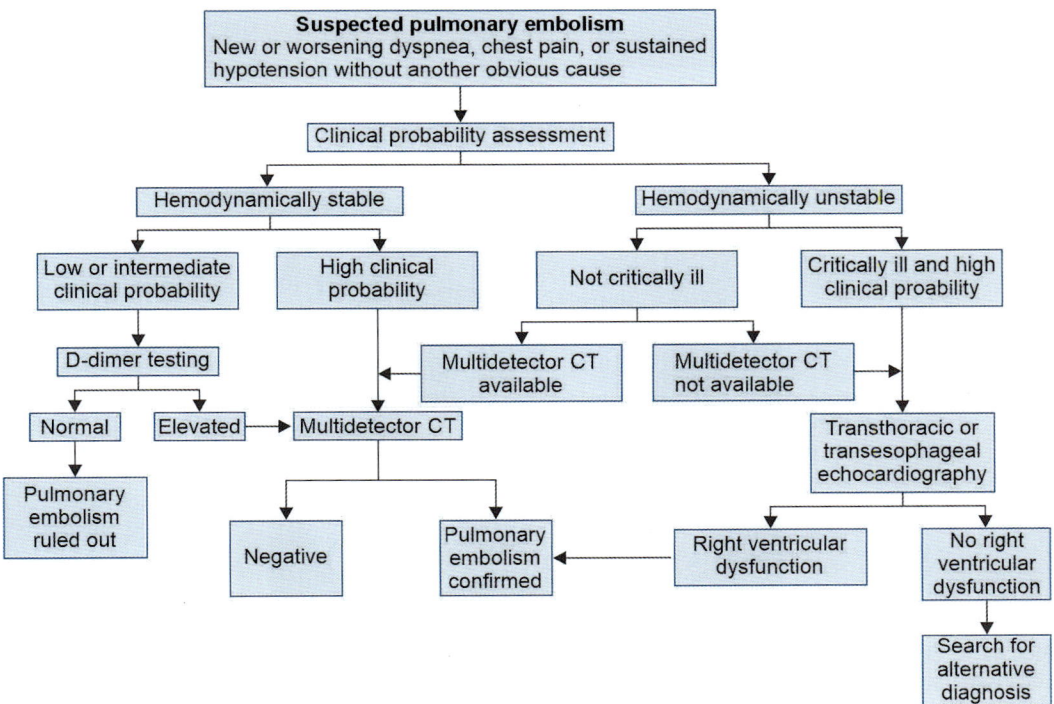

FLOWCHART 4C.1: Diagnostic algorithm for pulmonary embolism.
(CT: computed tomography)

Pulmonary Embolism

Pulmonary embolism has variable presentation and should be suspected in any patient complaining of new onset or worsening dyspnea, chest pain, or prolonged hypotension without an obvious etiology **(Flowcharts 4C.1 and 4C.2)**.

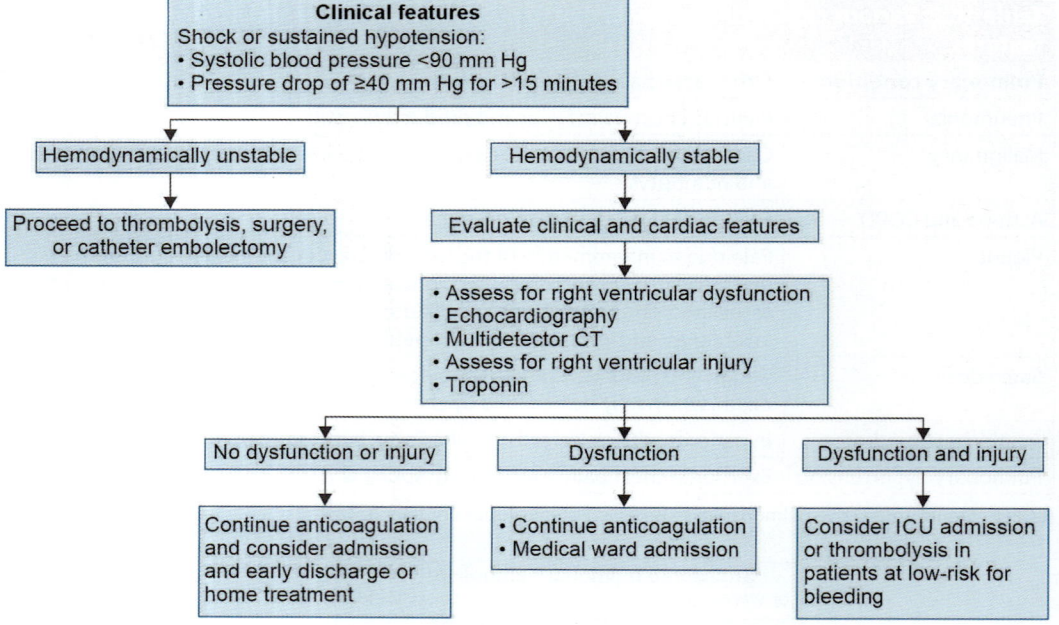

FLOWCHART 4C.2: Management of pulmonary embolism.
(CT: computed tomography; ICU: intensive care unit)

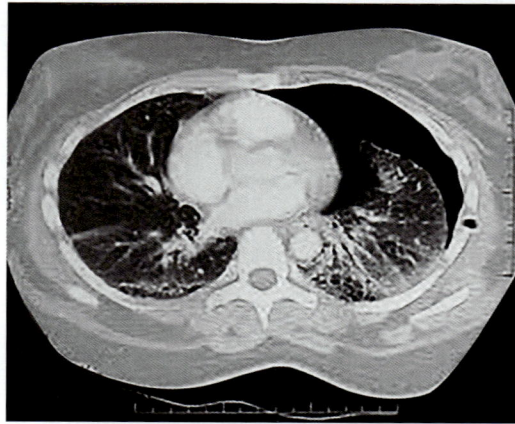

FIG. 4C.2: Computed tomography (CT) scan of thorax showing left-sided pneumothorax with underlying collapsed lung. CT scan can overestimate the size of the pneumothorax.

Pneumothorax (Figs. 4C.2 and 4C.3)

Patients with spontaneous pneumothorax present with sudden onset of pleuritic chest pain and dyspnea. Hemodynamic instability suggests a tension pneumothorax, which can be life threatening.

Pneumothorax can be primary or secondary.

CHAPTER 4: Clinical Approach and Analysis of Respiratory Symptoms

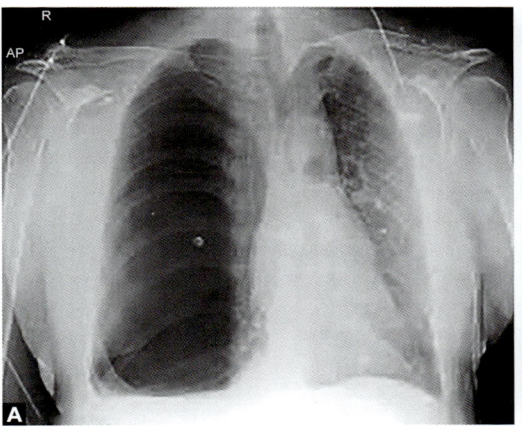 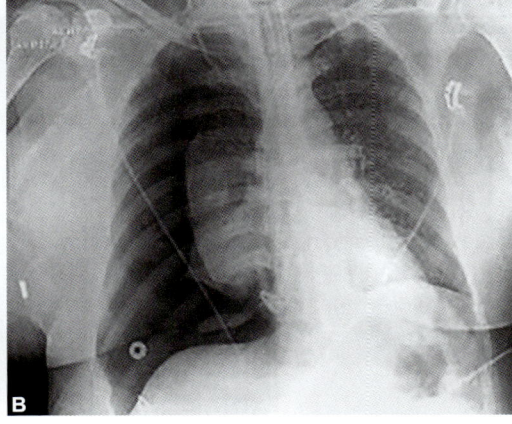

FIGS. 4C.3A AND B: (A) Right sided giant bulla; (B) Right sided pneumothorax.

Primary Spontaneous Pneumothorax

- It is seen in patients without underlying lung disease.
- It typically occurs in tall and thin males. Smoking, male gender, and Marfan's syndrome are major risk factors.
- Patients are usually young (typically in their 20s), present with sudden onset dyspnea, and pleuritic chest pain at rest.
- Physical findings include decreased chest excursion, decreased breath sounds, and hyperresonance.
- Arterial blood gas (ABG) may be normal or may suggest type 1 respiratory failure. Hypercapnia is uncommon due to adequate ventilation of contralateral lung.

Secondary Spontaneous Pneumothorax

- It is seen in patients with underlying lung disease.
- Any lung disease can predispose; however, COPD is most common and a major risk factor.
- *Pneumocystis carinii* pneumonia, cystic fibrosis, and tuberculosis are also common causes.
- Physical presentation is similar to primary spontaneous pneumothorax, but ABG is typically abnormal due to the underlying lung disease.

Gastrointestinal Causes of Chest Pain (Box 4C.1)

Certain gastrointestinal conditions can also give rise to chest pain. Gastroesophageal reflux disease (GERD) is a common cause of noncardiac chest pain. Esophageal perforation, although rare, is a life-threatening etiology of chest pain.

Esophageal Rupture: Diagnosis and Management

- Early chest radiographs show mediastinal or free peritoneal air.
- Hours to days later, widening of the mediastinum and pleural effusion can be seen.

> **BOX 4C.1** **Gastrointestinal causes of chest pain.**
>
> *Chest pain of gastrointestinal etiology*:
> - *Esophageal rupture and perforation*: Spontaneous perforation of the esophagus results from a sudden increase in intraesophageal pressure, usually caused by straining or vomiting. It is also called Boerhaave syndrome
> - It can also be iatrogenic, as a result of instrumentation done in the gastrointestinal tract
> - *Gastroesophageal reflux disease*: It is described as squeezing or burning type, located substernally and radiates to back, neck, jaw, or arms and mimics the pain of myocardial ischemia. It usually resolves spontaneously or with antacids
> - *Esophagitis*: It can be medication induced
> - *Other causes*: Esophageal motility disorders and hiatus hernia

- CT scan shows esophageal edema, extraesophageal air, and periesophageal fluid.
- Esophogram will characteristically show the extravasation of contrast.
- There is no role for endoscopy which introduces more air into the mediastinum.

■ MUSCULOSKELETAL CAUSES OF CHEST PAIN

- Chest pain due to musculoskeletal etiology is very common, besides gastrointestinal causes. Pain can be mild-to-severe but seldom life-threatening.
- Can occur due to various causes such as isolated musculoskeletal chest pain syndrome, the most common cause of which being costochondritis and lower rib pain syndromes, or it can be due to rheumatoid arthritis and fibromyalgia.
- Rib fractures associated with pleuritic chest pain that is localized and reproducible with palpation. There is often a description of an associated injury.
- Chest wall trauma should be evaluated carefully because there could be an association of injury to the underlying lung parenchyma and major.

■ PSYCHIATRIC CAUSES OF CHEST PAIN

Chest pain is a common complaint among patients with psychiatric disorders, especially in panic attack and panic disorders. But such pain should also be evaluated carefully as such patients may develop or have coexisting coronary heart disease (CHD).

Depression and somatization syndrome are other psychiatric conditions wherein patients may present with chest pain.

■ OTHER CAUSES OF CHEST PAIN

Box 4C.2 summarizes other causes of chest pain.

BOX 4C.2   Other causes of chest pain.

- *Substance related*: Cocaine use can result in myocardial ischemia (most common), besides aortic dissection, coronary artery aneurysm, myocarditis, cardiomyopathy, and arrhythmias
- Chest pain due to cocaine use can also be due to pulmonary toxicity ("crack lung"), pneumothorax and pneumomediastinum, and pulmonary vascular disease
- Methamphetamine toxicity may cause similar features
- *Referred pain*: For example, from abdominal organs (biliary colic) or from cervical disk disease
- It occurs because the same spinal cord segment supplies the dermatomal areas of chest wall as well as parietal pleura or peritoneum
- *Herpes zoster*: Pain is usually preceded by the characteristic rash, and dysesthesia is usually present in the affected dermatome
- Similarly, postherpetic neuralgia may also cause chest pain
- Trauma and domestic violence

■ CASE VIGNETTE

A 40-year-old lady presented with low-grade fever, dry cough, pleuritic chest pain in right side and that was followed by shortness of breath for 2 weeks. She had fullness of right hemithorax, diminished movement of right hemithorax, trachea shifted to left, apical impulse in left anterior axillary line, percussion notes dull on fourth space in midclavicular line, all over midaxillary line, and infrascapular area below seventh space in scapular line; breath sound absent in mammary, axillary, infra-axillary and infrascapular areas. There may be egophony or bronchial breath sound at the upper border of dullness. She was a housewife, she was nonsmoker, she was married with 2 healthy sons, and she denied past history of lung disease.

Q1. What is your diagnosis?
Ans. Diagnosis should include anatomical/pathological diagnosis such as "right-sided pleural effusion", etiological diagnosis "tuberculous", and complications if any.

Q2. What are the points in favor of the diagnosis?
Ans. Points in favor are pleuritic chest pain, dyspnea, and low-grade fever; fullness of right hemithorax, diminished movement of right hemithorax, trachea shifted to left, apical impulse in left anterior axillary line, percussion notes dull on fourth space in midclavicular line, all over midaxillary line and infrascapular area below seventh space in scapular line; and breath sound absent in mammary, axillary, infra-axillary, and infrascapular areas. There may be egophony or bronchial breath sound at the upper border of dullness.

Q3. What is the differential diagnosis?
Ans.
- Consolidation—without mediastinal shift, bronchial breath sound, and crackles
- Collapse—mediastinal shift to same side and absence of breath sound
- Hydropneumothorax—presence of horizontal fluid level, immediate shifting dullness, and succussion splash

Q4. What are the conditions where there is:
a. **No mediastinal shift?**
b. **Mediastinal shift to same side in pleural effusion?**

Ans. Effusion with collapse, encysted effusion, mesothelioma, and bilateral effusion.

Q5. What is the sternomastoid sign?

Ans. Prominence of sternomastoid due to shifting of trachea—suggests trachea shifted toward the side of sternomastoid sign.

Q6. What is the importance of examination of other systems?

Ans. Cardiovascular system to rule out cardiac failure or pulmonary HTN; abdominal examination to rule out ascites, pancreatitis; and lymphoreticular system to rule out lymphoma, leukemia.

Q7. What are the causes of:
a. **Pleural effusion?**

Ans.
- Transudative—congestive cardiac failure (CCF), nephrotic syndrome, ascites, Miegs' syndrome, and hypothyroidism
- Exudative—tuberculosis, malignancy, parapneumonic, connective tissue diseases, lymphoma, and pancreatitis
- Exudative effusion is defined as when any of the three criteria is present: (1) pleural fluid protein/serum protein > 0.5, (2) pleural fluid lactate dehydrogenase (LDH)/serum LDH > 0.6, and (3) pleural fluid LDH > two-thirds than the normal upper limit of serum LDH.

b. **Hemorrhagic pleural effusion?**

Ans. Malignancy, connective tissue diseases, lymphoma, tuberculosis, pulmonary thromboembolism, patient with anticoagulation therapy, traumatic, and leaking aneurism.

c. **Chylous pleural effusion?**

Ans. Triglyceride level > 110 mg/dL. Trauma, lymphoma, and metastasis.

d. **Bilateral pleural effusion?**

Ans. Transudative effusions, tuberculosis, lymphoma, and connective tissue diseases.

e. **Drug-induced pleural effusion?**

Ans. Nitrofurantoin, amiodaron, methysergide, bromocriptine, dantrolene, etc.

Q8. What are the causes of chest pain:
a. **Is it pleurisy?**

Ans. It is a pinpricking/stabbing chest pain usually occurs in lateral part of chest, increases with coughing and deep inspiration.

b. Is it musculoskeletal?

Ans. It is localized chest pain that patients can pinpoint. The degree of pain may vary depending on the cause of chest pain. There may be local tenderness. Pain may increase during chest wall movement. Severe, persisting, and progressive pain may suggest malignant involvement of chest wall.

c. Is it nerve root irritation?

Ans. Pain usually radiates through the course of the nerve, in the intercostal space from back to front. There may be manifestations of spinal disease including spinal tenderness. In herpes zoster, pain is followed by rashes in the intercostal space.

d. Is it esophageal?

Ans. It is retrosternal, poorly localized, usually from above downward and increases with deglutition. It may be associated with acidity and heartburn. Sometimes it is associated with anorexia, nausea, and vomiting.

Q9. What is empyema thoracis?

Ans. It is collection of pus in pleural space. It is characterized by manifestation of pleural effusion, sometimes associated with high fever, toxicity, and intercostal tenderness. Effusion may be encysted.

Q10. What is hemothorax?

Ans. It is the collection of blood in pleural space. Hemothorax can be differentiate from hemorrhagic effusion by the ratio between hematocrit values of pleural fluid and blood (>50%). History is suggestive of chest trauma or rupture aneurysm/AV malformation.

Q11. What is chylothorax?

Ans. Collection of chyle in pleural space. It can be differentiated from pseudochylous effusion resulting from chronic empyema, by measuring triglyceride level > 110 mg/dL.

Q12. What is subpulmonic effusion:

a. How to diagnose?

Ans. It is the collection of fluid between the diaphragm and lungs. It can be diagnosed by chest X-ray finding of raised hemidiaphragm with highest point shifted laterally. Previously lateral decubitus X-ray was used, but now ultrasonography (USG) can easily diagnose it.

Q13. How to diagnose minimal pleural effusion:

a. What are the investigations?

Ans. Collection of excess fluid in pleural fluid that hardly obliterates pleural angle. Lateral decubitus X-ray (X-ray taking anteroposteriorly in placing the patient in lateral decubitus position for about 30 minutes) is helpful to detect minimum effusion. Trendelenburg position may improve the yield. Nowadays, USG is used to diagnose minimum effusion.

Q14. What are indications of thoracocentesis?

Ans. All cases of exudative pleural effusion should be aspirated (under USG guidance) for diagnostic purpose and therapeutic purpose (as much as possible) to prevent pleural fibrosis. Transudative pleural effusion should be aspirated if there is any uncertainty or confusion in diagnosis.

Q15. What are the indications of chest drain insertion?

Ans. Following conditions need intercostal tube drainage: empyema thoracis, complicated parapneumonic effusion (where organism can be isolated, pH < 7.2, and glucose < 60 mg/dL), and malignant pleural effusion where pleurodesis is planned/sometimes in huge effusion.

Q16. What are the indications of pleurodesis?

Ans. Where there is a recurrent collection of fluid that causes respiratory distress. Malignant pleural effusion where there is no intraluminal obstruction [seen by fiberoptic bronchoscopy (FOB)], so that lung can expand to obliterate pleural space. Recurrent pleural effusion in chronic pancreatitis, ascites, or chylous effusion.

■ CONCLUSION

Musculoskeletal and gastrointestinal conditions are the most common etiologies presenting with chest pain, but a clinician should always have an eye to identify the life-threatening etiologies, viz., acute coronary syndrome, aortic dissection, pulmonary embolism, tension pneumothorax, pericardial tamponade, and mediastinitis.

Such patients tend to appear anxious and distressed and may be diaphoretic and dyspneic and often have unstable vital signs and should be referred to the ED immediately.

While the clinical history and physical examination are the most important aspect of any disease evaluation, they are often not sufficient in distinguishing cardiac from noncardiac chest pain or life-threatening conditions from not so serious conditions.

Initial work-up should include an ECG and a chest radiograph, and further work-up and imaging can be decided by the clinician based on the suspicion of the most likely cause of the chest pain.

Atypical presentations also often occur, especially in the elderly, terminally ill and patients with other comorbidities, and it is important to guard against premature diagnostic closure based upon the history.

SUGGESTED READINGS

1. Harrison's Principles of Internal Medicine. 21st Edition. 2023.
2. Pleural Diseases. Richard W Light. 6th Edition, 2013.
3. Manual of Practical Medicine. R Alagappan. 7th edition, 2023.
4. Macleod's Clinical Examination. 15th edition, 2023.

D. CLINICAL APPROACH TO DYSPNEA

Supriya Sarkar, Nandini Chatterjee, Biva Bhakat

■ INTRODUCTION

Unlike cardiac activities, respiratory activities can be controlled voluntarily. Yet we are not aware of our breathing as we take breathing for granted. But when we cannot breathe anything else matters. Dyspnea is classically described as unusually uncomfortable awareness of breathing. Dyspnea may be described as chest tightness or constriction, increased work or effort of breathing, air hunger, need to breathe, urge to breathe, cannot get a deep breath, unsatisfying breath, heavy breathing, rapid breathing, or breathing more. We must be convinced about the symptoms of dyspnea. For example, the catch of breath may be due to pleuritic chest pain, or heaviness of chest may be due to accumulation of pleural fluid and those should be differentiated from dyspnea. It is always useful to understand what patient means rather than what patient describe.

■ DEFINITION OF DYSPNEA

The American Thoracic Society defines dyspnea as a "subjective experience of breathing discomfort that consists of qualitatively distinct sensations that vary in intensity. The experience derives from interactions among multiple physiological, psychological, social, and environmental factors and may induce secondary physiological and behavioral responses".

Dyspnea is a symptom and that must be distinguished from the signs of increased work of breathing. Signs of increased work of breathing include increased rate and depth of respiration; the use of accessory muscles of respiration; intercostal, suprasternal, and supraclavicular suction, etc. As dyspnea is a subjective symptom, some patients may malinger, some may complain disproportionately increased dyspnea compared with his disease, and some patient may not complain even they have signs of increased work of breathing (probably they ignore it or may be habituated with it or may accommodate dyspnea with life-style modification).

■ ETIOLOGY OF DYSPNEA

Dyspnea may occur due to increased work of breathing as a result of airway obstruction, stiff lung, or hyperinflated lung; increased respiratory activity as a result of increased need of ventilation; and stimulation of receptors within lungs, pulmonary vessels, and extravascular structures. Cardiovascular diseases may cause dyspnea by accumulation of fluid in lungs. Some noncardiac/nonrespiratory conditions may also cause dyspnea. Finally, dyspnea may be psychological in origin.

Dyspnea in Airway Diseases

Both asthma and chronic obstructive pulmonary disease (COPD) can cause dyspnea by expiratory airflow obstruction and dynamic hyperinflation of the lungs and chest wall, and thereby increasing the work of breathing. Patients with acute bronchoconstriction may complain of a sense of tightness of chest. Ventilation-perfusion mismatch in obstructive airway diseases may cause hypoxemia, and thereby increases respiratory effort.

Classically dyspnea in COPD is persistent (without symptomless period), progressive (increases its intensity relentlessly) with periods of exacerbations (periods of increased symptoms). On the other hand, dyspnea in asthma is usually episodic in nature with symptom-free intervals. Dyspnea of chronic asthma may have the same characteristics of that of COPD. Dyspnea of airway diseases is usually associated with wheeze (a music wheezy sound heard by naked ears).

Dyspnea of Lung Parenchymal Diseases

Diseases involving interstitium and lung parenchyma due to several mechanisms (infections, occupational dust exposures, autoimmune disorders, or by unknown mechanisms) cause the stiffness of the lung. As a result, lung compliance (distensibility of lungs) decreases, and thereby the work of breathing increases. Hypoxemia due to ventilation-perfusion mismatch increases ventilatory drive. Stimulation of pulmonary receptors is also responsible in the pathogenesis of dyspnea in mild-to-moderate interstitial lung diseases.

Diseases of the Chest Wall and Pleura

Diseases of chest wall (kyphoscoliosis), weakness of respiratory muscles (myasthenia gravis or Guillain–Barré syndrome), and the stiffness of chest wall (scleroderma) increase the effort of breathing. Similarly, pleural diseases (effusion or pneumothorax) cause dyspnea by increasing the work of breathing and by stimulating pulmonary receptors (due to underlying atelectasis).

Dyspnea due to Diseases of Cardiovascular System

Left ventricular diseases resulting from coronary artery diseases, hypertensive heart diseases, and nonischemic cardiomyopathies cause pulmonary interstitial edema and thereby stimulates pulmonary receptors. Dyspnea may be augmented by hypoxemia (as a result of ventilation-perfusion mismatch) and increased ventilatory drive. Constrictive pericarditis and cardiac tamponade increase intracardiac pressure and pulmonary vascular pressures and thereby cause dyspnea.

Pulmonary thromboembolic diseases and primary diseases of the pulmonary circulation (primary pulmonary hypertension and pulmonary vasculitis) can cause dyspnea. The underlying mechanism is thought to be due to stimulation of receptors in pulmonary vessels. Hypoxemia and hyperventilation may augment that process.

Other Causes of Dyspnea

Anemia is associated with dyspnea and that may be due to stimulation of metaboreceptors. Dyspnea may be observed in hyperthyroidism as a result of increased metabolic activities and in hypothyroidism as a result of pleural or pericardial effusion.

APPROACH TO DYSPNEA

Firstly, we should identify different expressions of dyspnea as dyspnea may be expressed in different words according to patients' understanding. It is also important to be sure whether the patient is actually complaining of dyspnea. Expressions of other symptoms may mimic that of dyspnea. For example, a catch of breath may be due to pleuritic chest pain. It is also important to recognize dyspnea even when the patient is not complaining about it. A patient with arthritis may have limited activities and thereby he/she cannot recognize his/her symptoms. A patient with chronic dyspnea may adapt that problem by modifying his/her lifestyle.

Secondly, the respiratory origin of dyspnea should be to differentiate from dyspnea arising from other diseases. Anemia, hyperthyroidism, or hypothyroidism can be easily identified clinically as well as with simple laboratory tests.

Psychological Dyspnea

Psychological dyspnea is usually identified by a detailed history, patients' background, and meticulous observation of patients' behavioral pattern. But in some cases, it is difficult to recognize and then it is important to rule out organic diseases before diagnosing it as functional. It is also important to remember that psychological factors may precipitate attacks of dyspnea in organic diseases, for example, attacks of asthma may be precipitated by psychological stress.

Distinguishing Cardiovascular Dyspnea from Respiratory Dyspnea

The differentiation is often difficult and sometimes may be impossible. Yet an endeavor in this regard is always beneficial in clinical medicine. Differentiating dyspnea from respiratory diseases and cardiac diseases is an important step. The differentiation is often difficult as cardiac diseases and causes dyspnea mainly by accumulation of fluid in lungs. Cardiac origin of dyspnea should be suspected if there is a history suggestive of cardiac disease, history of hypertension, ischemic heart disease, the presence of palpitation, precordial chest pain, and history suggestive of paroxysmal nocturnal dyspnea. On the other hand, the presence of wheeze, cough with expectoration, hemoptysis, and nonprecordial chest pain are suggestive of respiratory origin of dyspnea. Wheeze may be found in left ventricular failure due to accumulation of fluid in the peribronchovascular spaces. Cough may be found in both conditions, but expectoration (mucoid and mucopurulent) is suggestive of respiratory disease, and pink frothy expectoration is suggestive of left ventricular failure. Frank hemoptysis is always suggestive of respiratory diseases except mitral valvular diseases.

High blood pressure may suggest cardiac origin, but it is nonspecific. Physical findings such as gallop rhythm, murmur, abnormal heart sounds, and fine basal crackles are suggestive of cardiac origin of dyspnea. Right ventricular gallop, murmur arising from tricuspid, and pulmonary valves may occur in cor pulmonale and are indicative of respiratory cause of dyspnea. Basal crackles are also found in respiratory diseases, particularly in diffuse parenchymal lung diseases.

Cardiopulmonary exercise test may be an effective tool in differentiating respiratory from cardiac origin of dyspnea. Respiratory origin is evident when at peak exercise the patient demonstrates hypoxemia or develops bronchospasm. Cardiac origin is suggested if heart rate becomes more than 85% of predicted maximum; if anaerobic threshold occurs early; blood pressure is extremely high or low; and O_2 consumption per heart rate falls or there is appearance of ischemic changes in electrocardiogram (ECG).

A detailed history taking has no substitute in the analysis of dyspnea. The onset of dyspnea is important as sudden onset usually indicates a vascular phenomenon (acute myocardial infarction and pulmonary thromboembolism) or pneumothorax. In children, sudden onset of dyspnea may occur in foreign body inhalation. Longer duration of dyspnea usually suggests obstructive airway diseases, interstitial lung diseases, chronic heart failure, or cardiomyopathy. Shorter duration of dyspnea may occur in infective diseases, pleural diseases, or acute cardiac diseases. Dyspnea may increase rapidly in tension pneumothorax, acute myocardial infarction, or gradually in pleural effusion or cardiomyopathy. Episodic dyspnea (with symptom-free intervals) usually suggests asthma, bronchospasm, intermittent myocardial ischemia, pulmonary embolism, etc. Acute increase in dyspnea in patients with relentlessly progressive dyspnea is suggestive of exacerbations of COPDs or interstitial lung diseases.

Dyspnea with wheeze usually suggests obstructive airway diseases. Nocturnal dyspnea can occur in left ventricular failure (due to increased venous return) and asthma (due to presence of allergens in bed). Exertional dyspnea is nonspecific, and it only gives an early indication of respiratory or cardiac diseases. Orthopnea occurs in conditions such as congestive cardiac failure, gastroesophageal reflux diseases, and obesity. Platypnea (dyspnea in an upright position that relieves in supine position) occurs in left atrial myxoma or hepatopulmonary syndrome. Smoking history may be associated with both COPD and ischemic heart disease.

A meticulous physical examination may give important clues to the diagnosis. General surveys should focus on pallor, cyanosis, jaundice, clubbing, neck vein, edema, etc. Signs of dyspnea such as tachypnea; the use of accessory muscles of respiration; supraclavicular and intercostal retractions; and tripod position (sitting with one's hands braced on the knees) are important to note. Different breathing patterns (Cheyne–Stokes breathing, Biot's breathing, Kussmaul's breathing, etc.) should be appreciated. Palsus paradoxus may be found in COPD or asthma. Examination of thorax (symmetry of hemithorax, movement of thorax, mediastinal position, percussion notes, breath sounds, added sounds, and vocal resonance) should be carefully done to diagnose the pathological changes of lungs, pleura, or thoracic cage. Engorgement of neck vein and its pulsatility are important and reflect right sided cardiac events and diseases of superior vena cava. Cardiac examination should include examination of blood pressure, pulses, jugular veins, abnormalities of heart sounds, and murmurs. Abdomen should be carefully examined for paradoxical movement. Raynaud's phenomenon may suggest collagen vascular diseases.

Investigations should depend on clinical clues and clinical settings. Investigations depend on the suspected origin of dyspnea. Routine blood examination, thyroid function tests, liver function tests, and lipid profile will eliminate anemia, thyroid disorders, hepatopulmonary syndrome, and risk for cardiovascular diseases.

When cardiac cause of dyspnea is suspected then investigation should start with ECG and echocardiography. Special cardiac investigations such as 24 hours Holter monitoring or cardiac angiography should be done on a case-to-case basis. When respiratory causes are suspected then investigations should start with chest X-ray posteroanterior (PA) view, spirometry, and sputum examination. High-resolution computed tomography (HRCT) of thorax should be done if preliminary investigations suggest interstitial lung disease, parenchymal lung disease, or airway disease. Contrast-enhanced computed tomography (CECT) of thorax should be done for pleural diseases, lung malignancies, and mediastinal diseases. Pleural fluid examination is an essential step for pleural effusion. It should be remembered that the most common cause of bilateral pleural effusion is congestive cardiac failure. Measurement of diffusion capacity of lung for carbon monoxide (DLCO) should be done for interstitial lung diseases and obstructive airway diseases. Bronchoprovocation test is rarely required for the diagnosis of asthma when symptoms are intermittent, and spirometry is normal.

When no clue is available from history and clinical examination then apart from routine blood biochemistry, chest X-ray PA view, ECG, echocardiography, and HRCT of thorax should be done to start with. Next step will be determined by results of preliminary investigation results.

It is important to assess the severity of dyspnea. Generally, dyspnea is classified as stage I (dyspnea occurring with more than habitual exercise); stage II (with habitual exercise); stage III (with less than habitual exercise); and stage IV (dyspnea occurring at rest). Modified Medical Research Council (mMRC) dyspnea scale **(Box 4D.1)** is widely used and standardized. Patients' descriptions of dyspnea are graded as "I only get breathlessness with strenuous exercise" (mMRC Grade 0); "I get short of breath when hurrying on the level or walking up in a slight hill" (mMRC Grade 1); "I walk slower than people of my age on the level because of breathlessness, or I have to stop for breath when walking on my own space on the level" (mMRC Grade 2); "I stop for breath after walking 100 meters or after few minutes on the level" (mMRC Grade 3); and "I am too breathless to leave the house or I am breathless when dressing or undressing" (mMRC Grade 4). COPD assessment score (CAT score) is an important tool for assessing dyspnea and other symptom **(Fig. 4D.1)**.

BOX 4D.1 | **Modified Medical Research Council scale for dyspnea.**

- Modified Medical Research Council (MRC) dyspnea scale
- Please tick in the box that applied to you (one box only) (Grades 0–4)
- *Modified Medical Research Council (mMRC) Grade 0*: I only get breathless with strenuous exercise
- *mMRC Grade 1*: I get short of breath when hurrying on the level or walking up in a slight hill
- *mMRC Grade 2*: I walk slower than people of same age on the level because of breathlessness, or I have to stop for breath when walking on my own pace on the level
- *mMRC Grade 3*: I stop for breath after walking 100 meters or after few minutes on the level
- *mMRC Grade 4*: I am too breathless to leave the house, or I am breathless when dressing or undressing

CAT assessment

For each item below, place a mark (x) in the box that best describes you currently. Be sure to only select one response for each question.

	Score	
I never cough	0 1 2 3 4 5	I cough all the time
I have no phlegm (mucus) in the chest at all	0 1 2 3 4 5	My chest is completely full of phlegm (mucus)
My chest does not feel tight at all	0 1 2 3 4 5	My chest feels very tight
When I walk up a hill or one flight of stairs I am not breathless	0 1 2 3 4 5	When I walk up a hill or one flight of stairs I am very breathless
I am not limited doing any activity at home	0 1 2 3 4 5	I am very limited doing activity at home
I am confident leaving my home despite my lung condition	0 1 2 3 4 5	I am not at all confident leaving my home because of my lung condition
I sleep sound	0 1 2 3 4 5	I do not sleep sound because of my lung condition
I have lots of energy	0 1 2 3 4 5	I have no energy at all

FIG. 4D.1: Chronic obstructive pulmonary disease (COPD) assessment score for assessment of respiratory limitations.
(CAT: Chronic obstructive pulmonary disease assessment test)

■ CASE VIGNETTE 1

An 18-year boy, while taking his breakfast, suddenly had right-sided pleuritic chest pain following a bout of cough. That was followed by dyspnea that was maximum at the onset and gradually decreasing. There was decreased movement and fullness of right hemithorax, trachea, and apical impulse shifted toward left, tympanitic notes on right hemithorax with absent breath sound and vocal resonance. He was a nonsmoker and denied any past history of lung disease.

Q1. What is your diagnosis?
Ans. Right-sided primary spontaneous pneumothorax.

Q2. What are the points in favor?
Ans. Sudden onset of pleuritic chest pain followed by dyspnea; fullness of right hemithorax, diminished movement of right hemithorax, trachea shifted to left, apical impulse in left anterior axillary line, percussion note hyperresonance/tympanitic in the hemithorax; breath sound, and vocal resonance are absent over the hemithorax. Amphoric breath sound may be heard in open pneumothorax.

CHAPTER 4: Clinical Approach and Analysis of Respiratory Symptoms

Q3. What is the clinical presentation?
Ans. Primary spontaneous pneumothorax presents with sudden onset of pleuritic chest pain followed by dyspnea. Secondary pneumothorax presents with sudden deterioration of previous manifestations. Deterioration of hypoxemia in ventilated patient.

Q4. How to diagnose subcutaneous emphysema?
Ans. Swelling of face, neck and chest wall, crepitus during palpation/percussion, and crepitus sound during auscultation.

Q5. How to elicit coin sound?
Ans. Patient is asked to hold a coin over chest wall. The doctor has to percuss over the coin with another coin and auscultate with stethoscope over area of lung exactly opposite to the coin.

Q6. What are causes of:
a. Pneumothorax?
b. Recurrent pneumothorax?

Ans. Rupture of apical pleural bleb in primary and rupture of bullae, cyst in secondary pneumothorax. Trauma due to accident or iatrogenic trauma.

Primary spontaneous pneumothorax has a chance to recur, chance of first time recurrence is about 16%, second time about 64%. Causes such as lymphangioleiomyomatosis (LAM) and COPD may present with recurrent pneumothorax.

Q7. What are the types of pneumothorax?
Ans. Pneumothorax is divided into traumatic (accidental or iatrogenic) and spontaneous (primary and secondary).

Primary spontaneous pneumothorax is due to rupture of apical pleural bleb. Secondary spontaneous pneumothorax due to—secondary to lung diseases such as COPD, asthma, and LAM. Practically all lung diseases may have pneumothorax. Traumatic pneumothorax due to accidental trauma or iatrogenic after some procedures or ventilator induced, etc.

Another classification described is closed (dyspnea maximum at onset then gradually reducing), open (dyspnea usually less, usually presents with hydropneumothorax, amphoric breath sound may be heard over the junction of air and fluid), and tension pneumothorax (presents as respiratory emergency, dyspnea maximum usually with hemodynamic instability and respiratory failure).

Q8. What are the causes of:
a. Dyspnea with chest pain?
b. Dyspnea with acute onset?

Ans. Pneumothorax, pleural effusion, ischemic heart disease/acute myocardial infarction, lung malignancies with effusion, or lymphangitic spread.

Q9. How to investigate the case?
Ans. Chest X-ray and HRCT of thorax to see underlying lung disease are usual investigation. Sputum examination for suspected TB, ABG analysis for patient in ventilator, etc., may be required in special situations. Chest X-ray during expiration will give better diagnostic yield than usual X-ray in full inspiration.

Q10. How to treat the case?

Ans. Conservative management with oxygen and rest in mild asymptomatic closed pneumothorax. Aspiration of air in mild symptomatic closed pneumothorax. Most of the cases require intercostal tube insertion and water seal drainage that to be followed by pleurodesis if not contraindicated.

Thoracoscopy with stapling of blebs and pleural ablation is indicated for recurrent primary spontaneous pneumothorax. All secondary spontaneous pneumothorax needs tube thoracostomy. Thoracoscopy/thoracotomy may be required for treatment of primary lung condition followed by pleural ablation/pleurodesis.

Traumatic pneumothorax, following procedures usually treated with oxygen inhalation, sometimes with aspiration and rarely required tube thoracostomy. Ventilator-induced pneumothorax is treated with tube thoracostomy.

Tension pneumothorax needs immediate drainage with a wide bore needle in the anterior chest wall at second intercostal space followed by tube thoracostomy.

■ CASE VIGNETTE 2

A 30-year man presented with sudden onset left-sided pleuritic chest pain and dyspnea he had a past history of pulmonary TB, treated with anti-TB drugs 5 years back. There was decreased movement and fullness of left hemithorax, trachea, and apical impulse shifted toward right, tympanitic notes in the left midclavicular line up to fourth space, dullness in midaxillary line, resonant notes in left supra and interscapular areas and dullness in left infrascapular line in scapular line, absent breath sound, and vocal resonance in left hemithorax. Shifting dullness was present, and succussion splash was present.

Q1. What is your diagnosis?

Ans. Left-sided hydropneumothorax secondary to tuberculosis.

Q2. What are the points in favor?

Ans. In addition to manifestations of pleural effusion, there are presence of horizontal fluid level (not space wise but by drawing line through upper level of dullness midclavicular, midaxillary, and scapular line); shifting dullness (immediate) and succussion splash.

Q3. How is shifting dullness elicited?

Ans. Percuss in the midaxillary line to delineate the upper border of dullness in sitting position; place the finger at that place and make the patient lye in the opposite lateral decubitus posture without removing the finger; percuss over the area to elicit resonance sound to show fluid is replaced by air; and then make the patient sit and percuss over the area to elicit dullness to show air is replaced by fluid. Shifting dullness may be elicited in the midclavicular line and spinal line with the same method.

Q4. Is shifting dullness found in pleural effusion?

Ans. Yes, but not immediately, it will take minutes to elicit that. When present in pleural effusion, it signifies a better prognosis as the underlying lung is assumed to be healthy.

Q5. What is succussion splash?

Ans. Place the stethoscope over the air-fluid junction at midaxillary line, and sudden jerk is applied to patient to elicit the splashing sound. It should be avoided, as it may induce entry of fluid to lung through bronchopleural fistula.

Q6. What is tidal percussion?

Ans. Percussion over the lower border of lung resonance during full inspiration and full expiration to elicit diaphragmatic movement.

Q7. How to differentiate with:
a. **Pleural effusion?**
b. **Pneumothorax?**

Ans. Same findings except dullness/stony dullness in effusion and hyperresonance to tympanitic sound in pneumothorax.

Q8. What are the investigations?

Ans. Chest X-ray, CT of the thorax, and pleural fluid manometry (to differentiate among types of pneumothoraxes, other investigation as per cause of hydropneumothorax).

Q9. What is the treatment?

Ans. Intercostal tube insertion with water-seal drainage; treatment of underlying causes such as antituberculosis drug (ATD) in TB, respiratory physiotherapy, and antibiotics if bronchopleural fistula persists then pleural ablation surgery or pleurectomy may be tried. Other options include closure of opening surgically through video assisted thoracoscopic surgery (VATS) or intrabronchially with glue. When the underlying lung is grossly damaged then consider pleuropneumonectomy.

■ CONCLUSION

Dyspnea may arise from a wide variety of respiratory, cardiac, hematological, metabolic, and psychological diseases. Identification of the causes of dyspnea is an essential step. Detailed history, meticulous clinical examination, and routine investigations will identify the etiology in most of the cases. Sometimes special investigations are required. Symptomatic management should go along with specific management of etiological disease. In terminally ill patients, assurance and opioids may alleviate symptoms.

SUGGESTED READINGS

1. Alan MF, Stephan K, David O. Respiratory Emergencies (Vol. 1). Hodder Arnold. Indian Edition, 2007, Jaypee Brothers Medical Publishers(P) Ltd. New Delhi. Chapter: 'Dyspnea: pathophysiology, diagnosis, diagnosis and quantification. pp. 3-16.
2. Joseph L, Richard MS. Harrison's Pulmonary and Critical Care Medicine. 2nd edition. MaGraw Hill Education (India) Private Limited, New Delhi. 2013. Chapter Dyspnea. pp. 7-13.

E. CLINICAL APPROACH TO CYANOSIS

Subhasis Mukherjee, Nandini Chatterjee

■ INTRODUCTION

Cyanosis means a bluish discoloration of skin and/or mucous membrane due to presence of an increased quantity of deoxygenated hemoglobin or of hemoglobin derivatives in the small blood vessels. The word cyanosis is derived from cyan, which appears to come from kyanós, the Greek word meaning "blue".

The cyanosis should be examined ideally in daylight or with artificial light sources with spectral composition nearly similar to the sunlight. Cyanosis should be looked for in areas of the body which have minimal melanin pigmentation, good perfusion, and abundance of capillary bed in close proximity to skin surface. Common areas where cyanosis is looked for are lips, ears, trunk, nail bed, hands, conjunctiva, and perioral area and the mucous membrane inside oral cavity and undersurface of the tongue—though tongue is the most sensitive area, the lips are more specific in detecting cyanosis.

■ PATHOPHYSIOLOGY OF CYANOSIS

Bluish discoloration of skin and mucous membrane in cyanosis results from an increased concentration of reduced deoxygenated hemoglobin in the capillaries. It probably happens due to the fact that as deoxygenated hemoglobin is less red in color, it absorbs more red color; so, after subtraction of the red spectral waves, there is predominance of the blue spectrum in the reflected light. It usually requires 4–6 g/dL of deoxygenated hemoglobin in the subpapillary capillaries for cyanosis to become evident, and this value is translated into a corresponding value of 3.4 g/dL deoxygenated hemoglobin in arterial blood. Newer researches have proposed that the above mentioned values are probably an overestimate and in reality, manifestation cyanosis can occur with a deoxyhemoglobin concentration of 2 g/dL. Manifestation of cyanosis depends on the absolute value of reduced hemoglobin concentration, so cyanosis becomes apparent at a higher partial pressure of arterial oxygen (PaO_2) and arterial oxygen saturation (SaO_2) value in persons with normal or higher hemoglobin concentration compared to those with anemia **(Fig. 4E.1)**.

Increased deoxygenated hemoglobin or in other words reduction in SaO_2 can be due to several factors such as reduced partial pressure of alveolar oxygen (PAO_2), ventilation-perfusion mismatch (V–Q mismatch), presence of shunts, hypoventilation, and impaired cardiac output. All these conditions ultimately result in impaired arterial oxygenation and give rise to central cyanosis.

On the other hand, anemia (anemic hypoxia), circulatory collapse (stagnant hypoxia), local arterial or venous obstruction, hypothermia, and histotoxic hypoxia result in a low SaO_2 and low or normal PaO_2 in spite of a normal PaO_2 and normal cardiac function; hence, these states give rise to cyanosis known as peripheral cyanosis.

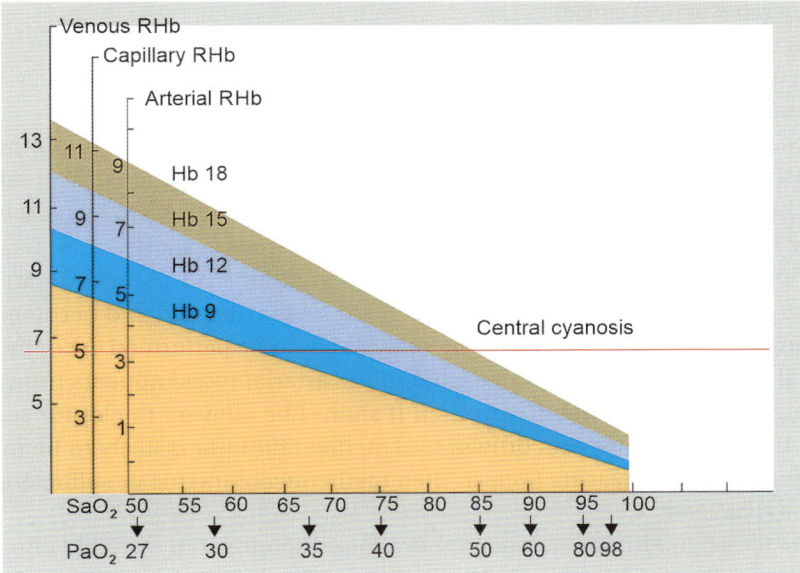

FIG. 4E.1: Relationship between hemoglobin concentration and threshold of appearance of cyanosis. (Hb: hemoglobin; RHb: reduced hemoglobin)

Sometimes, cyanosis may result even with a normal PaO_2 due to presence of excess amounts of abnormal variants of hemoglobins such as methemoglobin and sulfhemoglobin.

CAUSES OF CYANOSIS

Central Cyanosis

- *Respiratory causes*:
    - Pneumonia
    - Pulmonary thromboembolism
    - Acute severe asthma
    - Acute exacerbation of chronic obstructive pulmonary disease (COPD)
    - Acute respiratory distress syndrome (ARDS)
    - Tension pneumothorax
    - Pulmonary arteriovenous malformations
    - Acute exacerbation of idiopathic pulmonary fibrosis
    - Cor pulmonale
- *Cardiac causes*:
    - Congenital cyanotic heart diseases such as tetralogy of Fallot.
    - Other acyanotic heart diseases with reversal of shunts
    - Left ventricular failure
    - Myocardial infarction

- *Central nervous system causes*:
    - Intracranial hemorrhage
    - Drug overdose
    - Generalized tonic–clonic seizure
- Presence of excessive abnormal hemoglobin derivatives such as methemoglobin (>1.5 g/dL) and sulfhemoglobin (>0.5 g/dL) in blood (enterogenous/pigment cyanosis). It has to be kept in mind that in these conditions, cyanosis appears to be present clinically, but there is normal PaO_2. So, these are also called spurious cyanosis.
- One simple bedside approach to assess these conditions is to obtain an arterial blood sample and look at its color. If the arterial blood seems dark red and becomes bright red on shaking in air, subsequent blood gas analysis has to be performed to confirm presence of arterial hypoxemia. On the other hand, if the arterial blood appears brown and does not change color on shaking in air, then it should be allowed to clot for separation of plasma. If the plasma appears brown, too, methemalbumin is likely to be present. But, after separation, if the plasma is clear, then methemoglobinemia or sulfhemoglobinemia should be suspected.
- *Other causes*: High altitude, congenital cyanosis [hemoglobin M (HbM) Boston due to permanent mutation in the α-codon], etc.

Peripheral Cyanosis

Peripheral cyanosis is found in all cases of central cyanosis. In addition, following conditions can give rise to cyanosis of the peripheral sites without any primary problem of oxygenation of blood in the lungs:
- Reduced cardiac output (e.g., heart failure and hypovolemia)
- Cold exposure
- Arterial obstruction (e.g., peripheral vascular disease and Raynaud phenomenon)
- Venous obstruction (e.g., deep vein thrombosis)

■ TYPES OF CYANOSIS

Central Cyanosis

Central cyanosis is caused by defective oxygenation of blood due to mostly some pulmonary or cardiac problem. It is always associated with arterial hypoxemia and needs immediate attention and management.

Peripheral Cyanosis

Peripheral cyanosis is noted in all causes of central cyanosis. In addition, isolated cyanosis in the peripheral sites with sparing of central sites such as tongue, inner margin of lips, and oral mucosa are seen in conditions with decreased arterial perfusion such as cardiogenic shock, peripheral vascular disease, and reflex arteriolar narrowing in cold weather. It can also be seen in sluggish circulatory states as in congestive cardiac failure and venous thrombosis.

Differential Cyanosis

Differential cyanosis is presently cyanosis of the lower limbs, but not in the upper limbs and the head. This can be seen in patients with a patent ductus arteriosus with reversal of shunt.

Pseudo or Spurious Cyanosis

Pseudocyanosis is a bluish tinge of the skin and/or mucous membranes in absence of hypoxemia or peripheral vasoconstriction. This condition is mostly related to metals (e.g., silver nitrate, silver iodide, silver, and lead) or drugs (e.g., phenothiazines, amiodarone, and chloroquine hydrochloride).

■ CLINICAL APPROACH TO A PATIENT WITH CYANOSIS

To simplify the clinical approach, it should be remembered that the following four basic issues must be addressed while evaluating a patient with cyanosis:
1. Timing of onset of cyanosis—congenital or acquired
2. Type of cyanosis—central or peripheral
3. Associated with clubbing or not—presence of clubbing narrows the differential diagnosis toward presence of a cyanotic heart disease
4. Result of arterial blood gas (ABG) and pulse oximetry

Clinical Examination

A detailed clinical history, particularly onset, duration, history of exposure to offending drugs or chemicals, past history of similar episodes, etc. should be taken. Cyanosis should be sought for in broad daylight and in both peripheral as well as central sites to have a clinical clue regarding central or peripheral etiology of cyanosis. Pulse, blood pressure, pallor, clubbing, respiratory rate and type of respiration, engorgement of neck veins, and generalized skin conditions are to be especially looked for on general survey. General clinical signs of hypoxemia such as tachycardia, tachypnea, confusion, and agitation may be present but are nonspecific. Systemic examination needs thorough examination of respiratory, cardiovascular, peripheral vascular system, and central nervous system.

The combination of cyanosis and clubbing usually indicates the presence of cyanotic heart disease or pulmonary arteriovenous malformation. The presence of isolated cyanosis without other clinical signs of hypoxemia or pulmonary or cardiological disease should arouse suspicion regarding etiologies such as methemoglobinemia and sulfhemoglobinemia.

Differentiation between Central and Peripheral Cyanosis

Table 4E.1 shows the difference between central and peripheral cyanosis.

Pulse Oximetry and CO-oximetry

As cyanosis is a subjective sign, pulse oximetry should always be done in all cases for objective assessment of SaO_2. Although, pulse oximetry is a very handy bedside tool to substantiate

CHAPTER 4: Clinical Approach and Analysis of Respiratory Symptoms

Table 4E.1: Difference between central and peripheral cyanosis.		
	Central cyanosis	**Peripheral cyanosis**
Site of involvement	Involves both skin and mucous membranes. For example, involvement of tongue, inner margin of lips, mucosa of gums, soft palate, and cheeks are specific for central cyanosis	Involves skin only, mucous membrane is not involved. So, tongue and mucous membranes are not involved in peripheral cyanosis
Temperature of extremities	Extremities remain warm	Extremities are cold
Pulse volume	Pulse volume remains normal to high	Pulse volume becomes low due to circulatory stasis
Dyspnea	Dyspnea is always present	Patient may not be dyspneic
Response to application of local heat (Lewis test)	Cyanosis does not change	Cyanosis is decreased or disappears
Response to 100% oxygen for 10 minutes (hyperoxia test)	Cyanosis is decreased except in case of shunt or refractory hypoxemia	Cyanosis remains unaltered

hypoxemia, it lacks sensitivity in certain conditions such as pigmented skin and nails, use of nail polish, cold and clammy extremities, and methemoglobinemia.

Modern new generation pulse oximeters using eight wavelengths and CO-oximeters when available can measure abnormal hemoglobins such as carboxyhemoglobin and methemoglobin and can readily discriminate between true cyanosis and methemoglobinemia.

Arterial Blood Gas Analysis

The analysis of ABG can confirm the presence of hypoxemia and also can assess the severity of hypoxemia. ABG should be done in all patients with cyanosis.

Other investigations should be guided on the basis of clinical judgment.

■ LIMITATIONS

Although cyanosis is a bedside clinical indicator of arterial hypoxemia, it has certain limitations as a clinical prediction tool. It lacks sensitivity as well as specificity in detecting arterial hypoxemia. As cyanosis is a subjective tool, it is observer dependent.

The detection of cyanosis is also influenced by skin color—it is easily appreciable in persons with fair complexion but sometimes difficult to detect in people with dark complexion.

So, cyanosis must always be confirmed by an objective assessment tool such as pulse oximetry or ABG analysis. Cyanosis also varies with hemoglobin concentration as explained earlier.

■ CASE VIGNETTE

A 60-year-old diabetic female developed shortness of breath and drowsiness after 4 days of high fever and was rushed to the emergency. On examination (O/E), the vitals were as: pulse

130 beats/min, BP 90/60 mm Hg, respiratory rate 38 breaths/min, and SPO_2 82%. The patient also had cyanotic tongue and chest bilateral crepitations.

She had been suffering from fever dry cough for last 6 days and was found to be COVID-19 positive.

Q1. How to diagnose ARDS?
Ans. ARDS is characterized by hypoxemia with PaO_2/fraction of inspired oxygen (FiO_2) ratio <300; bilateral lung infiltrate, having a definite etiological factor and exclusion of cardiac failure or fluid overload.

Q2. What are the causes of ARDS?
Ans. Infections (pulmonary and extrapulmonary) including septicemia, chest trauma, aspiration of gastric content, inhalation of toxic fume, near drowning, pancreatitis, fat embolism etc.

Q3. What are the types of cyanosis?
Ans. Central (deoxygenated blood in artery—usually found in heart and lung diseases) and peripheral [deoxygenated blood in venous or capillary circulation—usually found in local diseases and congestive cardiac failure (CCF)]. Enterogenic cyanosis has also been described.

Q4. What are the causes of cyanosis?
Ans. The causes of central and peripheral cyanosis are different. Respiratory disorder such as severe pneumonia, acute exacerbation of asthma or chronic obstructive airway disease, pulmonary thromboembolism or cardiac disorder such as cyanotic cardiac diseases or acyanotic cardiac diseases with reversal of shunts or methemoglobinemia, etc.

Q5. How to investigate the case?
Ans. Investigation for cyanosis includes a detailed history and clinical examination, and investigations should be directed accordingly. For lung diseases, chest X-ray, ABG, CT scan (type of CT depends on whether parenchyma, pleura, and mediastinum are to be focused), spirometry, sputum examination; for heart disease, ECG, echocardiography, Doppler study of lower limbs, etc., and hematological examination.

Q6. How to treat the case?
Ans. Oxygen therapy along with treatment of the primary disease.

Q7. What are the types of respiratory failure?
Ans. Type I and type II.

Q8. What are the ABS characteristics of type I and type II respiratory failures?
Ans. PaO_2 is <60 mm Hg in both conditions, partial pressure of carbon dioxide ($PaCO_2$) is less than normal in type I and raised in type II respiratory failure.

Q9. What are the causes of type I respiratory failure?
Ans. All lung diseases except COPD causes type I failure such as asthma, pneumonia, interstitial lung disease (ILD), and ARDS.

CHAPTER 4: Clinical Approach and Analysis of Respiratory Symptoms

Q10. What are the causes of type II respiratory failures?

Ans. COPD, ventilatory failure due to diseases of respiratory centers, nerves, neuromuscular junction, muscles and chest wall. Type I respiratory failures will ultimately end up into type II failure in terminal stages.

Q11. How to recognize impending respiratory failures?

Ans. Serious diseases, bilateral disease, high respiratory rate, signs of dyspnea such as the use of accessory muscles, intercostal and suprasternal suction, and paradoxical movement of abdominal wall. Hypoxemia usually causes irritations, whereas hypercapnia usually causes drowsiness, early morning headache, etc.

To summarize, cyanosis is an important bedside clinical tool to assess hypoxemia and tissue hypoxia. It can be used as a reversible clinical sign to assess response to oxygen therapy. Cyanosis is a subjective clinical tool and it must be supported by objective tools like pulse oximetry and arterial blood gas (ABG) analysis. However, when interpreting cyanosis in the clinical context, its limitations must be always kept in mind.

■ CONCLUSION

Cyanosis is a crude but useful initial bedside indicator of hypoxemia that can arise due to multiple etiologies. Although it is not very sensitive or specific, in appropriate clinical setting and with experienced eye, and especially when substantiated by pulse oximetry and ABG, it can be a useful tool for assessment of hypoxemia in the emergency.

SUGGESTED READINGS

1. Anderson, D M. Mosby's Medical, Nursing & Allied Health Dictionary, 6th edition. Missouri, USA: Mosby; 2002. p. 1324.
2. Lundsgaard C, Van Slyke DD. Cyanosis. Medicine. 1923;2:1-76.
3. Lundsgaard C, Van SD, Abbott ME. Cyanosis. Can Med Assoc J. 1923;13:601-4.
4. Martin L, Khalil H. How much reduced hemoglobin is necessary to generate central cyanosis? Chest. 1990;97:182-5.
5. Goss GA, Hayes JA, Burdon JG. Deoxyhaemoglobin concentrations in the detection of central cyanosis. Thorax. 1988;43:212-3.
6. Finch CA. Methemoglobinemia and sulfhemoglobinemia. N Engl J Med. 1948;239:470-8.
7. Mansouri A. Review: methemoglobinemia. Am J Med Sci. 1985;289:200-91.
8. McMullen SM, Patrick W. Cyanosis. Am J Med. 2013;126:210-2.
9. Barker SJ, Curry J, Redford D, Morgan S. Measurement of carboxyhemoglobin and methemoglobin by pulse oximetry: a human volunteer study. Anesthesiology. 2006;105(5):892-7.
10. Comroe JH Jr, Botelho AB. The unreliability of cyanosis in the recognition of arterial anoxemia. Am J Med Sci. 1947;214(1):1-6.

CHAPTER 5

General Examination

Jyotirmoy Pal, Pradip Kumar Choudhury, Subhodeep Gupta, Tanuka Mondal, Uddalok Chakraborty

■ INTRODUCTION AND FIRST IMPRESSION

Clinical examination consists of both history taking and general and systemic examination.

Look at patient and first impression will help physician to have an initial assessment of particular system involved.

Physical examination will start as soon as you see your patient—two situation may occur, either patient is entering in your clinic or you are entering in a patient's ward or room.

Patient Entering in Your Clinic

Look the way the patient is entering your room. Patient's look—anxious look, emotionless look, and apathetic look including gait—will give you first impression. Gait abnormality usually occurs in neurological, musculoskeletal, or psychiatry disorder. Difficulty in walking may be due to dyspnea or morbid obesity. Observe whether patient can walk with or without support including visual or hearing abnormality.

Next shake your hand and introduce yourself. From shaking hand following information can be obtained.

Handshake

Introduce yourself and shake hand. This will not only give you a lot of information but also make the doctor-patient relationship friendly.
- Cold, sweating—anxiety neurosis
- Hot, sweating—hyperthyroidism
- Cold, dry—Raynaud's phenomenon, heart failure
- Delayed relaxation of hand—myotonic dystrophy
- Deformed hand—rheumatoid arthritis

Appearance and Clothing

- During introduction of each other, observe language, speech, mood, and other psychological well-being.
- Clothing whether well-dressed or not appropriate for age and sex gives clue to mental well-being. Dirty clothing, facial, or urinary soiling may be noted in immobile, dementic, or mentally ill patients. Tattoos on arm or forearm are found in HIV and hepatitis B and C patients.
- Odor from mouth or body is to be noted by physicians at first sight.

Odors

- *Fetor hepaticus*: Mousy smell of volatile amines is found in chronic liver disease (CLD).
- *Ketones*: A sweet smell due to acetone is found in diabetic ketoacidosis (DKA).
- *Foul smell or putrid smell*: Lung abscess
- *Foul smelling belching*: Gastrointestinal reflux disease
- *Uremic fetor*: In chronic kidney disease
- *Halitosis*: Bad breath due to decomposition of food. It is found in gingivitis, stomatitis, wedging of teeth, tumor of nasal sinus, etc.
- Tobacco, alcohol, and *Cannabis*: They can be identified with particular odor.

You are Entering Patient's Ward or Room

Observe decubitus of the patient, distressed or comfortable at bed, sitting, lying supine or semirecumbent position, or any other particular posture. Whether patient looking toward you or apathy will help you for initial assessment.

■ APPROPRIATE SETTING FOR EXAMINATION

The primary duty of a physician is to ensure privacy. Talk quietly, friendly, and make a good rapport with the patient. Good communication skill will help in revealing more information from patient. This is more important for children, elderly, and mentally ill patients.

Room should be warm, good illumination, good curtain, and lady attendant.

Explain to the patient what you want to do and take proper permission. Avoid unnecessary exposure.

■ EXAMINATION OF HIGHER FUNCTION OR COGNITION

Cognitive assessment at first impression and also beginning of examination has immense importance. To conduct different clinical examination, proper cognition is needed.

Useful and commonly used tool is mini–mental state examination (MMSE).

Mini–mental State Examination

It is commonly used tool to assess the cognitive state of patient **(Fig. 5.1)**.

It is basically a screening test to differentiate between normal and persons with impaired cognition.

CHAPTER 5: General Examination

Patient's Name: _____ Date: _____

Instructions: Ask the questions of the order listed.
Score one point for each correct response within each question or activity.

Maximum score	Patient's score	Question
5		"What is the year? Section? Date? Day of the week? Mouth?"
5		"Where are we now: State? Country? Town/City? Hospital? Floor?"
3		The examiner names three unrelated objects clearly and slowly, then asks the patient to name all three of them. The patient's response is used for scoring. The examiner repeats them until patient learns all them, if possible. Number of trials: _____
5		"I would like you to count backward from 100 by sevens" (93, 86, 79, 72, 65, …). Stop after five answers. Alternative: "Spell WORLD backwards." (D-L-R-O-W)
3		"Earlier I told you the names of three things. Can you tell me what those were?"
2		Show the patient to simple objects, such as a wristwatch and a pencil, and ask the patient to name them.
1		"Repeat the phrase: 'No ifs, ands, or buts.'"
3		"Take the paper in your right hand, fold it in half, and put it on the floor." (The examiner gives the patient a piece of blank paper)
1		"Please read this and do what it says." (Written instruction is "Close your eyes")
1		"Make up and write a sentence about anything." (This sentence must contain a noun and a verb)
1		"Please copy this picture." (The examiner gives the patient a blank piece of paper and ask him/her to draw the symbol below. All 10 angles must be present and two must intersect) 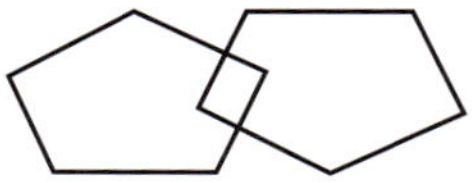
30		**Total**

FIG. 5.1: Mini–mental state examination chart.

Cut-off Values

Single cut-off:
- <24—abnormal

Education:
- <21—abnormal for eighth standard
- <23—abnormal for high school standard
- <24—abnormal for college graduate

Severity:
- 24–30—no impairment
- 19–23—mild impairment
- 10–18—moderate impairment
- 0–9—severe impairment

Advantage:
- Simple procedure, takes 10–15 minutes in outpatient department (OPD)
- Mainly verbal response, no sophisticated tools required
- Can be documented

Disadvantage:
- Age and education dependent
- Cannot be applied in a person below eighth standard of education
- Patient with physical disability such as hearing problem and limb weakness can interfere result
- In right hemispheric lesion, result can be normal.
- Cannot differentiate between focal and diffuse lesions
  Inspite of all these, it is reasonably good tool to assess cognitive function.
  Another comprehensive and short tool is Mini-Cog examination.

Mini-Cog Examination

Step 1: Ask to repeat three unrelated objects, e.g., pen, television, and cricket.
Put score: 0–3

Step 2: Ask to draw a clock and set time in it.
Put score: 0–2

Total score maximum 5
Score less than 3—signs of cognitive impairment.

Key Areas of Cognitive Assessment

Key areas of cognitive assessments are:
- Level of consciousness
- Orientation
- Memory
- Language
- Praxis
- Attention and orientation
- Calculation, visual-constructional abilities, intelligence, abstract thinking, and insight

Consciousness

State of awareness of self and surroundings.
    Level of consciousness is to be assessed at the beginning. Also whether it is fluctuating or progressively increasing is to be noted.

Alteration of consciousness is divided into two categories: Disorder of arousal and disorder of cognition.
1. *Disorder of arousal* can be categorized as alert, drowsy, stupor, and coma.
2. *Disorder of cognition* can be acute or chronic. Example of acute cognitive disorder is delirium, and examples of chronic cognitive disorders are dementia, delusion, and inattention.

Attention: Ability to focus on specific stimuli to exclusion of others

Confusion: Inability for clear and coherent thought and speech

Arousal: Responsiveness to action

Alert: Normal state of arousal

Drowsy: Baseline unresponsiveness, but on application of stimuli, arousal occurs and behaves appropriately.

Stupor: State of baseline unresponsiveness that requires repeated application of vigorous stimuli to achieve arousal, but on arousal it behaves inappropriately.

Coma: Complete unresponsive to arousal

Delirium: Acute confusional state with fluctuating attention

Dementia: Chronic confusional state with loss of higher mental function—such as judgment capacity, memory, language, but unlike delirium not associated with altered consciousness

Orientation

Patient's orientation to time, place, and person should be asked directly by giving leading questions.
- Name:
- Age:
- Time:
    - Date/hour: Conscious, alert patients do a correct statement.
    - Month/year: Oriented person at least tells year correctly. Long-standing hospital admission or home bound patient frequently misses date and month.
    - Morning/evening/night: Intensive care patients frequently do this mistake.
- *Place*: Where are you, home or in hospital?
- *Person*: Identification of relative, doctor, or nurse?
- Name and address of village

Language

- *Spontaneous*:
    - Fluent—flows rapidly and effortlessly: Broca's are normal.
    - Nonfluent: Utter single word, phrase, and frequent pause, e.g., Broca's aphasia
- *Comprehension*: *Yes/no answer to command*:
    - Pointing to object in response to command (e.g., take a book in your hand)
    - Impaired in Wernicke's aphasia
    - To differentiate from apraxia yes/no answer to command to apply (that do not require motor activity)

- *Repetition*: Severely impaired in conduction aphasia
- *Naming object*: Parts, pictures, color, etc.
- Reading
- Writing
- Calculation
- *Paraphasia*: The presence of errors in speech output. Ex-patient utters fork for spoon.
- *Neologism*: Utter new words that never exist.
- *Circumlocution*: To make word meaningful, the patient uses long phrase, e.g., pen: Cannot say it is pen, but say it is an instrument to write on paper.

Memory

Immediate/working:
- Utter three unrelated objects such as ball, fish, and book, and ask to repeat. Any mistake is abnormal.
- Slowly and clearly tell seven digits. Patient should repeat at least five numbers.

Normal human brain can retain 5–9 meaningful items for 18–20 seconds without rehearsal. Area responsible for working memory is prefrontal area.

Recent: Ability to retrieve specific items after a few minutes (usually 5 minutes) or hours; responsible areas are hippocampus and parahippocampus of medial temporal lobe.
- Give some information, few objects or numbers. Then give some other task to distract attention. After 5 minutes tell patient to repeat the same. Any error is abnormal.
- You can ask menu of morning breakfast.

Remote:
- Consolidation of long-term memories occurs at synaptic level and via protein synthesis in lateral temporal region, hippocampus, and neocortex.
- Assessed from patient's personal history. Name of village where he born, past history of schooling, travel abroad, etc.

Amnestic syndrome: Impaired recent memory but preserved working and long-term memory
- *Cause*: Bilateral hippocampal damage

Confabulation: Patient fills up gap of memory loss with information not supplied by memory system.

Praxia

Inability to perform well-organized voluntary activity in spite of having normal motor and sensory function.
- Ask to take a pen from table, and write own name.
- Take a shirt, wear, and put button.

Attention and Concentration

Attention is tested by observing distractibility such as response to noise which may be real or unreal (hallucination).

Concentration is tested by:
- Repetition of certain words
- Back calculation, e.g., 20 minus 2, further minus 2
- Summation of numbers

Calculation, Visual–constructional Ability, Abstract Thinking, and Insight

It means capacity of patient to understand patient's problem. It requires intelligence, which is tested by a combination of education, occupation, general knowledge, abstract thinking, foresight, and understanding.

For example, what is similarity between orange and cricket ball. Visual-constructional ability is tested by asking drawing a clock, copying a cube, etc.

With these tests, preliminary localization can be made:
- Lesion in reticular activating system—coma
- Diffuse lesion in hemisphere—coma vigil and persistent vegetative state
- Less severe diffuse abnormality of association cortex—dementia and delirium
- Memory impairment—medial temporal and prefrontal region
- Insight and judgment—frontal lobe
- Calculation defect—left parietal region
- Visual-constructional inability—right parietal region
- Broca's aphasia—left frontal lesion
- Wernicke aphasia—left temporal lesion
- Apraxia—left parietal lesion
- Constructional apraxia—right parietal lesion
- Multiple focal lesions affecting cognitive function—dementia

■ POSTURE AND DECUBITUS (TABLE 5.1)

Table 5.1: Different posture in clinics.	
At will without difficulty	**Healthy person**
Orthopnea	Lying flat in bed worsens the breathlessness as in pulmonary edema and left ventricular failure (LVF)
Comfortable in lying flat with shallow respiration	Peritonitis (often legs drawn up)
Rolls forward	Renal colic
Neck bent backward	Meningitis
Platypnea	Breathlessness on sitting upright while comfortable on lying down Example: Pleural effusion, arteriovenous malformation, atrial septal defect with pulmonary hypertension, and cirrhosis of liver
Trepopnea	Feeling uncomfortable on lying on one lateral side while feeling comfortable on lying on another lateral side as in collapsed lung (In this situation if the patient lies on better lung side, ventilation perfusion ratio will be better in dependent lung, so patient will feel comfortable)
Kyphosis	Exaggerated anterior curvature of spine
Scoliosis	Exaggerated lateral curvature of spine

PALLOR

The pallor or paleness is the manifestations of various clinical conditions. Therefore, though pallor may be misleading but commonly suggest anemia.

Clinical Presentation of Anemia

The sign and symptoms of anemia depend upon the severity of anemia. Mild chronic anemia usually presents with weakness and fatigue on exertion. Moderate anemia is associated with weakness, fatigue, dizziness, breathlessness, and tachycardia. Severe anemia presents with breathlessness, confusion, and features of postural hypotension (i.e., presyncope or syncope). Patient is unable to do his or her daily activities normally. In case of acute blood loss (>40%, i.e., >2 L blood in an average sized adult) signs of hypovolemic shock including confusion, dyspnea, sweating, hypotension, and tachycardia appear. Such patient needs immediate volume replacement and blood transfusion.

The pallor or anemia is best seen in the:
- *Lower palpebral conjunctiva*: We try to assess hemoglobin (Hb)% concentration in capillaries—via nonkeratinized mucous membrane.
- Lips, tongue, and buccal mucous membrane **(Figs. 5.2 and 5.3)**
- Nail beds
- Palm and palmar crease

Method or Examination of Anemia

During examining pallor or anemia following points to be remembered:
- Pallor of the palmar creases of the hands suggests Hb may be <7 g/dL.
- Angular stomatitis and koilonychia (spoon-shaped nails)—iron deficiency anemia
- Pallor from vasoconstriction occurs during a faint or from fear.

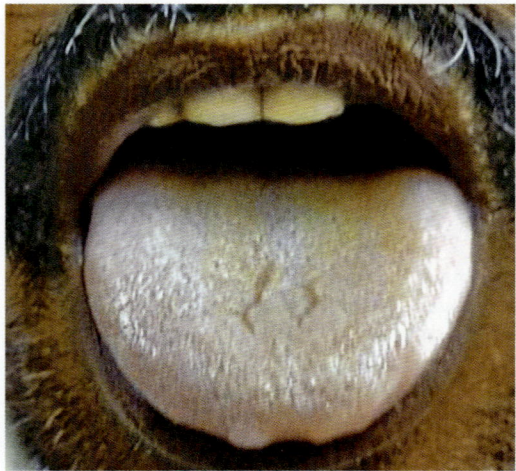

FIG. 5.2: Detection of anemia: Patient is asked to protrude the tongue after opening the mouth widely.

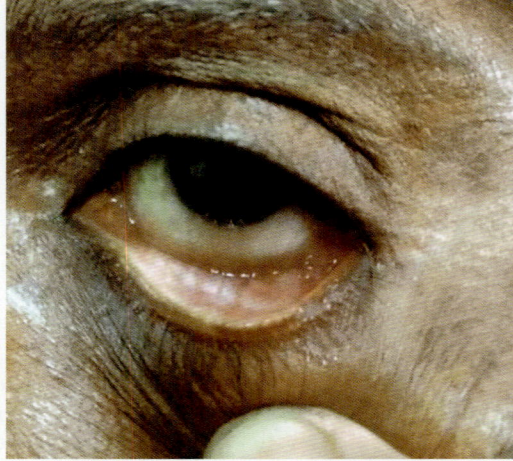

FIG. 5.3: Detection of anemia: Lower palpebral conjunctiva is exposed by dragging the lower eyelid downward while patient is asked to look upward.

CHAPTER 5: General Examination

- Vasodilatation may produce a pink complexion, even in anemia.
- Perimenopausal women may have transient pink flushing, especially of the face, due to vasodilatation, which may be accompanied by sweating.
- Facial plethora is caused by increased Hb concentration with elevated hematocrit (polycythemia).
- Blue sclera is associated with iron deficiency anemia.
- History of dyspepsia, change in bowel habit, and heavy menstrual periods should be taken for investigating anemia.
- Nutritional status, prolonged illness, history of blood loss, e.g., hematuria, hemoptysis, hematemesis, melena, and worm infestation should be enquired.

Classification of Anemia

Anemia has been classified in **Box 5.1**.

BOX 5.1 **Types of anemia.**

Microcytic anemia [mean corpuscular volume (MCV): <80 fL]
- Chronic blood loss
- Iron deficiency anemia
- Anemia of chronic disease
- Thalassemia
- X-linked sideroblastic anemia
- Lead poisoning
- Rheumatoid arthritis
- Hodgkin's lymphoma
- Myelofibrosis with myeloid metaplasia

Macrocytic anemia (MCV: >96 fL)
- Megaloblastic marrow due to vitamin B12 or folate deficiency
- Excess alcohol consumption
- Liver disease
- Hypothyroidism
- Hydroxyurea treatment

Normocytic anemia (MCV: 80–96 fL)
Intrinsic causes:
- Idiopathic aplastic anemia
- Paroxysmal nocturnal hemoglobinuria-associated aplastic anemia
- Myelodysplastic syndrome
- Congenital dyserythropoiesis

Extrinsic causes:
- Acute blood loss
- Chronic kidney disease
- Endocrine disorders
- Anemia of chronic disease
- Immune-mediated red cell aplasia
- Marrow infiltrative disorders
- Hemolytic anemia
- Drug toxicity
- Radiation toxicity

CYANOSIS

Cyanosis is bluish discoloration of skin and mucous membrane due to increased amount of deoxygenated Hb in circulation. Normally capillary blood has 2.5 g% of reduced hemoglobin. Deoxyhemoglobin should be more than or equal to 5.0 g% for developing cyanosis. Increased blood level of methemoglobin (>1.5 g%) and sulfhemoglobin (>0.5 g%) can also cause cyanosis. Cyanosis in anemic patient is a red flag sign. Physiological cyanosis may be found in polycythemic patient.

Method of Examination

- Ask the patient to protrude the tongue—look at lips and undersurface of tongue.
- Look at fingers, ear lobules, and toes to observe bluish discoloration.
- Examine whether extremity is warm or cold and observe the change of bluish discoloration with warming of extremities and oxygen inhalation.

Types of Cyanosis (Table 5.2)

- *Peripheral cyanosis*:
    - Seen in outer surface of lip, fingers, toes, and ear lobules
    - On warming, cyanosis disappears.
    - Pathologically tongue is not affected in peripheral cyanosis.
    - Localized reduction of blood flow, vasoconstriction, excess extraction of oxygen due to reduced perfusion or prolonged stasis
    - Causes: Exposure to cold, heart failure, and Raynaud's phenomenon **(Fig. 5.4)**
- *Central cyanosis*:
    - Found in inner surface of lip, tongue, and buccal mucosa
    - *Pathophysiology*:
        - Improper oxygenation of blood in lung
        - Admixture of venous and arterial blood
        - Occurs when oxygen saturation falls below 80–85% **(Fig. 5.5)**

Table 5.2: Types of cyanosis.		
	Central cyanosis	**Peripheral cyanosis**
Mechanism	Improper oxygenation of blood in lung or admixture of venous and arterial blood	Localized vasoconstriction or reduction of arterial flow
Cyanosis	Generalized	Localized
Extremity	Warm	Cold
Application of warmth	Cyanosis does not disappear	Cyanosis disappears
Oxygen inhalation	Cyanosis may (lung cause) or may not disappear (congenital right to left shunt)	Cyanosis disappears
Tongue	Affected	Not affected

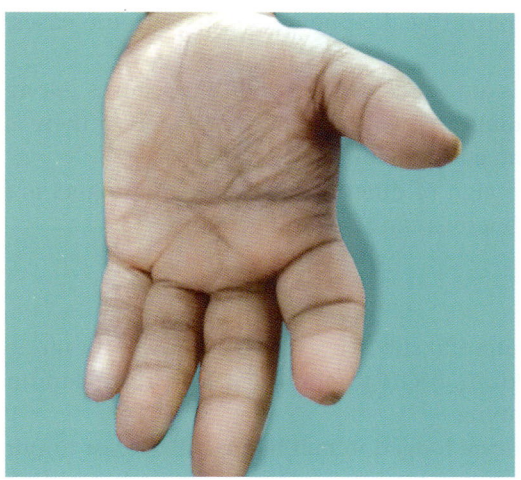

FIG. 5.4: Peripheral cyanosis.

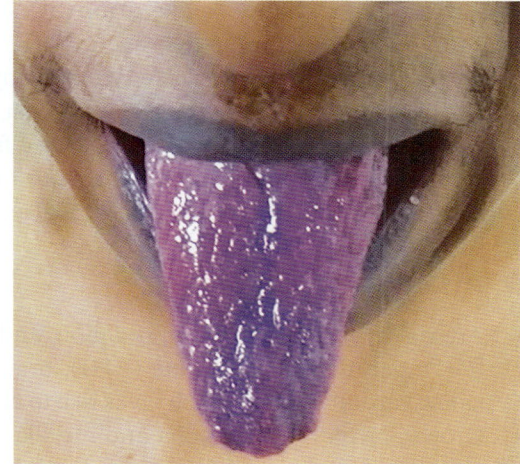

FIG. 5.5: Central cyanosis.

- *Causes*:
    - Respiratory: Chronic obstructive pulmonary disease (COPD), pneumonia, severe bronchial asthma, massive pulmonary embolism, and diffuse parenchymal lung disease
    - Cardiac: Cyanotic congenital heart disease, heart failure, and cardiogenic shock
    - Others: Polycythemia and high altitude
- *Mixed cyanosis*: Left ventricular failure
- *Differential cyanosis*: Cyanosis is present in lower limb, absent in upper limb, e.g., patent ductus arteriosus (PDA) with reversal of shunt and coarctation of aorta below the origin of subclavian artery at the level of ligamentum arteriosum.
- *Reverse differential cyanosis*: Cyanosis is present in upper limb, absent in lower limb, e.g., transposition of great vessels with preductal coarctation or narrowing of aorta (reverse flow from PDA to aorta).
- *Enterogenous cyanosis*: Discoloration of skin due to the presence of abnormal pigments in blood, e.g., hereditary hemoglobin M (HbM) disease, sulfhemoglobinemia, and methemoglobinemia. It is not associated with dyspnea or any other respiratory symptom.

Age of Cyanosis and Common Etiology

- *At birth*: Transposition of the great arteries
- *2–5 months of age*: Tetralogy of Fallot
- *Middle age*: Ventricular septal defect (VSD) and atrial septal defect (ASD) with Eisenmenger syndrome
- *Old age*: Cor pulmonale

■ CLUBBING

Clubbing is the swelling of soft tissue of terminal phalanges with resultant nail bed convexity due to proliferation of connective tissue due to various stimuli. Subsequently nail becomes more convex in both anteroposterior and transverse diameter. In advanced cases, the size of nail increases and looks like drumstick or parrot beak appearance. In extreme cases, hypertrophic osteoarthropathy is seen.

Hypertrophic pulmonary osteoarthropathy is almost associated with lung causes. Along with clubbing of the finger's distal end of wrist, joints are swollen and become tender. There is subperiosteal new bone formation separated from cortex of long bones.

It can be congenital or familial or can be a sign of different diseases. The fingers are commonly and usually symmetrically involved, but toes can also be affected.

Mechanism of Clubbing

- Arterial hypoxemia, vagal stimulation, and humoral substances such as growth hormone (GH), parathyroid hormone (PTH), bradykinin, 5-OH tryptamine, and prostaglandin cause vasodilatation, which gives rise to clubbing.
- Growth factors from platelet and megakaryocyte lodged in nail bed capillaries or tumor necrosis factor—due to infection or inflammation—can cause increased capillary permeability, increased fibroblastic activity, arterial smooth muscle proliferation in nail bed, and thus clubbing (most acceptable theory).

Method of Examination

- Put finger of patient at your eye level.
- Look at nail bed, nail, and distal phalanges.
- Measure distal phalangeal diameter (DPD) and distal interphalangeal diameter (IPD).
- Measure nail bed angle (Lovibond's angle) **(Fig. 5.6)**.
- Put corresponding finger back to back and look for any visible window between two nail beds (Schamroth's window sign) **(Fig. 5.7)**
- Place two thumbs under the pulp of distal phalanges and press the nail alternately by index fingers to observe the movement of nail for fluctuation **(Fig. 5.8)**.

Interpretations

Clubbing is present:
- If IPD/DPD ratio is less than 1
- If nail bed angle (Lovibond's angle) is more than 190° (normal <180°)

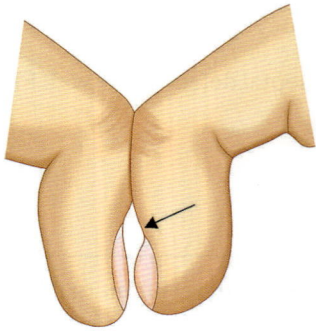

FIG. 5.6: Lovibond's angle.

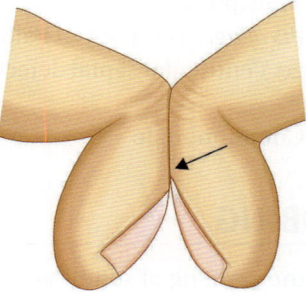

FIG. 5.7: Schamroth's window sign.

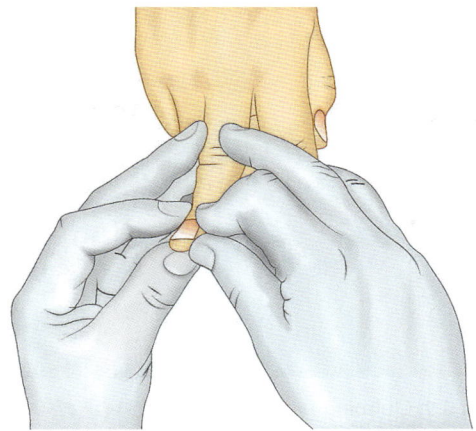

FIG. 5.8: Movement of nail for fluctuation.

- If Schamroth's window sign is absent
- If fluctuation test is positive (less reliable sign, as feeling is subjective)

Grades

- *Grade I*: Loss of Lovibond's angle and/or Schamroth's window sign with or without positive fluctuation test
- *Grade II*: Positive fluctuation test with parrot beak appearance
- *Grade III*: Positive fluctuation test with drum stick appearance
- *Grade IV*: Grade III feature with hypertrophic osteoarthropathy

Causes

- *Pulmonary*:
    - Bronchogenic carcinoma
    - Bronchiectasis
    - Lung abscess
    - Empyema thoracis
    - Interstitial lung disease
    - Mesothelioma
    - Cystic fibrosis
- *Cardiac*:
    - Congenital cyanotic heart disease
    - Infective endocarditis
- Cirrhosis of liver
- Inflammatory bowel disease (IBD)
- Idiopathic
- Thyrotoxicosis (thyroid acropachy)
- The most common cause of clubbing in the elderly is bronchogenic carcinoma.
- The most common cause of clubbing in the young is bronchiectasis **(Fig. 5.9)**.

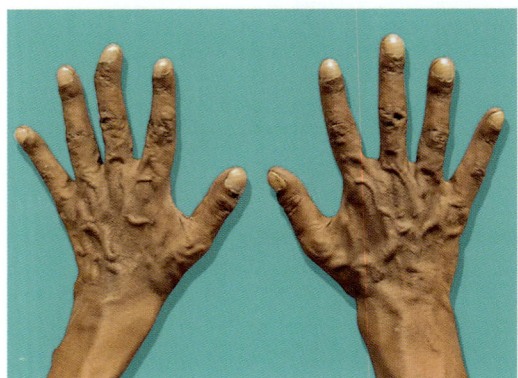

FIG. 5.9: Clubbing.

Differential Clubbing

Clubbing in toes and not in fingers, as is seen in:
- PDA with reversal of shunt
- Infected abdominal aortic aneurysm
- Coarctation of abdominal aorta

Unilateral Clubbing

It is seen in (proximal vascular condition):
- Arteriovenous shunt for dialysis
- Axillary artery aneurysm
- Bronchial AV aneurysm
- Aneurysm of ascending aorta

Clubbing of Single Finger

Causes include:
- Trauma
- Chronic tophaceous gout
- Sarcoidosis
- Thyrotoxicosis (thyroid acropachy—more on radial side of hand)

Reversible Clubbing

Clubbing occasionally becomes reversible in idiopathic or familial variety and after vagotomy.

■ EDEMA

The accumulation of fluid in extravascular space or in interstitial area is called edema. Capillary membrane separates fluid between vascular and extravascular space. The movement of fluid through capillaries depends on hydrostatic pressure, oncotic pressure, and capillary permeability **(Flowchart 5.1)**.

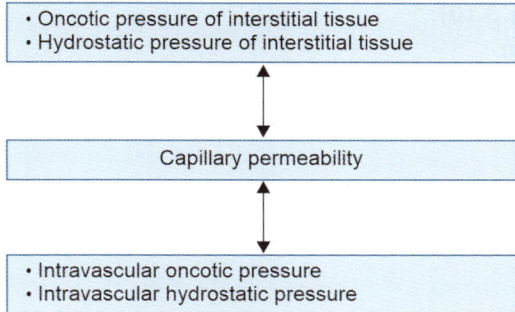

FLOWCHART 5.1: Movement of fluid.

Causes of Edema

- *Generalized*:
  - Volume overload (increased hydrostatic pressure):
    - Heart failure
    - Nephrotic syndrome
    - CLD
  - Hypoproteinemia (decreased oncotic pressure): Nephrotic syndrome, malabsorption syndrome, and CLD.
  - *Localized*:
    - Inflammation: Other features of inflammation may be present (raised temperature, tenderness, and redness will be present), due to increased permeability and due to release of vasoactive amines.
    - Lymphatic obstruction: In chronic condition, fibrous tissue proliferates and affected area becomes nonpitting. For example, Milroy's disease, radical mastectomy, and filariasis.
    - Deep vein thrombosis and venous incompetence: Increased hydrostatic pressure due to venous obstruction
  - *Pitting*:
    - Heart failure
    - Nephrotic syndrome
    - CLD
    - Hypoproteinemia
  - *Nonpitting*:
    - Filariasis
    - Myxoedema
    - Chronic venous stenosis
- *Postural edema*: Due to lack of muscle movement, common in lower limb of inactive person

Signs and Symptoms of Edema

Symptoms:
- Swelling of whole body or localized swelling
- Breathlessness

- Puffiness of face **(Fig. 5.10)**
- Increased weight gain

Signs:
- *Earliest sign*: The concavity of area between medial malleolus and tendo-Achilles is obliterated.
- *Method*: Press with finger 5 cm above medial malleolus for 10 seconds. After releasing pressure, pit should persist more than 5 seconds **(Fig. 5.11)**.

Other areas are:
- Dorsum of foot
- Sacrum in bedridden patient (pushing on the back produces a dimple in the skin)
- Arm edema-lower limb is dependent, so edema is more common in the lower limb. But it is possible in upper extremity due to local inflammation or lymphatic obstruction.
- Edema in acute venous obstruction—shiny skin and pitting edema
- Edema in chronic venous obstruction—darkened, discolored, stained skin with multiple ulceration, and nonpitting edema.
- Edema in lymphatic obstruction—nonpitting edema, Peau d'orange appearance **(Fig. 5.12)**

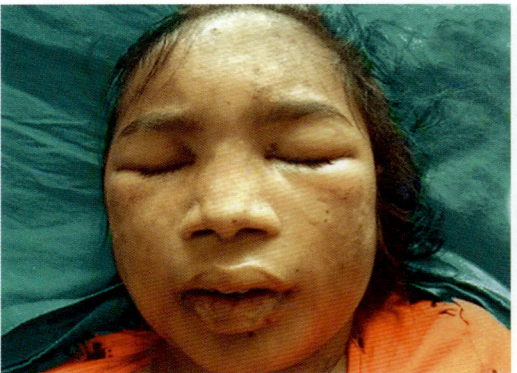

FIG. 5.10: Symptoms of edema.

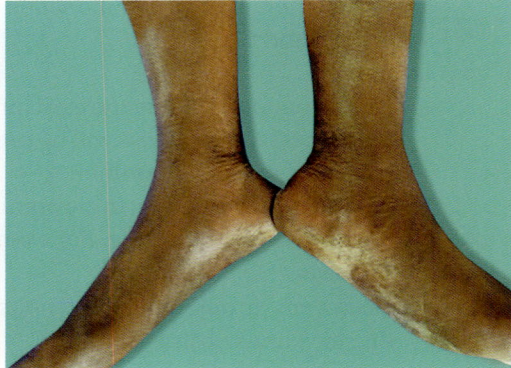

FIG. 5.11: Signs of edema.

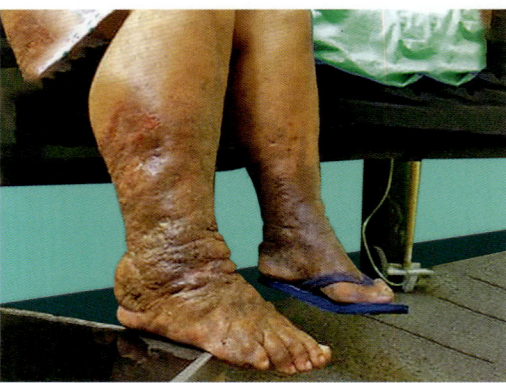

FIG. 5.12: Edema in lymphatic obstruction.

- Review serial body weight and urine output. Usually, 10–15% body weight should increase before appearance of edema.
- Check edema in sacral area in bedbound patient.
- Examine and measure jugular venous pressure (JVP).
- Examine feet whether involved or not (in obese patient edema present in ankle but not in feet).

■ JAUNDICE

- Yellowish discoloration of skin, sclera, and mucous membrane due to hyperbilirubinemia
- If serum bilirubin is more than 2–2.5 mg/dL, clinically jaundice appears.
- If icterus is present, but urine is normal colored, it indicates unconjugated hyperbilirubinemia, as unconjugated bilirubin binds to albumin and cannot get filtered in renal glomeruli.
- If icterus present also urine is dark colored, it indicates conjugated hyperbilirubinemia **(Fig. 5.13)**.

Causes

Unconjugated hyperbilirubinemia:
- Increased production of bilirubin—increased hemolysis, e.g., spherocytosis, Glucose-6-phosphate dehydrogenase (G6PD) deficiency, paroxysmal nocturnal hemoglobinuria (PNH), and immune hemolysis
- *Congenital*: Gilbert's syndrome (unconjugated), Criglen–Najjar type I and II

Mixed hyperbilirubinemia:
- *Hepatocellular*:
    - Viral hepatitis
    - Drugs [antitubercular drug (ATD), phenytoin, alcohol, etc.]
    - Autoimmune hepatitis
    - CLD

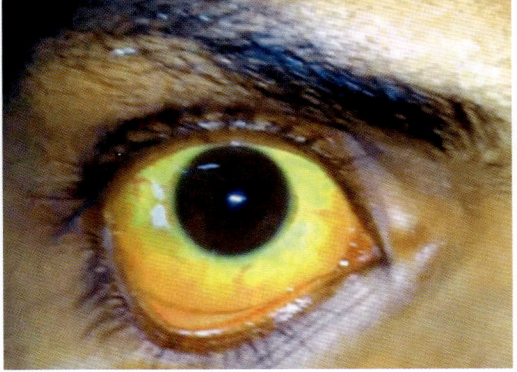

FIG. 5.13: Conjugated hyperbilirubinemia.

Cholestatic hyperbilirubinemia:
- *Intrahepatic cholestasis*:
    - Drugs—oral contraceptive pill (OCP), chlorpromazine, and erythromycin
    - Primary biliary cirrhosis
    - Pregnancy
- *Extrahepatic cholestasis*:
    - Neoplastic
    - Gallstones and worm

Differential Diagnosis

Hypercarotenemia—due to excess intake of carotene, tomatoes, etc. Hand and feet are yellow but not sclera.

◾ BLOOD PRESSURE (TABLE 5.3)

The arterial pressure cannot be measured with precision by means of sphygmomanometers yet the same imprecise method continues to be the accepted standard for the measurement of arterial blood pressure **(Figs. 5.14A and B)**. This indirect measurement of BP overestimates more accurate direct intra-arterial pressure by 10–20 mm Hg. Only 3% of the general practitioners and 2% of the nurses obtained blood pressure accurately by indirect method revealed in one study.

Table 5.3: Blood pressure.		
BP category	Systolic blood pressure (SBP)	Diastolic blood pressure (DBP)
Normal	<120 mm Hg	<80 mm Hg
Elevated	120–129 mm Hg	<80 mm Hg
Hypertension (I)	130–139 mm Hg	80–89 mm Hg
Hypertension (II)	>140 mm Hg	>90 mm Hg

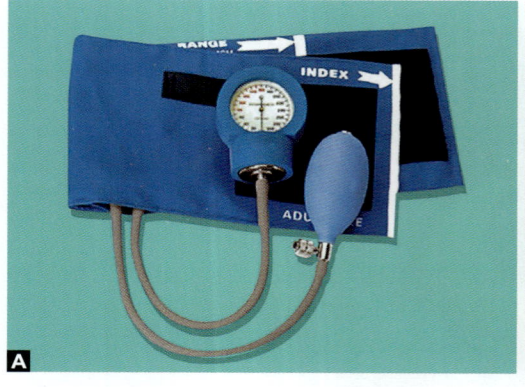 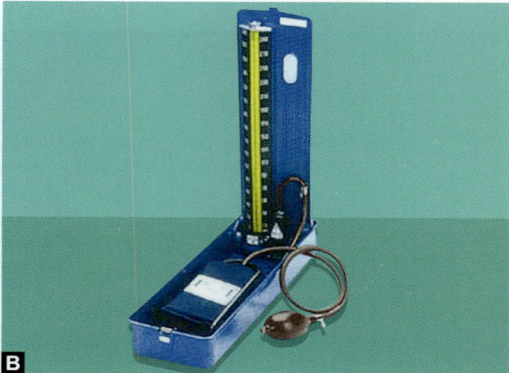

FIGS. 5.14A AND B: Sphygmomanometers.

Sphygmomanometry

The indirect blood pressure is measured with a device called a sphygmomanometer, (sphygmos is the Greek term for pulse, and manometer is a pressure measuring device) which consists of an inflatable bladder covered by a cloth sleeve and a gauge or column of mercury to measure pressure. The cloth sleeve is wrapped around the mid-arm or mid-thigh in an area that overlies a major artery and the bladder in the sleeve is inflated to compress the underlying artery. Turbulence of blood through compressed artery produces noise that is picked up by the stethoscope, which is known as Korotkoff sounds. These sounds are used to record BP.

Size of Cuff

The length of the cuff should be at least 80% of mid-arm circumference (MAC), and width should be at least 40% of MAC **(Table 5.4)**.
- Smaller cuff overestimates blood pressure.
- Larger cuff underestimates blood pressure.

Method of Estimation

Patient should sit comfortably or in supine position for 5–10 minutes. If the patient is in the sitting position, the arm and the back should be supported. Otherwise, the reading of diastolic blood pressure (DBP) can be falsely elevated. Manometer should be at the same level of the cuff on the patient's arm and mid-arm at heart level. The cuff should be wrapped over the mid-arm so tightly that one finger can be inserted between cuff and arm with difficulty. Palpate radial artery and inflate cuff to a pressure of 20 mm Hg above the level at which radial pulse becomes impalpable. Put stethoscope over brachial artery at antecubital fossa. Do not place the head of the stethoscope under the cuff as this creates sounds during cuff deflation that will interfere with detection of the Korotkoff sounds. Deflate the cuff at the rate of 2 mm Hg/s till the first sound is audible. This is the first Korotkoff sound and correlates with systolic blood pressure (SBP). The rate of cuff deflation should not exceed 2 mm Hg/s. More *rapid deflation* leads to *underestimation of the SBP* and *overestimation of DBP*. With further lowering of pressure, second and third Korotkoff sounds appear and then diminution of turbulence (so called muffling sound and it is the fourth Korotkoff sound) occurs. Finally, the sound disappears that is fifth Korotkoff sound which correlates with DBP.

Table 5.4: Sizes of cuff.		
	Blood pressure cuff	
Mid-arm circumference	**Size**	**Dimensions**
22–26 cm	Small adult	12 × 24 cm
27–34 cm	Adult	16 × 30 cm
35–44 cm	Large adult	16 × 36 cm
45–52 cm	Adult thigh	16 × 42 cm

Auscultatory GAP

In 20–25% of elderly hypertensive patients, Korotkoff sound appears at systolic pressure and disappears at an interval between systolic and diastolic pressure. If the first appearance of sound is missed, SBP may be falsely recorded at a lower level. To eliminate this effect, the first palpatory method should be applied.

Interpretation

The BP should be recorded as: 128/84 mm Hg, supine, right arm.
- In aortic regurgitation (AR), pregnancy, and arteriovenous (AV) fistula due to hyperdynamic circulation turbulence persists for longer period, so DBP is further lowered. In such cases along with SBP (e.g., 120 mm Hg), two DBPs are recorded, one at muffling sound (e.g., 80 mm Hg) and second at disappearance of Korotkoff sound (e.g., 60 mm Hg), and it is written as 120/80/60 mm Hg. Some obstetricians record the DBP at muffling sound only.
- Difference between SBP and DBP is called pulse pressure. If someone's BP is 120/80 mm Hg, then his/her pulse pressure will be 120–80 mm Hg = 40 mm Hg. If pulse pressure is more than 50 mm Hg, it is called wide pulse pressure. Wide pulse pressure is common in elderly person due to arteriosclerosis, hyperthyroidism, etc.
- Ideally blood pressure should be measured in both arms, and higher value should be taken for future reference.
- Difference of blood pressure between standing and supine position gives an assessment of baroreceptor function. If SBP falls more than 20 mm Hg and DBP falls more than 10 mm Hg from supine to standing position, it is called orthostatic hypotension or postural hypotension (a feature of autonomic dysfunction). To detect orthostatic hypotension, BP is measured within 3 minutes of standing from supine position in both arms.
- Home monitoring or ambulatory blood pressure (ABP) monitoring is more accurate method which can eliminate white-coat effect.
- *White-coat hypertension*: Elevated clinic BP but normal home BP
- *Masked hypertension*: Normal clinic BP but elevated home BP
- *Nocturnal hypertension*: No night time reduction in BP (dipping)
- Blood pressure should be taken ideally in multiple occasions, at least 2–3 times.
- Normally, the difference of SBP between two arms is 5–10 mm Hg. If the gap is more than 10 mm Hg (but DBP should be same in both upper arm), it indicates subclavian artery obstruction.

Pseudohypertension

Palpation of radial artery in absence of pulse-signs of atherosclerosis. In this case, both SBP and DBP can be overestimated. It is called pseudohypertension, and intra-arterial recorder gives correct measurement.

Mean Arterial Pressure

The mean arterial pressure (MAP) is the *principal driving force for systemic blood flow*. The MAP is often derived from the SBP and DBP as follows:

$$MAP = \tfrac{1}{3} SBP + \tfrac{2}{3} DBP = \tfrac{1}{3} (SBP + 2\, DBP)$$

CHAPTER 5: General Examination

However, this relationship is reliable when the diastole accounts for two-thirds of the cardiac cycle, which occurs only when the heart rate is 60 beats/min; a rarity in critically ill patients. Therefore, the calculation of MAP is not advised in critically ill patients.

Ankle-brachial Pressure Index

Ratio of highest pedal artery pressure to the highest brachial artery pressure is the ankle-brachial pressure index (ABPI).

In healthy individuals, ABPI is 0.97–1.1, when patient is supine.

Typical value of intermittent claudication is less than 0.9, and critical limb stenosis is less than 0.4.

Ambulatory Blood Pressure Monitoring

Ambulatory blood pressure monitoring involves measuring BP at regular intervals (usually every 20–30 minutes) over a 24-hour period while patients undergo normal daily activities, including sleep. The portable monitor is worn on a belt connected to a standard cuff on the upper arm and uses an oscillometric technique to detect systolic, diastolic, and mean BP as well as heart rate. When complete, the device is connected to a computer that prepares a report of the 24 hour, daytime, night time, and sleep average systolic and diastolic BP, and heart rate. ABP monitoring is safe. Occasionally *edema or petechiae of the upper arm or bruising under the inflating cuff may occur.* It *may disturb sleep* during the night potentially *requiring retesting* if there are poor nocturnal BP measurements. ABP monitoring may be inaccurate in patients with *irregular heart rate and arrhythmias.*

Indications: In suspected:
- White-coat hypertension (elevated clinic BP but normal home BP)
- Masked hypertension (normal clinic BP but elevated home BP)
- Nocturnal hypertension or no nighttime reduction in BP (dipping)
- Resistant hypertension
- Patients with a high risk of future cardiovascular events
- Episodic hypertension.

Ambulatory blood pressure monitoring may also be useful for:
- Titrating antihypertensive therapy
- Borderline hypertension
- Hypertension detected early in pregnancy
- Suspected or confirmed sleep apnea
- Syncope or other symptoms suggesting orthostatic hypotension

Instruction to the patient: Patients should be instructed about:
- Not to wet the device. The patient should attend after bathing.
- The patients should take all their usual medications.
- When the cuff starts to inflate, the patient should stop moving and talking, keep the arm still and relaxed, and breathe normally.
- They should avoid activities such as vigorous exercise.
- A brief diary is important to record timing of activities, sleep, taking of medicines, posture, and symptoms (e.g., dizziness) that may be related to BP.

Working mechanism: ABP monitors use cuff oscillometry. The cuff is inflated until the pressure occludes flow within the brachial artery. As the pressure is released, blood begins to flow, causing fluctuations (oscillations) in the arterial wall that are detected by the monitor. These oscillations increase in intensity, then diminish and cease when blood is flowing normally. The monitor defines the maximal oscillations as mean arterial BP and then uses an algorithm to calculate systolic and diastolic BP. The correct cuff size is essential and in very large patients, a conical shaped cuff is necessary. Measure BP in both arms and if the SBP difference is less than 10 mm Hg, use the nondominant arm. If the SBP difference is greater than 10 mm Hg, use the arm with the higher pressure. If there are fistulas or previous axillary clearance in one arm, the monitor must be fitted on the other arm. To ensure validity, at least three readings should be recorded simultaneously using a calibrated sphygmomanometer connected to the ABP monitoring device by a Y connector. Average readings for ABP and sphygmomanometer should not differ by more than 5 mm Hg. The devices are usually programmed to take readings at set intervals; 15–30 minutes during the day and every 30–60 minutes at night, to obtain numerous readings, while limiting interference with activity or sleep.

Result and interpretation: The BP must be interpreted carefully with reference to diary information and the timing of medicines. Reference "normal" ABP values for nonpregnant adults are:
- *24-hour average* less than 115/75 mm Hg (hypertension threshold 130/80 mm Hg)
- *Daytime* (*awake*) less than 120/80 mm Hg (hypertension threshold 135/85 mm Hg)
- *Nighttime* (*asleep*) less than 105/65 mm Hg (hypertension threshold 120/75 mm Hg)

Ambulatory BP values above "normal" and below thresholds are considered "high normal". Nighttime (sleeping) average BP should both be at least 10% lower than daytime (awake) average. BP load (percentage of time that BP readings exceed hypertension threshold during 24 hours) should be less than 20%. Blood pressure variability, maximum systolic BP, and morning BP surge should also be taken into account (and targeted by treatment). Treatment targets based on ABP are lower than the targets for clinic BP readings (e.g., for clinic BP of 140/90 mm Hg, daytime ABP equivalent is 136/87 mm Hg). Importantly, ABP monitoring can be effectively used to manage antihypertensive treatment **(Figs. 5.15 and 5.16)**.

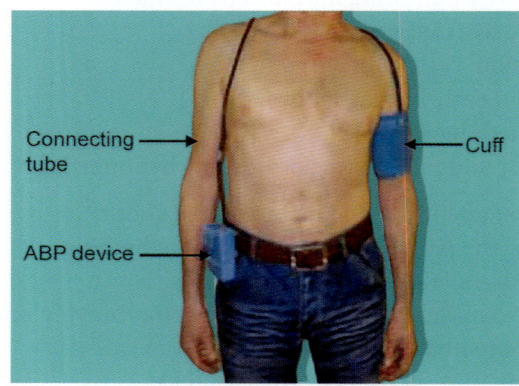

FIG. 5.15: Ambulatory BP (ABP) monitors fitted to a patient.

CHAPTER 5: General Examination

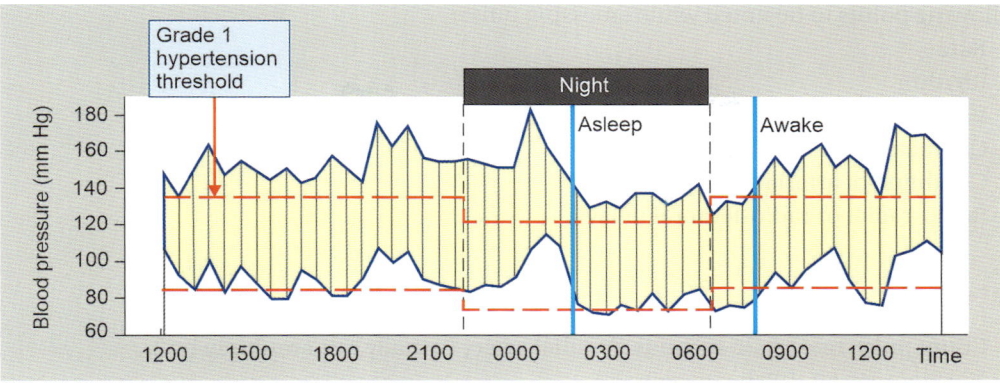

FIG. 5.16: Ambulatory blood pressure report.

Fallacy

- Cannot detect postural hypotension as the measurements occur at a fixed interval. However, diary information and event data with high variability of BP often give clues about orthostatic hypotension.
- The test may be negative or inconclusive due to insufficient valid readings (patient removes or inactivates device or sleep disturbances) necessitate repeat test.

■ PULSE

When the left ventricle contracts, it ejects blood in the systemic arterial circulation, called pressure wave, that is felt as pulse in a superficial artery. Pulse wave is not synonymous with blood flow as pulse wave is faster than blood flow. So pulse can be felt even when there is no blood flow in the artery. Pulse wave depends on: heart rate, stroke volume, left ventricle outflow tract obstruction, and arterial elasticity and resistance **(Fig. 5.17)**.
- *Percussion wave*: Impact of rapidly ejected volume from left ventricle to aorta
- *Tidal wave*: Second smaller wave reflected from periphery
- *Dicrotic wave*: Elastic recoil from peripheral arteries

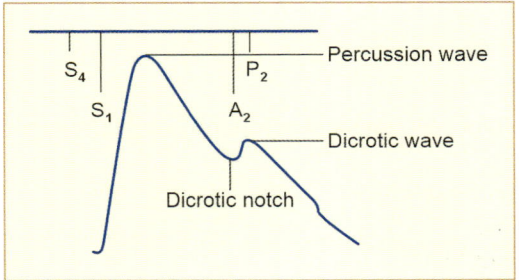

FIG. 5.17: Flow of pulse wave.

Following points to be noted while assessing pulse:
- Rate
- Rhythm
- Volume
- Character
- Condition of arterial wall
- Radio-radial or radio-femoral delay.

Rate

- Count pulse rate for 30 seconds in radial artery (usually) and multiply by 2.
- *Normal rate*: 60–100 beats/min
- If heart rate less than 60 beats/min—bradycardia
- If heart rate more than 100 beats/min—tachycardia
- In case of bradycardia and tachycardia, pulse rate should be counted for 1 minute to minimize error.

Causes of Tachycardia

- *Sinus rhythm*:
    - Exercise
    - Pain
    - Excitement or anxiety
    - Fever
    - Hyperthyroidism
    - Medication: Sympathomimetics, e.g., salbutamol and vasodilators
- *Arrhythmia*:
    - Atrial fibrillation
    - Atrial flutter
    - Supraventricular tachycardia
    - Ventricular tachycardia

Causes of Bradycardia

- *Sinus rhythm*:
    - Sleep
    - Athletic training
    - Hypothyroidism
    - Medication: Beta-blockers, digoxin, verapamil, and diltiazem.
- *Arrhythmia*:
    - Carotid sinus hypersensitivity
    - Sick sinus syndrome
    - Second-degree heart block
    - Complete heart block

Rhythm

- Pulse should be regular with minor variation during respiration
- During inspiration, heart rate increases, during expiration, heart rate decreases
- Irregularly irregular pulse—atrial fibrillation
- Regularly irregular pulse—second-degree atrioventricular block and multiple ectopics

Pulse Deficit

In atrial fibrillation, due to variability of pulse rates, pulse volume also varies, so some cycles are not perceived at radial artery.

Pulse deficit is calculated by counting radial pulse and subtracting this from apical pulsation (done by auscultation):
- Pulse deficit more than 10—atrial fibrillation
- Pulse deficit less than 10—multiple ectopics

Common causes of atrial fibrillation:
- Hypertension
- Heart failure
- Myocardial infarction
- Thyrotoxicosis
- Alcohol-related heart disease
- Mitral valve disease
- Infection, e.g., respiratory and urinary
- Following cardiothoracic surgery.

Volume: Stroke volume is reflected as pulse volume.
- *Low pulse volume*: Left ventricular failure (LVF), hypovolemia, and peripheral arterial disease
- *High pulse volume*:
  - *Physiological*: Exercise and pregnancy
  - *Pathological*: High-output state such as fever, anemia, AR, Paget's disease, and thyrotoxicosis.

Character

Pulsus parvus et tardus: Slow rising pulse with a reduced peak, e.g., aortic stenosis (AS) **(Fig. 5.18)**.

Pulsus bisferiens: Increased pulse with double systolic peak, separated by a distinct dip, e.g., AS + AR **(Fig. 5.19)**.

Pulsus alternans: Beat-to-beat variation in pulse volume with regular rhythm, e.g., heart failure **(Fig. 5.20B)**.

Collapsing pulse (water hammer pulse) **(Fig. 5.20A)**: Peak of pulse wave arrives very quickly and then descents rapidly (due to regurgitation), giving a collapsing feeling. This fall can be exaggerated by raising the arm above the level of the heart, e.g., severe AR.

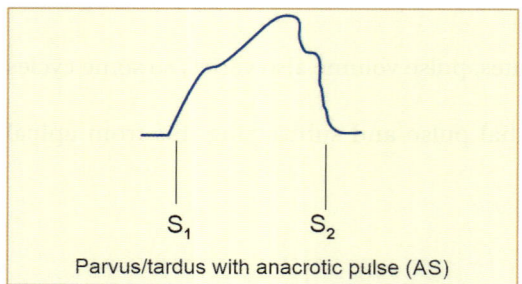

FIG. 5.18: Pulsus parvus et tardus.

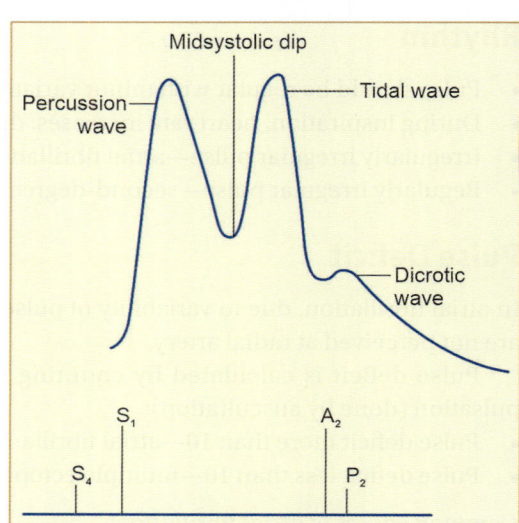

FIG. 5.19: Pulsus bisferiens.

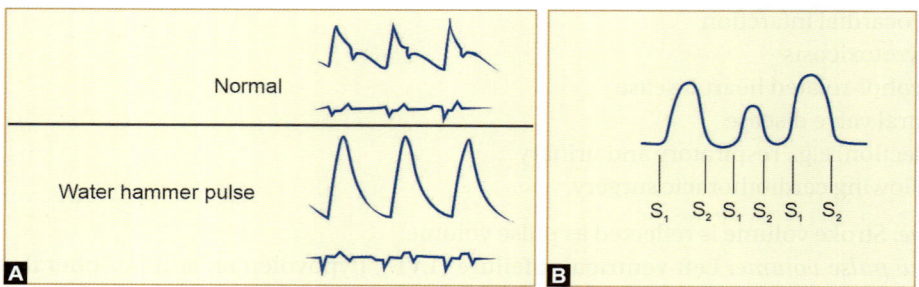

FIGS. 5.20A AND B: (A) Collapsing pulse; (B) Pulsus alternans.

Pulsus paradoxus: This is an exaggeration of the normal physiological cause of pulse volume. During inspiration, venous return increases in right heart, so septum is pushed toward left ventricle, hence stroke volume decreases. Opposite happens during expiration. If patient has cardiac tamponade, intrapericardial pressure is very high, so increased volume of blood in right ventricle pushes intraventricular septum to the left, causing further decrease in stroke volume, i.e., SBP. If difference of SBP and DBP between expiration and inspiration is more than 20 mm Hg, it is called pulsus paradoxus.

Dicrotic pulse: Two peaks, one at systolic and one at diastolic. This is seen in fever, endotoxic shock, and cardiac tamponade **(Fig. 5.21)**.

Surface Marking and Points of Palpation of Artery

- *Carotid*: Angle of jaw, anterior to sternocleidomastoid muscle
- *Brachial*: Medial to biceps tendon at antecubital fossa
- *Radial*: Lateral to insertion of flexor carpi radialis tendon at wrist
- *Femoral*: At mid-inguinal point (midpoint of anterior superior iliac spine and symphysis pubis)

CHAPTER 5: General Examination

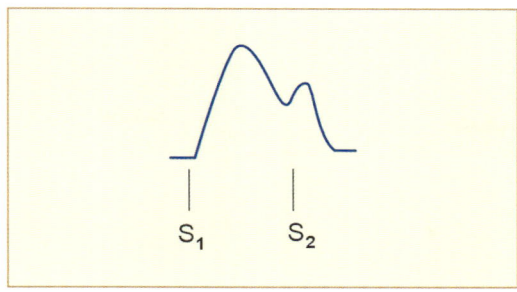

FIG. 5.21: Dicrotic pulse.

Table 5.5: Duration at which pulse wave arrives after systole.	
Artery	Duration at which pulse wave arrives after systole
Carotid	30 msec
Brachial	60 msec
Femoral	75 msec
Radial	80 msec

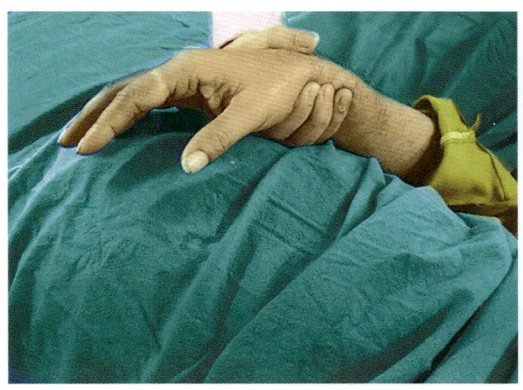

FIG. 5.22: Radial pulse.

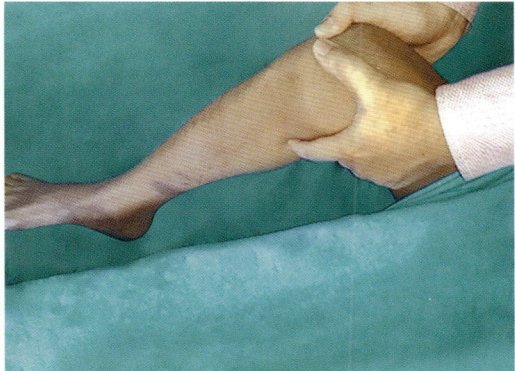

FIG. 5.23: Popliteal pulse.

- *Popliteal*: It lies posteriorly at deep knee crease.
- *Posterior tibial*: 2 cm below and posterior to medial malleolus
- *Dorsalis pedis*: In the groove between 1st and 2nd metatarsal and lateral to tendon of extensor hallucis longus **(Table 5.5)**

Radio-radial Delay

Palpate both radial artery simultaneously—asses difference in volume and any delay. Coarctation of aorta or stenosis of left subclavian artery produces radio-radial delay.

Radiofemoral Delay

Palpate radial and femoral pulse simultaneously to asses for any delay, e.g., coarctation of aorta.

Method of Palpation of Artery

Methods of palpation of artery are shown in **Figures 5.22 to 5.28**.

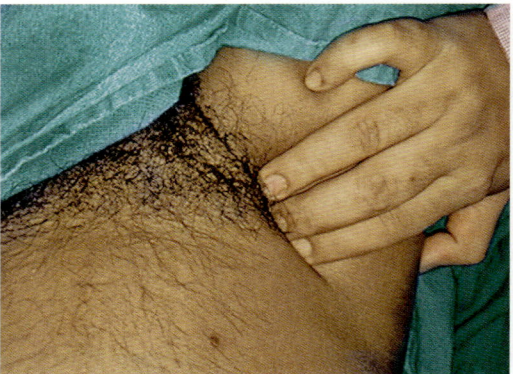

FIG. 5.24: Femoral pulse.

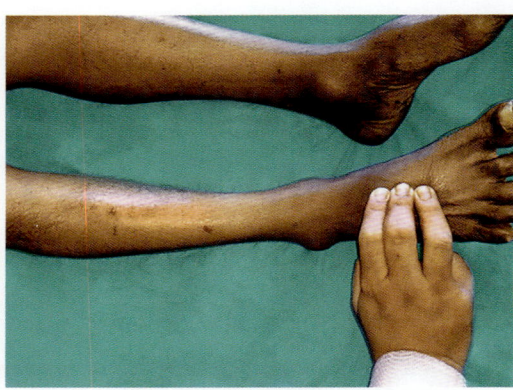

FIG. 5.25: Dorsalis pedis.

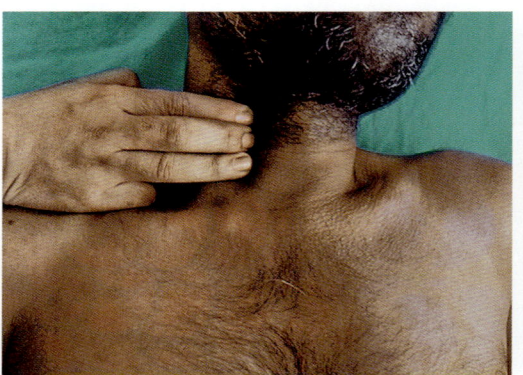

FIG. 5.26: Carotid pulse.

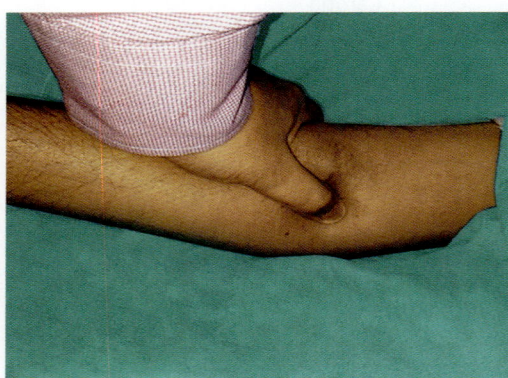

FIG. 5.27: Brachial pulse.

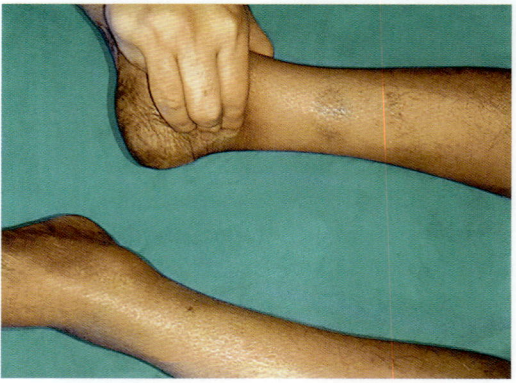

FIG. 5.28: Peroneal arterial pulse.

■ RESPIRATION

The process of taking up oxygen and removing carbon dioxide from cells of the body is known as respiration. Respiration takes place in two stages. The first stage is known as gas exchange, and the second as cellular respiration. Gas exchange occurs at two levels. The first level involves the transfer of oxygen and carbon dioxide between the atmosphere and the lungs by the process of breathing or ventilation. These involve: (1) Inspiration (inhalation of air or oxygen into the lungs) and (2) expiration (exhalation of air or carbon dioxide from the lungs). The second level involves the exchange of oxygen and carbon dioxide between the systemic blood and the metabolically active tissue. The movement of oxygen and carbon dioxide in and out of cells occurs by simple diffusion.

The rate at which breathing occurs (usually measured in breaths/min) is called the ventilation rate or respiratory rate. The normal respiratory rate for a healthy adult at rest is 12–18 breaths/min, regular with no apparent discomfort. Chest wall and abdomen expand and shrink during inspiration and expiration, respectively, and is symmetrical. The respiratory movements are predominantly abdominal in men and predominantly thoracic in women. Periodic deep breathing (sighs) less than 5 breaths/min is considered normal.

Measurement: The respiratory rate is measured when a person is at rest, and it is the number of breaths counted for 1 minute. Any of the following methods can be used to count the respiratory rate.
- Look at the chest to see the rise and fall of the chest or **(Fig. 5.29)**
- Place your hand on the person's chest to feel the rise and fall of the chest wall. One rise and one fall are counted as 1 breath.
- Try to listen the breath sounds. The patient should not be aware that you are counting his or her respiratory rate. The person's breathing is likely to change if he or she knows you are counting it. Count the respiratory rate while pretending to take the patient's pulse. Note the rate, intercostal sucking, wheeze, pattern, or any discomfort of respiration.

Normal resting breathing rate: Normal resting breathing rate is shown in **Table 5.6**.

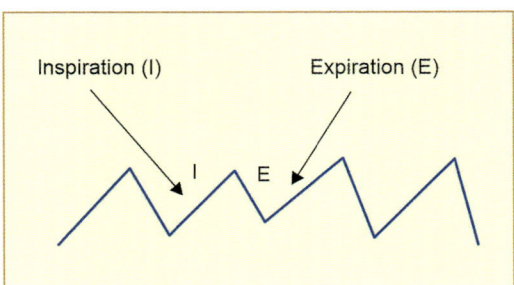

FIG. 5.29: Cycle of respiration.

Table 5.6: Normal resting breathing rate.	
Age	**Respiratory rate (breaths/min)**
0–3 months	35–55
3–6 months	30–45
6–12 months	25–40
1–3 years	20–30
3–6 years	20–25
6–12 years	14–22
>12 years	12–18

Pattern of respiration: Sighing respiration—breathing punctuated by frequent sighs should alert you to the possibility of hyperventilation syndrome—is a common cause of dyspnea and dizziness. Occasional sighs (<5 breaths/min) are normal **(Fig. 5.30)**.

Slow breathing (bradypnea): Slow breathing (rate <10 breaths/min) may be secondary to diabetic coma, drugs (e.g., narcotics such as morphine)-induced respiratory depression, myxedema, and increased intracranial pressure **(Fig. 5.31)**.

Rapid shallow breathing (tachypnea): Rapid shallow breathing (rate >20 breaths/min) has a number of causes including fever, anxiety, restrictive lung disease, pleuritic chest pain, and an elevated diaphragm **(Fig. 5.32)**.

Cheyne–Stokes breathing: Cyclical deepening and quickening of respiration, followed by diminishing respiratory effort and rate, sometimes associated with a short period of complete apnea that can last up to 30 seconds or longer, the cycle then being repeated. Children and aging people normally may show this pattern in sleep. Other causes include heart failure, uremia, drug-induced respiratory depression, strokes, traumatic brain injuries, brain tumors, carbon monoxide poisoning, and metabolic encephalopathy **(Fig. 5.33)**.

Obstructive breathing: In obstructive lung disease, expiration is prolonged because narrowed airways increase the resistance to air flow. Causes include asthma, chronic bronchitis, and COPD. With lips pursed patient controls expiration slowly which is also known as pursed lip breathing **(Fig. 5.34)**.

Rapid deep breathing (hyperpnea or hyperventilation): Rapid deep breathing has several causes, including exercise, anxiety, and metabolic acidosis. In the comatose patient, consider infarction, hypoxia, or hypoglycemia affecting the midbrain or the pons. Kussmaul breathing is a type of labored hyperventilation, which is rapid and deep breathing due to severe metabolic acidosis (e.g., DKA). Sometimes it may be rapid and shallow or deep and low with the features of "air hunger" **(Fig. 5.35)**.

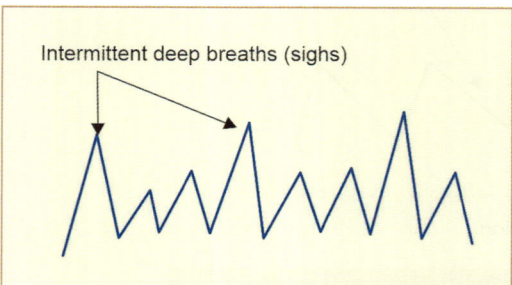

FIG. 5.30: Sighing respiration.

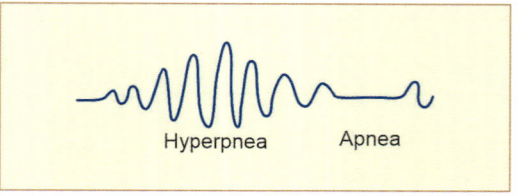

FIG. 5.33: Cheyne–Stokes breathing.

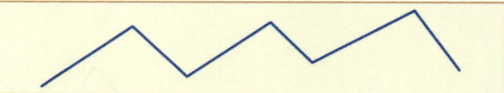

FIG. 5.31: Slow breathing.

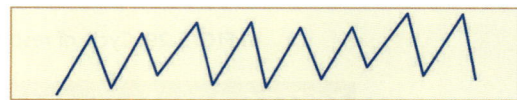

FIG. 5.32: Rapid shallow breathing.

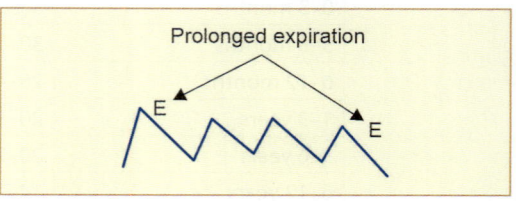

FIG. 5.34: Obstructive breathing.

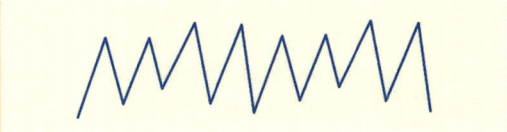

FIG. 5.35: Rapid deep breathing.

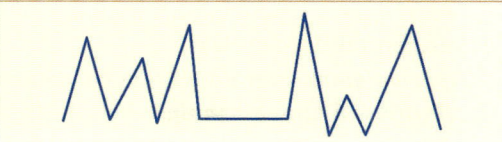

FIG. 5.36: Ataxic breathing.

Ataxic breathing (Biot's breathing): Ataxic breathing is characterized by unpredictable irregularity of shallow or deep breathing with increasing episodes of apnea. Causes include respiratory depression, brain damage typically at the medullary level by stroke [cerebrovascular accident (CVA)] or trauma, pressure on the medulla due to uncal or tentorial herniation, and prolonged opioid abuse **(Fig. 5.36)**.

Apneustic breathing: Apneustic breathing has a prolonged inspiratory phase followed by a prolonged expiratory phase. Apneustic breathing is caused by damage to the upper part of the pons.

Paradoxical breathing:
- *Abdominal paradox*: Instead of simultaneous chest and abdominal wall expansion with inspiration, there is a paradoxical movement of the chest wall inward and the abdomen outward during inspiration, which is known as abdominal paradox. This pattern of breathing is seen in diaphragmatic paralysis due to cervical spinal cord or phrenic nerve injury.
- *Thoracic paradox (flail chest)*: Flail chest occurs when three or more contiguous ribs are fractured in at least two locations. Paradoxical movement of this free-floating segment of chest wall is usually evident in patients with spontaneous ventilation. On the side of unstable chest wall, hemithorax retracts while the normal side expands with inspiration, which is known as thoracic paradox (flail chest).
- *Respiratory alternans*: A series of tidal breaths alternates between short periods of abdominal inward movement during inspiration followed by a period of chest wall inward movement during inspiration. This pattern of breathing is known as respiratory alternans and is seen in individuals being weaned from mechanical ventilation. This is associated with fatigue and indicates weaning should be stopped.

Abnormal respiration: Apnea—temporary cessation of breathing and, therefore, of the body's intake of oxygen and release of carbon dioxide. It is a serious and potentially life-threatening condition.

Types:
- *Deglutition apnea*: Apnea while swallowing
- *Central apnea*: Apnea during sleep that occurs when the respiratory center of the brainstem does not send normal periodic signals to the muscles of respiration. Observation of the patient reveals no respiratory effort (no movement of the chest and no breath sounds).
- *Obstructive apnea*: Absent or dysfunctional breathing that occurs when the upper airway is intermittently blocked during sleep. Observation of the patient reveals vigorous but ineffective respiratory efforts, often with loud snoring or snorting.

- *Mixed apnea*: Dysfunctional breathing during sleep that combines elements of obstructive and central sleep apneas.
- *Apnea of prematurity (AOP)*: A condition of the premature newborn, marked by repeated episodes of apnea lasting longer than 20 seconds. The diagnosis of AOP is one of the exclusions made when no treatable cause can be found. Increased frequency of apneic episodes directly relates to the degree of prematurity. AOP is not an independent risk factor for sudden infant death syndrome. Apneic episodes may result in bradycardia, hypoxia, and respiratory acidosis.
- *Sleep apnea*: The temporary absence of breathing during sleep. This common disorder affects about 10% of all middle-aged men and about 5% of middle-aged women in the United States and is classified according to the mechanism involved and by whether or not it is associated with daytime sleepiness. In obstructive sleep apnea, vigorous respiratory efforts are present during sleep but the flow of air in and out of the airways is blocked by upper airway obstruction. Patients with obstructive sleep apnea are usually middle-aged, obese men who make loud snorting, snoring, and gasping sounds during sleep. By contrast, central sleep apnea is marked by absence of respiratory muscle activity. Patients may exhibit excessive daytime sleepiness, but snorting and gasping during sleep are absent. Occasionally, life-threatening central apneas occur as a result of strokes. Mixed apnea begins with absence of respiratory effort, followed by upper airway obstruction. Whenever apneas are prolonged, oxygenation drops and carbon dioxide blood levels rise. Patients often awaken many times during the night or have fragmented sleep architecture. In the morning, many patients complain of headache, fatigue, drowsiness, or an unsatisfying night rest. In addition, these individuals often have hypertension, arrhythmias, type 2 diabetes mellitus, or signs and symptoms of right-sided heart failure. Although these findings may suggest the diagnosis, formal sleep studies in a laboratory are needed to document the disorder and to measure the effects of apneas on oxygenation and other physical parameters.

Apnea monitoring: Monitoring the respiratory movements, especially of infants, may be done by using an apnea alarm mattress or devices to measure the infant's thoracic and abdominal movements and heart rate. Apnea is usually detected by placing electrodes (linked to a cardiorespiratory monitor) on the skin overlying the abdomen and thorax of the patient.

Apnea test: A test used to determine whether a comatose person receiving life support has suffered brain death. The patient's ventilator is set to deliver no breaths per minute and the carbon dioxide level of the blood is allowed to raise 20–60 mm Hg. If apnea (no spontaneous breathing) occurs, brain death is confirmed. The test should not be performed if the person has recently received sedative, narcotic, or paralytic drugs; those drugs may suppress spontaneous breathing, falsely suggesting brain death.

Dyspnea (air hunger; breathlessness): The shortage of air results in labored or difficult breathing, sometimes accompanied by pain. It is normal when it is due to vigorous work or athletic activity and should quickly return to normal when the activity ceases.

- *Cardiac dyspnea*: Dyspnea due to inadequate cardiac output, i.e., from heart failure
- *Expiratory dyspnea*: Dyspnea associated with obstructive lung diseases such as asthma or chronic bronchitis. Wheezing is often present.
- *Inspiratory dyspnea*: Dyspnea due to interference with the passage of air to the lungs. Stridor may be present.
- *Paroxysmal-nocturnal dyspnea (PND)*: Sudden attacks of dyspnea that usually occur when patients are asleep in bed. The affected patient awakens gasping for air and tries to sit up (often near a window) to relieve the symptom. PND is one of the classic symptoms of left ventricular failure, although it may also occasionally be caused by sleep apnea or by nocturnal cardiac ischemia.

Hyperpnea: An increased respiratory rate or breathing that is deeper than that usually experienced during normal activity. A certain degree of hyperpnea is normal after exercise; it may also be caused by pain, a variety of respiratory diseases, fever, heart failure, certain drugs, panic attacks, or at high altitude.

Tachypnea: Respiratory rate >20 breaths/min.

Hypopnea: Decreased rate and depth of breathing.

Bradypnea: Respiratory rate <10 breaths/min.

Orthopnea: Labored breathing that occurs when lying flat and improves when standing or sitting up. This is one of the classic symptoms of heart failure (congestive heart failure and LVF), diaphragmatic paralysis, superior vena cava (SVC) syndrome, anterior mediastinal mass, although it occasionally occurs in other cardiac or respiratory illnesses.

Platypnea: The shortness of breath only when the patient is upright or seated but more comfortable in supine position. It is often seen in patients of cirrhosis (hepatopulmonary syndrome) in which small AV dilatations developed in the lower regions of the lungs. These dilated vessels cause a shunt that is aggravated by the upright position, resulting from greater blood flow through the lower areas of the lung due to gravity forces. Upon supine position, the gravity dependent pulmonary blood flow is redistributed to the posterior areas of the lungs that may be less affected by the vascular dilatations. Orthodeoxia often accompanies this condition in which oxygen desaturation experienced while upright and improves when supine.

Trepopnea: The shortness of breath when the patient lies on either the right or left lateral decubitus position. The symptom can be relieved by moving to the opposite lateral position. This suggests an underlying disease affecting one lung or pleural space more than the other; patients often prefer to lie with the less affected side dependent, which may allow greater pulmonary blood flow through the healthier lung. In contrast, the pleurisy, in which case patients may prefer to lie with the more affected side dependent to splint excessive respiratory movement.

FEVER

- Normal temperature ranges between 96.5 and 98.6°F.
- *Sites of measurement*: Mouth, axilla, ear, groin, and rectum
- Rectal temperature 0.6°F higher than normal temperature
- Axillary temperature 1°F lower than oral temperature

Definition

Oral temperature is above 98.6°F, or rectal temperature is above 100.5°F.

Diurnal variation: Lowest at morning and highest at evening

Physiology

Hypothalamus maintains a set point for temperature. Autonomic nervous system regulates blood flow from internal organs to skin and sweat glands.

Heat loss from body occurs by dilatation of cutaneous vessels and evaporation.

Heat gain occurs in body by constriction of cutaneous vessels. Constriction of vessels presents as chills for further generation of heat. Muscle contractions also occur that manifests as rigor.

Release of endogenous pyrogens increases set point of hypothalamus. So for increased demand of heat, first cutaneous vessels contract to decrease evaporation. If not adequate, then skeletal muscles contract vigorously.

Night sweats: *Exaggeration of physiological diurnal variation*—occur in chronic inflammatory conditions, malignancies.

Blunting of pyrexic response occurs in:
- Old age
- Chronic kidney disease
- Immunocompromised person

Pattern of Fever

- *Continuous fever*: Diurnal variation less than 2°F and temperature never touches the baseline, e.g., lobar pneumonia **(Fig. 5.37)**.
- *Remittent fever*: Diurnal variation more than 2°F and temperature never touches the baseline, e.g., typhoid fever **(Fig. 5.38)**.
- *Intermittent fever*: Temperature touches baseline in between two spikes, e.g., malaria **(Fig. 5.39)**.
- *Pel–Ebstein fever*: It is a type of fever lasting for 3–10 days followed by an afebrile period of 3–10 days, e.g., Hodgkin and other lymphomas.
- *Saddleback fever*: Initially fever lasts for 2–3 days followed by a remission lasting for 2 days and the fever reappears and continues for 2–3 days, e.g., dengue fever.
- *Cyclic neutropenia*: Cyclic neutropenia accompanied with fever occurs every 21 days.

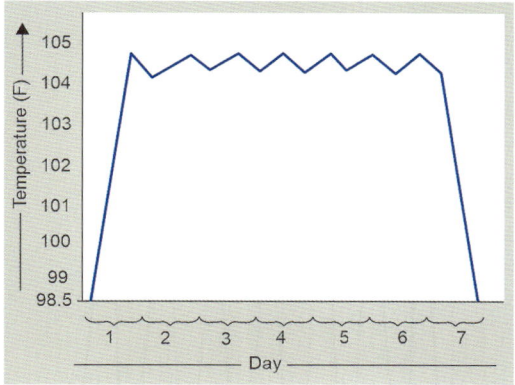

FIG. 5.37: Continuous fever.   FIG. 5.38: Remittent fever.

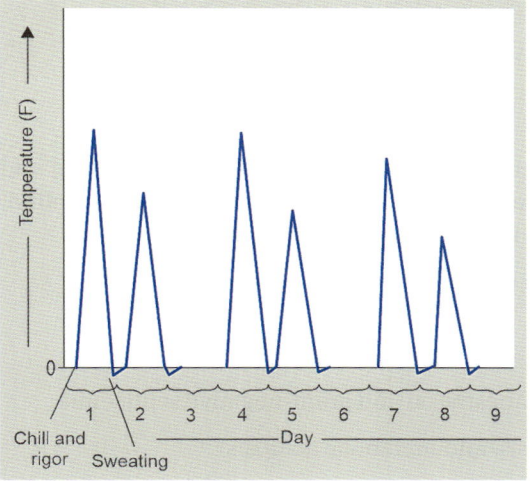

FIG. 5.39: Intermittent fever.

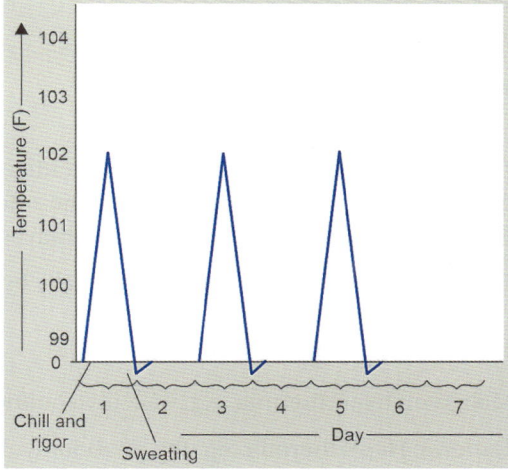

FIG. 5.40: Tertian fever.

Different types of intermittent fever:
- *Tertian fever*: Two fever paroxysms are separated by 1 day, e.g., *Plasmodium vivax* **(Fig. 5.40)**.
- *Quartan fever*: Two fever paroxysms are separated by 2 days, e.g., *Plasmodium malariae* **(Fig. 5.41)**.
- *Quotidian fever*: Fever everyday with temperature touching baseline in between, e.g., *Plasmodium falciparum* with *P. vivax* **(Fig. 5.42)**

Hectic fever: Fever with afternoon spikes, facial flushes, and wide variation of temperature, e.g., active tuberculosis, bacterial meningitis, abscesses, and encephalitis.

Relapsing fever: Febrile attack persisting for a few days, then attenuated for a few days, then again recurs, e.g., lymphoma, brucellosis, and typhoid.

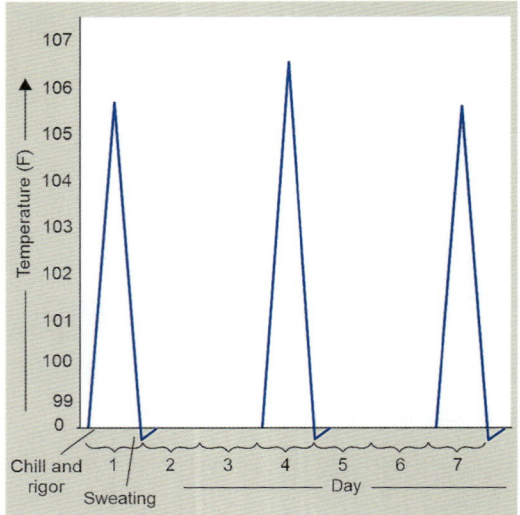

FIG. 5.41: Quartan fever.

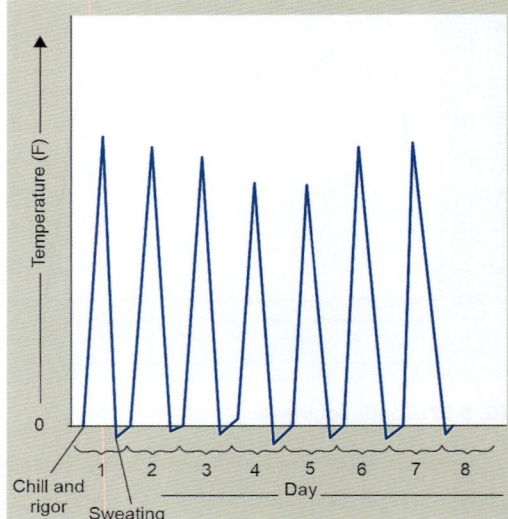

FIG. 5.42: Quotidian fever.

Drug fever: Febrile response that coincides temporarily with administration of a drug and disappears after discontinuation of the offending agent, e.g., amphotericin B, penicillin, methyldopa, bleomycin, etc. Relative bradycardia is the feature of drug fever.

Factitious fever: Fever produced artificially by a patient.

Malignant Hyperthermia

Malignant hyperthermia, e.g., succinylcholine anesthesia and gram-negative septicemia.

Features: Hyperthermia, rigidity, rhabdomyolysis, and metabolic acidosis

Heat stroke: Due to failure of thermoregulatory mechanism, core temperature rises rapidly. It mainly occurs due to lack of sweating, usually in elderly individuals, e.g., exposure to sun during summer time, CVA, and anticholinergic drug ingestion.

Pyrexia of unknown origin (PUO): Fever more than 3 weeks. Temperature above 101°F for at least two occasions, no diagnosis reached after three outpatient visits or at least 7 days in hospital.

Temperature-pulse dissociation: With each degree of temperature elevation, there should be an increase of 10 beats/min. If this does not occur, it is called *relative bradycardia*. For example, typhoid fever, drug-induced fever, legionellosis, brucellosis, leptospirosis, and meningitis with raised intracranial tension.

Hypothermia

Core temperature below 35°C (95°F). Occurs in:
- Elderly patients

- Drowning
- Cold weather
- Severe hypothyroidism
- Alcohol intoxication

JUGULAR VENOUS PRESSURE

It is a method of indirect assessment of central venous pressure (CVP).

Internal jugular vein (IJV) lies in straight line communication with right atrium. So IJV acts as manometer. Thus, it is a marker of CVP, intravascular volume status, and cardiac function.

Internal jugular vein lies between two heads of sternocleidomastoid, then in front of sternocleidomastoid, and finally in front of the ear. So to make it better visualize turn head to left and put resistance; two heads of sternocleidomastoid will be prominent and one can better appreciate.

External jugular vein (EJV) passes obliquely in front of sternocleidomastoid muscle, not in direct communication with right atrium, thereby not a reliable marker **(Fig. 5.43)**.

Method of Elicitation

- Place the patient at 45° angle on bed. In this position, upper level of venous column is best seen.
- Identify the sternal angle.
- Put two rulers; one horizontally at the top of the venous column and other vertically from sternal angle.

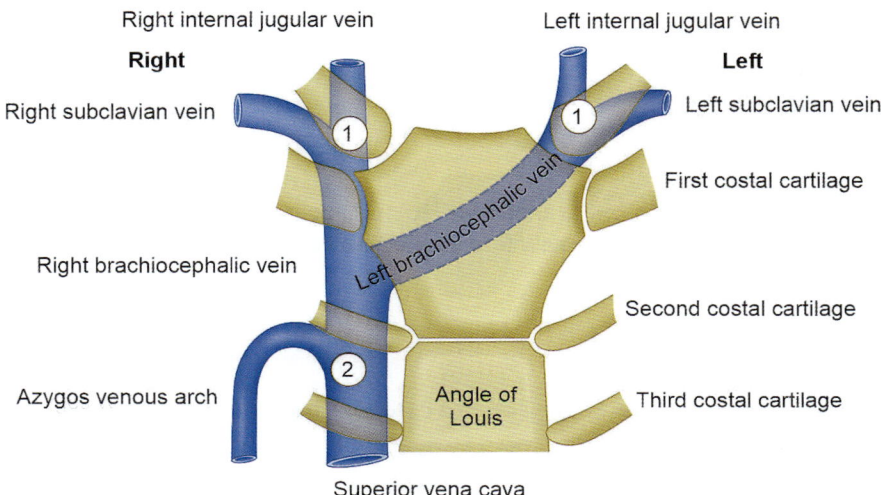

FIG. 5.43: Formation of superior vena cava (SVC): (1) Jugular vein; (2) Superior vena cava.

- Normally, the height from sternal angle is less than 3 cm.
- Distance between sternal angle and center of right atrium is 5 cm **(Figs. 5.44A and B)**.
- So, normal CVP is 8 cm of blood or H_2O.

Central venous pressure can be measured in sitting position with the legs dangling by the bedside. Normally, it lies just behind the clavicle. So, if venous column is visible above the level of clavicle, it signifies elevated venous pressure as the distance between the center of right atrium and the clavicle is at least 10 cm. It is to be noted that bedside estimation of JVP is done using cm of blood or H_2O. It is to be converted into mm Hg to provide better correlation with invasive hemodynamic measurements of cardiac chambers (1.36 cmH_2O = 1.0 mm Hg) **(Table 5.7)**.

Jugular Venous Pressure Waveform

- The "a" wave corresponds to right atrial contraction and precedes first heart sound (S1).
- The "c" wave corresponds to right ventricular contraction, causing the tricuspid valve to bulge toward the right atrium.
- The "x" descent follows the "c" wave and occurs as a result of the right ventricle, pulling the tricuspid valve downward during ventricular systole.
- The "v" wave corresponds to venous filling when the tricuspid valve is closed, immediately after second heart sound (S2).

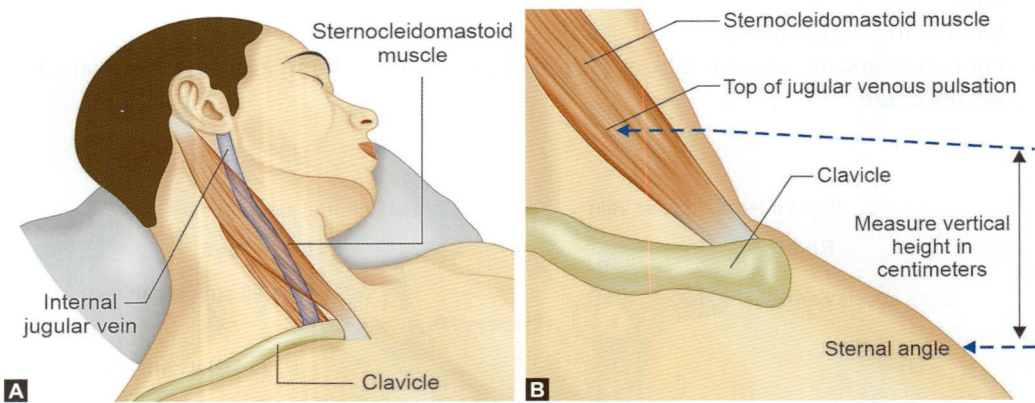

FIGS. 5.44A AND B: Carotid artery lies medial to internal jugular vein (IJV), the following **Table 5.6** will help to differentiate the two.

Table 5.7: Comparsion between jugular venous pressure and carotid pulse.	
Jugular venous pressure	**Carotid pulse**
Better seen	Better felt
Wavy	Pulsatile
If pressure is given at neck above clavicle, venous wave disappears	If pressure is given at neck above clavicle, carotid pulse will not disappear
Upstroke does not coincide with heart sound	Upstroke coincides with first heart sound

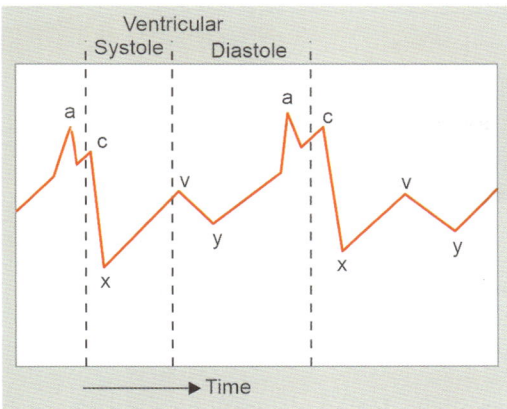

FIG. 5.45: Jugular venous pressure waveform.

- The "y" descent corresponds to the rapid emptying of the atrium into the ventricle following the opening of the tricuspid valve **(Fig. 5.45)**.

Abnormalities of JVP Waveform
- Elevated and nonpulsatile—SVC obstruction
- *Pulsatile*:
  - Giant *a* wave: Tricuspid stenosis; it is presystolic.
  - Cannon *a* wave (venous corrigan): Complete heart block, atrioventricular nodal reentrant tachycardia; occurs between S1 and S2.
  - Absent *a* wave: Atrial fibrillation
  - Large *v* wave: Tricuspid regurgitation
  - *cv* wave: Tricuspid regurgitation
  - Sharp *y* descent: Constrictive pericarditis; also known as Friedreich's sign.
  - Absent *y* descent: Cardiac tamponade
  - Slow *y* descent: Tricuspid stenosis
  - Prominent *x* descent: Constrictive pericarditis and cardiac tamponade
  - Absent *x* descent: Tricuspid regurgitation and atrial fibrillation

Anthem Sign
The patient lies supine on bed. Patient's right hand is put on chest at the sternal level as if putting the hand during observation of national anthem. In this posture, the hand is above the right atrial level. If venous engorgement is found, CVP is considered to be high.

Abdominojugular Reflux
If there is uncertainty about the status of JVP, put pressure over the right hypochondrium for 10 seconds. If venous column rises by 3 cm of water and remains so for at least 15 seconds even after the release of the pressure, it is called as "positive" abdominojugular reflux. It is a sign of impending heart failure **(Fig. 5.46)**.

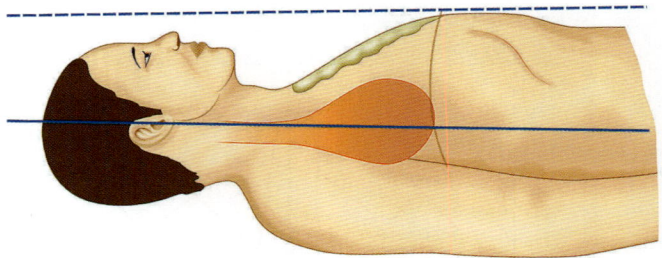

FIG. 5.46: Abdominojugular reflux.

Kussmaul's Sign

Physiologically, JVP column falls during inspiration as intrathoracic pressure decreases. In expiration, the exact opposite occurs. In constrictive pericarditis, during inspiration, blood is pulled into the thorax but due to fibrous pericardium, heart is unable to accommodate the blood, and thus we see elevated venous column even during inspiration. This is called "Kussmaul's sign".

Superior Vena Cava Obstruction

Anatomy

It is formed by the left and right brachiocephalic veins (also referred to as the innominate veins), which also receive blood from the upper limbs, eyes and neck, behind the lower border of the first right costal cartilage. It passes vertically downward behind first intercostal space and receives azygos vein just before it pierces the fibrous pericardium opposite right second costal cartilage, and its lower part is intrapericardial. And then, it ends in the upper and posterior part of the sinus venarum of the right atrium, at the upper right front portion of the heart.

Obstruction can happen at two sites:
1. Above azygos vein
2. Below azygos vein

Various collaterals are formed depending on the site of the obstruction:
- *Preazygos*: In this condition, mainly the right superior intercostal vein serves as the collateral pathway to drain into the azygos vein. So dilated veins are mostly found over chest wall and upper arm.
- *Azygos*: When the azygos vein is also obstructed, the collateral circulation establishes between SVC and IVC via minor communicating channels, i.e., internal mammary veins, superior and inferior epigastric veins to iliac veins, and finally into the IVC.
- *Postazygos*: In this case, the blood from the SVC is distributed into the azygos and hemiazygos and then into the IVC tributaries, i.e., ascending lumbar and lumbar veins. So dilated veins found over chest wall, abdomen, back, and groin.
- The most efficient collateral system is right superior intercostal and azygos circulation. For this reason, most of the patients with preazygos obstruction of SVC remain asymptomatic for a long period of time.

Causes

- Bronchogenic carcinoma, the most common (around 75%)
- Mediastinal tumor—thymoma and germ cell tumor
- Retrosternal thyroid
- Esophageal carcinoma
- Giant aneurysms of aorta
- Chronic fibrotic mediastinitis—idiopathic or secondary to tuberculosis, histoplasmosis, pyogenic infection, radiation, etc.

Features

- Puffiness of face (plethoric, edematous, suffused, and cyanosed)
- Periorbital edema, red and congested conjunctiva
- Swollen neck
- Nonpulsatile JVP
- Visible tortuous dilated vein over chest, neck, and upper limb
- Swelling of upper half of body including upper limbs

Mandatory Examinations to Search Etiology

- Lymph nodes in the neck
- Mediastinal percussion
- Thyroid examination (especially retrosternal thyroid)
- Clubbing
- Radiation mark in the neck
- Signs of Horner's syndrome
- Fundoscopy (dilated vessels, hemorrhage. Observe and exudates)

Pemberton's Sign

The Pemberton's maneuver is a physical examination tool used to demonstrate the presence of latent pressure in the thoracic inlet. The maneuver is achieved by having the patient elevate both arms until they touch the sides of the face. A positive Pemberton's sign is marked by the presence of facial congestion and cyanosis, as well as respiratory distress and stridor.

ORAL EXAMINATION

Normal Oral Cavity Dull Red in Color

- *Tonsil*: Both tonsils lie in pyriform fossa. Observe size, patches, and abscess.
- *Tongue*: Discussed later on
- *Teeth*: Broken, caries, malalignment, and abscess
- *Cheeks*: Ulcers
- *Hard palate*: High arch in Marfan's syndrome
- *Soft palate*: Ulcer, deviation, and swelling
- *Uvula*: Movement of uvula and deviation

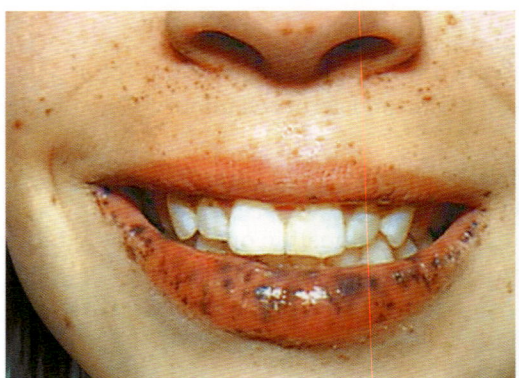

FIG. 5.47: Pigmentation around mouth.

- *Posterior pharyngeal wall*: Redness and thrush
- *Dryness of mouth*: Sjögren's syndrome

Gum

- *Hypertrophy*:
  - Epilepsy and pregnancy
  - Nifedipine and phenytoin
- *Ulcer*: IBD and Behçet's disease
- *Bleeding*: Bleeding diathesis and viral hemorrhagic fever
- *Inflammation*: Gingivitis and CLD

Mouth

- *Angular stomatitis*: Vitamin deficiency
- *Pigmentation around mouth*: Peutz–Jeghers syndrome **(Fig. 5.47)**
- *Telangiectasia over gum*: Osler–Weber–Rendu syndrome

■ TONGUE

Method

- *Ask the patient to put out the tongue to look for*:
  - Size—should fit comfortably in mouth, tip against lower incisor, and sublingual gland should not be displaced.
  - Shape—for ulcers and furrows
  - Fasciculation
  - Color—normally pink-red
  - Surface
  - Patches
- Ask whether tongue can fit in oral cavity and touch lower incisor.

- Ask to protrude the tongue straight for absence of deviation, color, texture, ulcer, patches, and fasciculation.
- Hold the tongue between index and thumb to observe for any mass or tenderness.

Findings

- *Macroglossia*:
  - *Pseudomacroglossia*—secondary to any condition, which pushes tongue to an abnormal position, looking large. For example, enlarged tonsil, oral cavity neoplasm, and low palate.
  - *True macroglossia*:
    - Congenital: Down's syndrome
    - Acquired: Hypothyroidism, acromegaly, and amyloidosis
- *Microglossia*: Pseudobulbar palsy
- *Fasciculation*: Motor neuron disease
- *Ulcer*:
  - *Aphthous ulcer*—painful ulcer, multiple in number, different in size, heal spontaneously, and can recur.
  - *Recurrent aphthous ulcer*—ulcerative colitis and Crohn's disease
  - *Single nonhealing ulcer*—possibly malignant
- *Color*:
  - *Beefy red tongue*—vitamin B12 deficiency
  - *Geographic tongue*—red ring and line frequently changing over time in vitamin B12 deficiency **(Fig. 5.48)**
  - *Glossitis*—smooth, reddened tongue due to atrophy of papillae in alcoholism, iron deficiency anemia, and vitamin deficiency
  - *Bald tongue of sandwich*—niacin deficiency
  - *Black tongue*—prolonged use of oral antibiotics
  - *Strawberry tongue*—scarlet fever.
- *Patches* **(Fig. 5.49)**:
  - Oral candidiasis—found in immunocompromised host and HIV, and steroid use can be scraped.

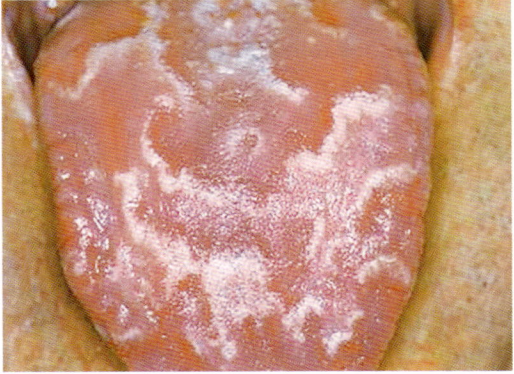

FIG. 5.48: Beefy red tongue.

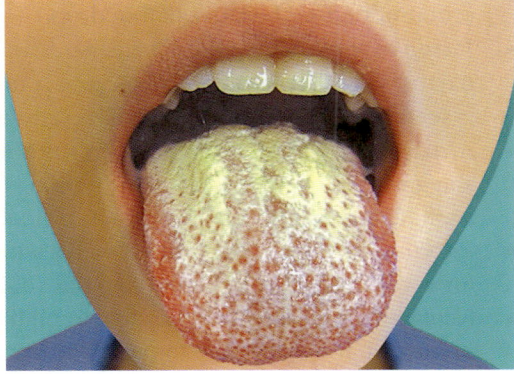

FIG. 5.49: Patches (oral candidiasis).

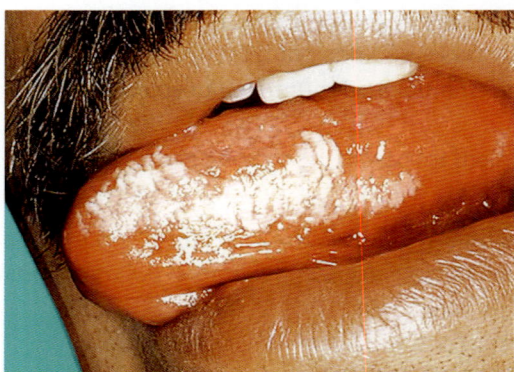

FIG. 5.50: Leukoplakia.

- *Leukoplakia* **(Fig. 5.50)**:
  - White patch cannot be scraped.
  - It is premalignant lesion.
- *Furrow*:
  - Transverse—benign
  - Longitudinal—found in syphilis
- *Tremor*: Anxiety and thyrotoxicosis

GAIT

It is important to look at the patient by the way he is entering the clinic. Gait can give a lot of information regarding the systems involved. Disorders can be due to musculoskeletal disorder, systemic disorder, and psychogenic.

Different Types of Gait

- *Hemiplegic gait*: The patient has unilateral weakness with affected arm flexed, abducted, and internally rotated while the affected leg is in extension with plantar flexion of foot and toes. The patient holds his arm to his side and drags his affected leg in a semicircle (circumduction) because of foot drop.
- *Paraplegic gait*: The patient has spastic lower extremities due to which he walks with narrow base, dragging both legs, and scraping the toes seen in cerebral palsy. *Scissors gait* is seen with extreme tightness of hip adductors.
- *Ataxic (cerebellar) gait*: Seen in cerebellar lesions and characterized with clumsy, staggering movements with wide base. *Titubation* or swaying back and forth is seen in such patients. It is also seen in acute alcohol intoxication.
- *Parkinsonism gait*: The patient walks with slow small steps with head and neck stooped forward. There may be associated pill-rolling movement of fingers.
- *Neuropathic gait*: It is also known as high steppage or equine gait and seen in foot drop. If unilateral, it may be due to peroneal nerve injury or L5 radiculopathy. If bilateral, it may be due to amyotrophic lateral sclerosis (ALS) and peripheral neuropathy due to diabetes.

- *Myopathic gait*: It is seen in weakness of hip girdle muscle leading to drop in pelvis of the contralateral side while walking (Trendelenburg sign). Waddling is seen if both sides are affected. It is seen in patients with myopathies.
- *Choreiform gait*: It is seen in basal ganglia disorders where irregular, jerky, involuntary movements of extremities are seen, which may increase on walking.
- *Stomping gait*: Patients lift their leg high up and hit it hard on the ground due to lack of proprioceptive sensation. It is seen in vitamin B12 deficiency or peripheral neuropathy due to uncontrolled diabetes.

SKIN LESIONS

- *Macule*: Flat, less than 2 cm in diameter, not raised from skin surface
- *Papule*: Small lesion less than 0.5 cm in diameter, raised above skin surface
- *Nodule*: 0.5–5 cm lesion, raised above skin surface
- *Mass*: Raised solid more than 5 cm diameter
- *Plaque*: Size more than 1 cm, flat topped, raised from surface, edge may be distinct or merged with surroundings
- *Vesicle*: Small fluid-filled lesion less than 0.5 cm in diameter
- *Pustule*: Vesicles filled with leukocytes
- *Bulla*: Fluid-filled raised lesion more than 0.5 cm in diameter
- *Wheal*: Raised erythematous, edematous papule or plaque due to vasodilatation
- *Telangiectasia*: Dilated superficial blood vessels
- *Erythroderma*: When majority of skin surface is red in color, it may be associated with scales, erosion, pustules, etc. For example, psoriasis, drug, and cutaneous T-cell lymphoma.
- *Exanthems*: Widespread rash due to toxins, drugs, micro-organisms or autoimmune diseases of which the following four are very common:
    i. Measles (Rubeola)
    ii. Rubella (German measles)
    iii. Erythema infectiosum
    iv. Roseola infantum
- *Urticaria*: Transient lesion composed of central wheal surrounded by erythematous halo or flare, often pleuritic. For example, exposure to drugs, allergen, and pollen grain.
- *Purpura* **(Fig. 5.51)**: Extravasation of red blood cells into dermis and as a result the lesion does not blanch with pressure:
    - Petechia means lesion less than 2 mm.
    - Purpura means lesion 3–10 mm.
    - Ecchymosis means lesion above 10 mm.
- *Nonpalpable*:
    - Trauma
    - Solar purpura
    - Steroid purpura
    - Clotting disorder (thrombocytopenia and clotting factor deficiency)
    - Vascular fragility (amyloidosis and serum)
    - Disseminated intravascular coagulation—warfarin and heparin induced

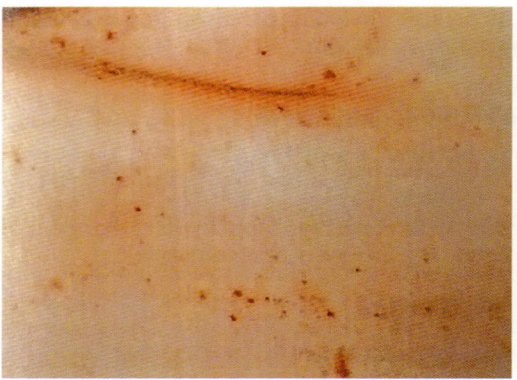

FIG. 5.51: Nonpalpable purpura.

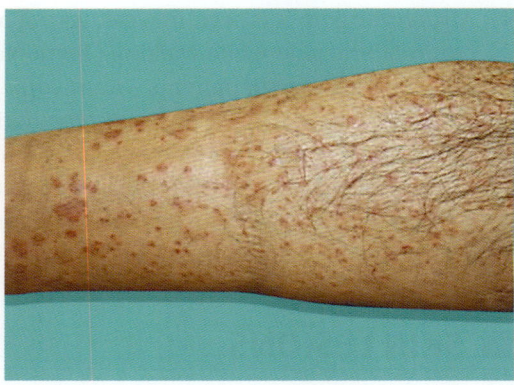

FIG. 5.52: Palpable purpura.

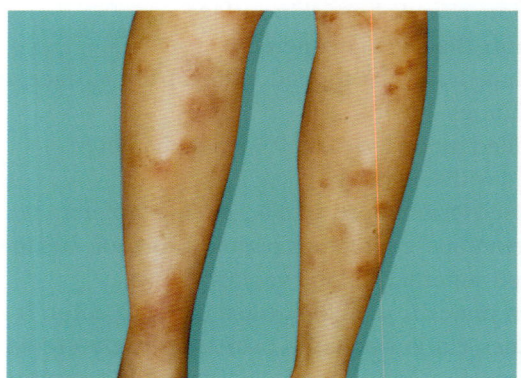

FIG. 5.53: Erythema nodosum appearing on lower limb around ankle and over shin.

- *Palpable (Fig. 5.52)*:
  ○ Vasculitis—polyarteritis nodosa (PAN)
  ○ *Embolic*:
    - Acute meningococcemia
    - Disseminated gonococcal infection

Erythema Nodosum

Features

- Site—usually lower limb around ankle and over shin **(Fig. 5.53)**
- Color—red to purple
- Shape—multiple, nodular, variable in size and shape, 2–6 cm in diameter
- Tender

Differential Diagnosis

- Drug rash
- Erythema multiforme

- Purpura
- Cellulitis
- Vasculitis [systemic lupus erythematosus (SLE) and PAN].

Pathogenesis

It is panniculitis (inflammation of subcutaneous fat), with infiltration of lymphocytes, histiocytes, giant cells, and immune complex deposition).

They are nonsuppurative, painful palpable nodular lesion in skin. Nodules are 2–6 cm in diameter, occur in crops over 2–3 weeks, resolve spontaneously, and leave a bluish stain in skin. They never ulcerate but may relapse.

Causes

- Idiopathic
- Tuberculosis
- Sarcoidosis
- Drugs—OCP, penicillin, salicylates, sulfonamide, etc.
- IBD (ulcerative colitis and Crohn's disease)
- Leprosy
- Protozoa (toxoplasmosis)
- Fungal (histoplasmosis).

■ PIGMENTATION

- Melanin
- Carotene
- Bilirubin
- Iron

Melanin

- Skin color is influenced by deposition of melanin.
- There are two types:
    i. Hypopigmentation
    ii. Hyperpigmentation

Hypopigmentation:
- *Albinism*: It is an inherited disorder having no melanin in skin.
- *Vitiligo*: It is bilateral symmetrical depigmentation, causes irregular patches over skin, more common on skin, neck, and extensor surface of limb. Often it is associated with autoimmune disorder **(Fig. 5.54)**.

Hyperpigmentation **(Fig. 5.55)**:
- Overproduction of melanin—situation such as excess melanotrophic secretion (Addison's disease and Nelson's syndrome)
- Pituitary overproduction causes pigmentation of skin particularly skin creases, bony prominences, buccal cavity, and lips.

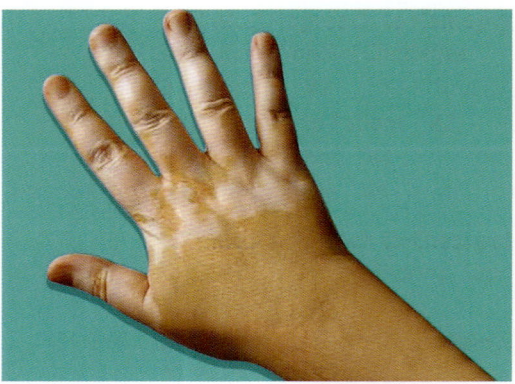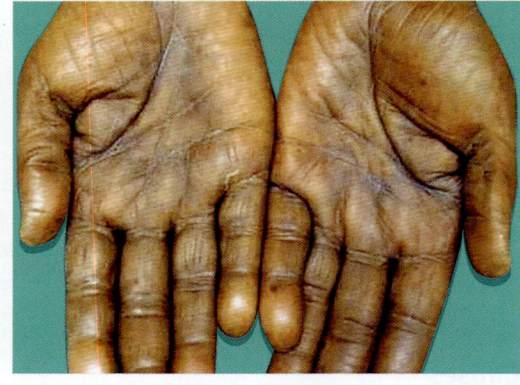

FIG. 5.54: Vitiligo.   **FIG. 5.55:** Hyperpigmentation.

- Melanoma—malignant condition of melanocytes
- Pregnancy and OCP use—may produce blotchy pigmentation on face, called chloasma.

Carotene

Hypercarotenemia:
- Causes yellowish discoloration of face, hands, feet but not sclera (distinguish from jaundice)
- Can occur after large intake of carrots and tomatoes

Bilirubin

Jaundice is detectable when serum bilirubin concentration is above 2–2.5 mg/dL. Sclerae, mucous membrane, and skin become yellow. In long-standing case, it turns to be yellowish green due to deposition of biliverdin.

Iron

Hemochromatosis: Iron deposition in skin causes stimulation of melanocytes and causes skin pigmentation.

Hemosiderin: It is an Hb breakdown product deposited in skin, due to extravasation of blood. It is found in chronic venous insufficiency.

GENERALIZED LYMPHADENOPATHY

Definition

Three or more anatomically noncontiguous areas of lymph node involvement. Areas commonly examined are:
- Cervical region
- Axillary region

- Inguinal region
- Para-aortic (in thin built person)
- Epitrochlear lymph nodes

Examination

The following points are to be mentioned during examination of a lymph node:
- Site
- Number
- Size and shape
- Tenderness
- Temperature
- Consistency
- Adhesion to surrounding structures
- Overlying skin condition and presence of sinus, ulcer, etc. **(Fig. 5.56)**

Different Patterns of Lymphadenitis

Patterns of lymph adenitis have been shown in **Table 5.8**.

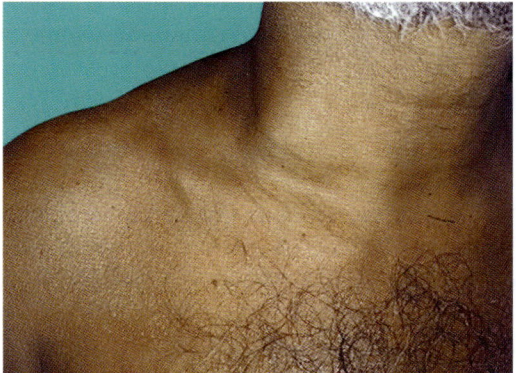

FIG. 5.56: Examination of a lymph node.

Table 5.8: Patterns of lymphadenitis.	
Pattern	**Significance**
Soft, cystic	Cold abscess
Stony hard	Calcified lymph node
Firm matted	Tuberculosis
Hard lymph node	Malignancy
Rubbery	Lymphoma
Tender and soft	Acute infection of both lymph nodes and surrounding tissues
Lymph nodes with goiter	Papillary carcinoma
Hard, immobile, and fixed to tissue	Malignancy

Causes

Following are the common causes of generalized lymphadenopathy:
- *Infection*:
  - Viral: Epstein-Barr virus, cytomegalovirus, HIV, and rubella
  - Bacterial: Disseminated tuberculosis, brucellosis, chlamydial lymphogranuloma venereum, and trachoma
  - Fungal: Histoplasmosis and coccidioidomycosis
  - Parasitic: Toxoplasmosis and filariasis
- Lymphoma
- Acute lymphocytic leukemia (ALL)
- Infectious mononucleosis
- Sarcoidosis
- Primary HIV syndromes
- Drugs such as phenytoin
- *Endocrine*: Hyperthyroidism
- *Neoplastic*: Secondaries from different primaries
- *Immunological*:
  - SLE
  - Juvenile rheumatoid arthritis (JRA)

Following are the common causes of generalized lymphadenopathy with fever:
- Lymphoma
- ALL and chronic lymphocytic leukemia
- Viral infection
- Sarcoidosis
- Disseminated tuberculosis
- Brucellosis

Following are the common causes of generalized lymphadenopathy with arthritis:
- JRA
- SLE
- Sarcoidosis
- Brucellosis
- Primary HIV syndrome

Following are the common causes of generalized lymphadenopathy with splenomegaly:
- Lymphoma
- Leukemia
- Sarcoidosis
- HIV
- Disseminated tuberculosis

Following are the common causes of generalized lymphadenopathy with matting or sinus:
- Tuberculosis
- Actinomycosis

Points to Remember

- Submandibular lymph node less than 1 cm normal in childhood
- Axillary lymph node less than 1.5 cm is normal.
- Inguinal lymph node less than 2 cm is normal in adult.
- Lymph node less than 1 cm suggests benign cause and more than 2.5 cm suggests malignant or granulomatous cause.
- Reactive lymph nodes are soft tender, expand quickly, and subside spontaneously.
- Epitrochlear, supraclavicular, and scalene lymph nodes are always pathological.
- If only left supraclavicular lymph node is enlarged, which is also known as *Troisier's sign*, it is possibly metastasis from carcinoma of stomach.
- *Epitrochlear lymphadenopathy is seen in*:
  - Lymphoma (non-Hodgkin's lymphoma)
  - Secondary syphilis
  - Sarcoidosis
  - Infection in hand or arm
- *Scalene lymphadenopathy is seen in*:
  - Lymphoma
  - Sarcoidosis
  - Tuberculosis
  - Metastasis from bronchogenic carcinoma
- *Unilateral axillary lymphadenopathy*:
  - Localized infection in upper extremity
  - Breast carcinoma
  - Lymphoma (non-Hodgkin's lymphoma)
  - Brucellosis.
- *Oblique shape (long axis > short axis)—usually benign*
  - Rounded (long axis < short axis)—chance of malignancy more

■ ANTHROPOMETRY

- Observe any abnormality in posture such as scoliosis and kyphosis.
- Measure height using vertical scale.
- Patient should stand erect on weight machine without shoes and wearing indoor garments only.
- Measure the waist by a measuring tape in between costal margin and iliac crest and take maximum distance.
- Measure arm span.

Weight

Weight is an important indicator of health status. Serial weight records have more significance.
- Calculate actual and ideal weight for age and sex.
- Calculate body mass index (BMI).

Weight Loss (Table 5.10)

- *Intentional weight loss*: Loss of total body mass as a result of effort to improve fitness and health
- *Unintentional weight loss*: Loss of body fat, fluids, muscle atrophy or combination of all these, due to medical problem. More than 5% weight loss in 6–12 months is significant. It may be due to the following reasons:
  - Malignancy
  - Chronic inflammation or infectious disease
  - Metabolic disorders (hyperthyroidism and diabetes mellitus)
  - Psychiatric illness

Weight Gain (Box 5.2)

- *Obesity*: It is a medical condition characterized by excessive accumulation and storage of fat in the body.

Table 5.9: Body mass index calculation.

BMI	Significance
<18.5	Underweight
18.5–24.99	Normal
25.0–29.99	Overweight
30.0–39.9	Obese
>40	Morbid obesity

Table 5.10: Weight loss.

Sarcopenia	Loss of muscle mass
Cachexia	Loss of weight, loss of muscle, and adipose tissue presenting with anorexia and weakness
Weight loss with anorexia	Seen in chronic infective or inflammatory illness
Weight loss with increased appetite	Seen in thyrotoxicosis and diabetes mellitus
Malnutrition	Undernutrition or overnutrition

BOX 5.2 | Weight gain.

- Increase in body weight due to increase in muscle mass, fat, fluids, and other factors
- Fluid—heart failure, nephrotic syndrome, and chronic liver disease
- Hormonal—Cushing's syndrome and hypothyroidism
- Drugs—OCP, steroids, beta blockers, etc.
- Psychiatric illness—depression

- *Causes*:
  - Increased food intake
  - Decreased exercise
  - Pathological conditions such as:
    - Hypothyroidism
    - Cushing's syndrome
    - Hypertension
    - Sleep apnea
    - Hyperlipidemia

Waist Circumference

- As per the World Health Organization (WHO) protocol, waist circumference should be measured at the midpoint between last palpable rib and highest point of iliac crest at mid-axillary line parallel to floor, after few breaths.
- Hip at the widest portion of buttock **(Fig. 5.57)**
- *Waist circumference cut of point*: Less than 94 cm (male) and less than 80 cm (female)
- *Waist-hip ratio*: Less than 0.9 (male) and less than 0.85 (female)
- Higher value increases cardiovascular (CV) risk and metabolic complications.

Arm Span

- *Measure height*: Crown to ground, person is erect, looking straight.
- *Measure arm span*: It is the distance between tips of outstretched middle fingers of both hands.
- Measure crown to symphysis pubis and from symphysis pubis to ground.
- *Age <5 years*: Arm span 1–2 cm smaller than body length
- *10–12 years*: Arm span = height
- *Adult*: Arm span >2 cm
- *Abnormal long arm span*:
  - Marfan syndrome
  - Klinefelter syndrome

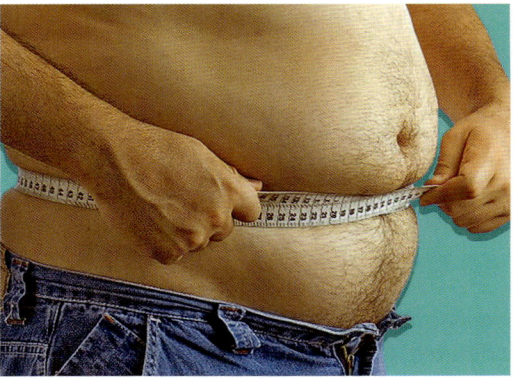

FIG. 5.57: Waist circumference.

- *Abnormal short arm span*:
  - Cretinism
  - Achondroplasia

Height

Measurement: Height is measured using a vertical scale and a rigid, adjustable arm-piece. In serial assessment of growth in children and adolescents, height is measured in nearest millimeter using a calibrated stadiometer.

Causes of loss of height in elderly:
- Collapse vertebrae due to osteoporosis
- Kyphosis.

Short stature: An adult height that is more than two standard deviations below the mean for age and gender.
- *Proportionate short stature*:
  - Familial
  - Chronic illness
  - Malnutrition
  - Chromosomal abnormality
  - Endocrine abnormality
  - Metabolic abnormality
- *Disproportionate short stature*:
  - *Short limb short stature*:
    - Achondroplasia
    - Hypochondroplasia
  - *Short trunk short stature*:
    - Mucopolysaccharidosis
    - Spondyloepiphyseal dysplasia

Long stature: Height beyond 97th percentile (over two standard deviations) of mean for age and sex. Causes may be:
- Marfan syndrome
- Hypogonadism
- Pituitary gigantism
- Familial

■ NUTRITION

Nutritional Assessment

Clinical

- *Body mass index (Quetelet's index)*:
  - Definition: BMI is defined as body weight (kg) divided by square of height (meter).
- *Weight*: Current weight, ideal weight calculation, and weight gain or loss

- *Dietary history*: 24-hour recall method/last 7 days, better than 24 days recall
- Underlying comorbidities
- Gastrointestinal function
- *General appearance*: Anemia, edema, puffiness of face, periorbital edema, skin changes, dry mucous membrane, petechiae, ecchymoses, glossitis, and angular stomatitis
- Atrophy and hypertrophy of muscles
- Loss of subcutaneous fat
- Oral ulcers and peripheral neuropathy

Triceps Skinfold Thickness

- Measured on posterior upper arm midway between the acromion and olecranon process
- Less than 3 mm—severe depletion of fat
- 8–10 mm—borderline fat store
- More than 10 mm—normal.

Method

Lift the fold placing the thumb and index finger around 3" apart. Fold is lifted 1 cm above the site to be measured. Caliper is to be placed 1 cm below the fingers and measured **(Fig. 5.58)**.

Mid-arm Circumference

- Measured by plastic tape between acromion and olecranon process of the nondominant arm **(Fig. 5.59)**
- MAC less than 12.5 cm—severe malnutrition
- 12.5–13.5 cm—moderate malnutrition
- More than 15 cm—normal

Nutritional Risk Index

- Nutritional risk index (NRI) = (1.489 × serum albumin g/L) + 41.7 (present weight/normal weight)

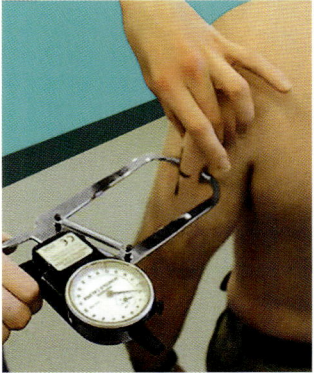

FIG. 5.58: Triceps skinfold thickness.

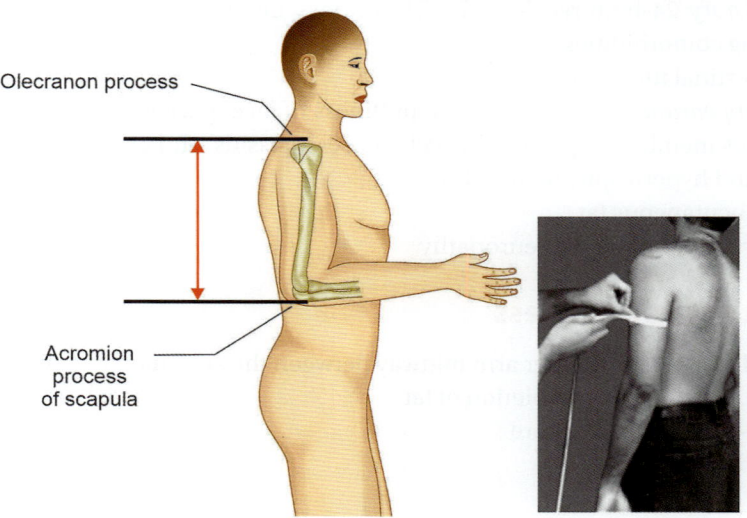

FIG. 5.59: Mid-arm circumference, measurement.

- NRI more than 100—normal
- 97.5–100—mild malnourishment
- 83.5–97.5—moderate malnourishment
- Less than 83.5—severe malnourishment

Laboratory Findings

- *Albumin*: It usually indicates liver, renal disease, or nutritional deficiency. Having long half-life cannot predict short-term nutritional deficiency.
- *Prealbumin*: It is produced by liver, released in blood, and carries certain hormones.
    - Half-life 2 days, much shorter than albumin
    - Sensitive marker in assessment of protein-energy malnutrition particularly short- term basis, before and after surgery, after critical illness, etc.
- Ferritin
- Transferrin
- Hemoglobin
- Cholesterol

Calculation of BMR/Calorie (Mifflin—St Jeor Equation)

- Basal metabolic rate (BMR) = 10 × weight (kg) + 6.25 × height (cm) – 5 × age (years) + 5 for Male
- 10 × weight (kg) + 6.25 × height (cm) – 5 × age (years) – 161 for female

Calorie calculation:
- *Sedentary*: BMR + 20%
- *Moderate work*: BMR + 30%
- *Heavy work*: BMR + 40%

CHAPTER 5: General Examination

Table 5.11: Water-soluble vitamins.	
Vitamins	**Deficiencies**
Vitamin B1 (thiamine)	Wernicke–Korsakoff syndrome and beriberi
Vitamin B2 (riboflavin)	Glossitis and angular stomatitis
Vitamin B3 (niacin)	Pellagra
Vitamin B6 (pyridoxine)	Polyneuropathy
Vitamin B7 (biotin)	Dermatitis and alopecia
Vitamin B9 (folic acid)	Megaloblastic anemia
Vitamin B12 (cobalamin)	Megaloblastic anemia and peripheral neuropathy
Vitamin C	Scurvy, gum bleeding, and easy bruising

Table 5.12: Fat-soluble vitamins.	
Vitamins	**Deficiencies**
Vitamin A	Night blindness and keratomalacia
Vitamin D	Rickets and osteomalacia
Vitamin E	Hemolytic anemia, skin disorder, and fertility problems
Vitamin K	Bleeding disorder

Vitamin Deficiency

Both fat-soluble and water-soluble vitamins are listed in **Tables 5.11 and 5.12**.

DIFFERENT TYPE OF NAILS IN CLINICAL MEDICINE

Koilonychia

It is due to thinning and softening of the nail plate, resulting in spoon-shaped nail.

Causes

- Iron deficiency anemia
- Hemochromatosis
- Raynaud's syndrome
- Porphyria
- Occupational
  - Motor mechanics
  - Rickshaw pullers
- Ischemic heart disease
- Syphilis
- Inherited—autosomal dominant

Beau's Line

They are transverse ridges in the nail plate due to temporary alteration of nail growth rate.

Causes

- Acute febrile illness
- Pneumonia
- Exanthemas—measles and mumps
- Myocardial infarction and pulmonary infarction
- Childbirth
- Drug reaction

Plummer Nail

Onycholysis of the nail (rat-bitten nail).

Causes

- Hypothyroidism and hyperthyroidism
- Raynaud's disease
- Porphyria
- Photo-onycholysis—doxycycline, chlortetracycline, and chloramphenicol

Lindsay Nail

It is characterized by proximal dull white portion and a distal pink or brown portion with a well-demarcated transverse line of separation.

Causes

It causes uremia.

White Nail

It is characterized by white color in the nail bed than the nail plate.

Causes

- Anemia
- Hypoalbuminemia (cirrhosis and nephrosis)
- Diabetes mellitus
- Congestive cardiac failure
- Rheumatoid arthritis
- Malignancy

Red Nail

It causes congestive cardiac failure.

Blue Nail

- Wilson's disease (copper deposits)
- Silver deposits

Black Nail

- Peutz–Jeghers syndrome
- Cushing's syndrome
- Addison's disease

Yellow Nail Syndrome

It is characterized by yellow finger and toe nails, clubbing and onycholysis. The other associated features are:
- Edema of finger, ankle, and face
- Infection—sinusitis, bronchitis, bronchiectasis, and pleural effusion
- Carcinoma of skin, larynx, and endometrium
- Lymphoma
- Agammaglobulinemia
- Psoriasis

Pitting over Nail

- Indentation over nail
- Seen in psoriasis and lichen planus

Onycholysis

Premature life time of nails

Leukonychia

- White discoloration of nails
- Seen in low albumin

Mees' Line

- Solitary transverse line
- Seen in arsenic poisoning

Paronychia

Infection adjacent to nail.

Onychomycosis

Fungal nail infection.

Blue-red Discoloration of Nail

Polycythemia.

Cherry-red Discoloration of Nail

Carbon monoxide poisoning.

Terry Nail

Distal half brown red and proximal half white pink [CLD, chronic kidney disease (CKD), and malnutrition).

■ EXAMINATION OF EYES

Eye

- *Exophthalmos*: Thyrotoxicosis, Graves' disease, alcoholism, and orbital malignancies **(Fig. 5.60)**.
- *Enophthalmos*: Horner's syndrome
- *Periorbital edema*: Renal disease and hypoproteinemia
- *Xanthelasma*: Hyperlipidemia **(Fig. 5.61)**
- *Ptosis* **(Fig. 5.62)**:
  - Congenital
  - Acquired:
    - Neurogenic:
      » Third nerve palsy
      » Horner's syndrome

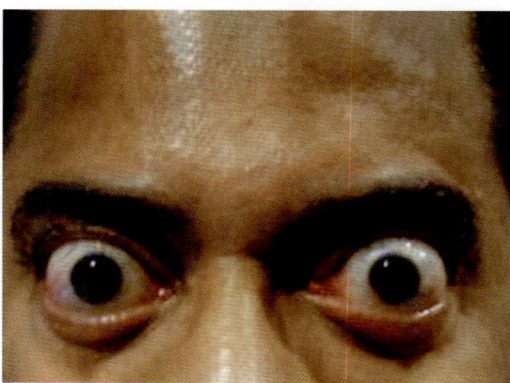

FIG. 5.60: Exophthalmos.

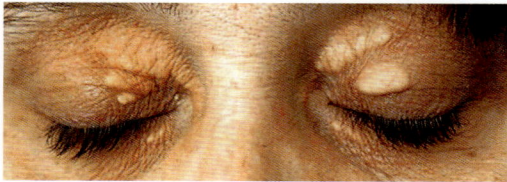

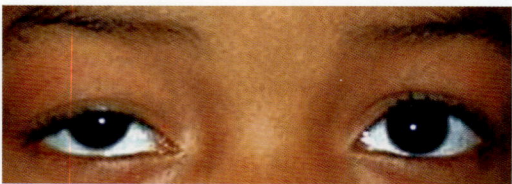

FIG. 5.61: Xanthelasma.

FIG. 5.62: Ptosis.

- » Ophthalmoplegic migraine
  - » Multiple sclerosis
  - *Myogenic*:
    - » Myasthenia gravis
    - » Ocular myopathy
    - » Oculopharyngeal muscular dystrophy
- *Dislocation of lens*: Marfan's syndrome and Ehlers–Danlos syndrome
- *Squint*: Definition—a malalignment of visual axes of the two eyes is called squint or strabismus.
  - *Paralytic squint*: Ocular deviation resulting from complete or incomplete paralysis of one or more extraocular muscles, acquired defect, diplopia present, and increase in direction of weak muscle.

    Causes: Neurogenic lesions (congenital absence of third/sixth cranial nerve nuclei, inflammatory lesions such as encephalitis, meningitis, neurosyphilis, peripheral neuritis, neoplastic lesions, vascular lesions, trauma, and demyelination)

    Myogenic lesions (congenital absence or hypoplasia of extraocular muscles, trauma, and myopathy)

    Neuromuscular junction lesions (myasthenia gravis)
  - *Nonparalytic squint (concomitant)*: Defective binocular vision, present from childhood, squint present in all direction, and no diplopia

Nystagmus

Definition
Regular and rhythmic to and fro involuntary oscillatory movements of the eyes.

Causes
- Physiological
- Congenital (ocular albinism, aniridia, Leber's congenital amaurosis, etc.)
- *Acquired*:
  - *Vertical*:
    - Upbeat—lesions of central tegmentum of brainstem
    - Downbeat—Cerebellar lesions, Arnold–Chiari malformation
  - *Horizontal*: Gaze evoked—CNS depressants such as alcohol, anticonvulsants, barbiturates, neurological lesions of brainstem, and posterior fossa
  - *Periodic alternating nystagmus*: Demyelination and vestibule-cerebellar disease
  - *Peripheral vestibular nystagmus*: Labyrinthitis, vestibular neuritis, etc.
  - *See saw nystagmus*: Upper brainstem lesion
  - *Ataxic nystagmus*: Disseminated sclerosis

Conjunctiva

- *Pallor*: Anemia, shock, heart failure, and hypopituitarism
- *Plethoric*: Polycythemia and SVC syndrome

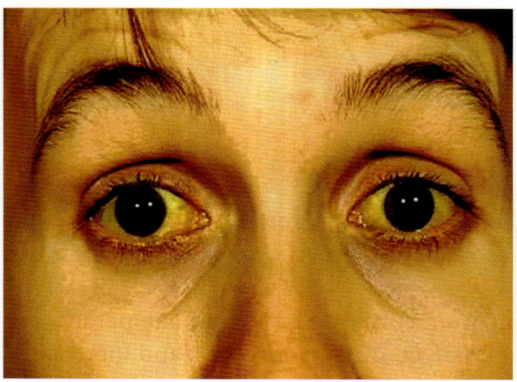

FIG. 5.63: Jaundice.

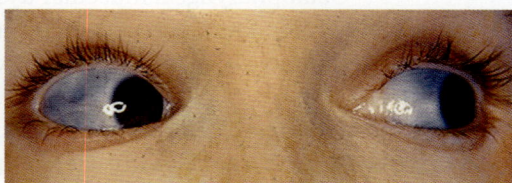

FIG. 5.64: Osteogenesis imperfecta.

- *Hemorrhage*: Bleeding diathesis, leptospira, viral hemorrhagic fever, trauma, and hypertension

Sclera

- *Yellow*: Jaundice **(Fig. 5.63)**
- *Blue*: Osteogenesis imperfecta **(Fig. 5.64)**
- *Red eyes*: Calcium deposition in sclera in CKD
- *Scleritis*: Dark, tender, white patches in sclera usually caused by infection and vasculitis

Lens

Cataract

- *Peripheral cortical cataract*: Incomplete black spikes from peripheries, e.g., diabetic cataract
- *Posterior subcapsular cataract*: Block-like opacities coming from center, e.g., steroid use
- *Nuclear cataract*: Aging cataract

Iris

Iritis—tuberculosis and sarcoidosis.

Pupil

- Size and symmetry (physiological and pathological anisocoria)
- *Hutchinson's pupil*: Raised intracranial tension
- *Constricted pupil (miosis)* **(Fig. 5.65)**:
  ○ *Causes*:
    – Drugs—parasympathomimetics
    – Poisoning—morphine, organophosphorus, phenol, and chloral hydrate

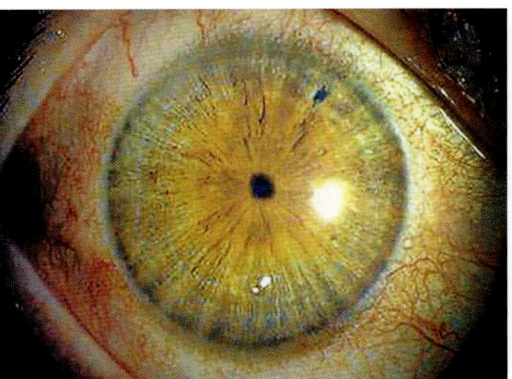

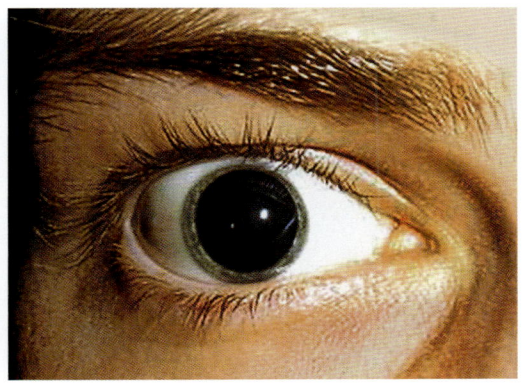

FIG. 5.65: Constricted pupil.

FIG. 5.66: Dilated pupil.

- Pontine hemorrhage
- Horner's syndrome
- Iridocyclitis
- *Dilated pupil (mydriasis)* **(Fig. 5.66)**:
  - *Causes*:
    - Drugs—sympathomimetics and parasympatholytics (atropine)
    - Acute congestive glaucoma
    - Third nerve palsy
    - Belladonna poisoning
    - Internal ophthalmoplegia
- *Argyll Robertson pupil*: Pupil is small in size, accommodation reflex is present, but light reflex is absent, e.g., neurosyphilis.
- *Adie's tonic pupil*: Reaction to light is absent, and accommodation reflex is slow and tonic. Affected pupil is larger, usually caused by postganglionic parasympathetic pupillomotor damage.
- *Marcus Gunn pupil*: Paradoxical dilatation of pupil in response to light, e.g., relative afferent pathway defect.

Cornea

- *Corneal arcus*: Hyperlipidemia and CKD **(Fig. 5.67)**
- *Corneal scar*: Postinfection and trauma
- *KF ring*: Wilson's disease (copper deposition around cornea) **(Fig. 5.68)**

Retina

- Retinal hemorrhage **(Fig. 5.69)**
- Tubercle
- Papilledema
- Disk atrophy

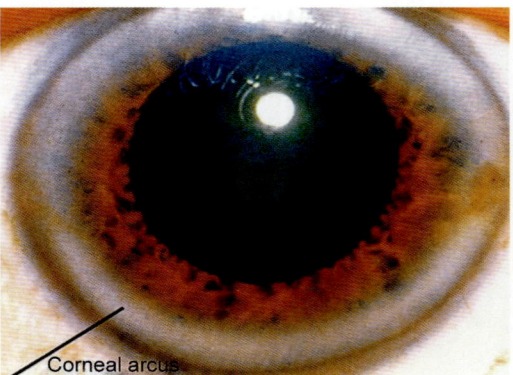

FIG. 5.67: Corneal arcus.

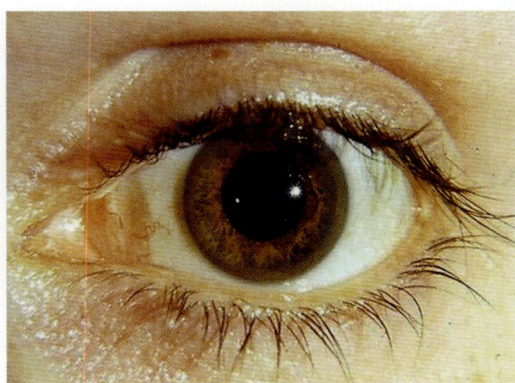

FIG. 5.68: Kayser–Fleischer (KF) ring.

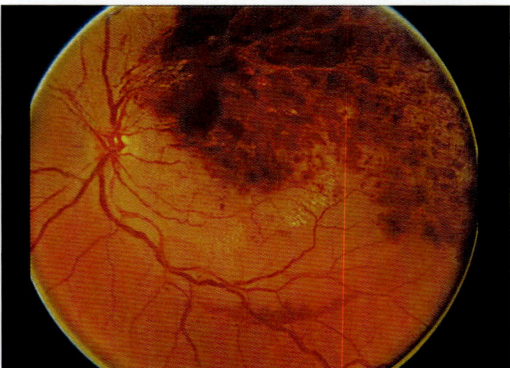

FIG. 5.69: Retinal hemorrhage.

■ FACE EXAMINATION

Facies

Congenital
- *Elfin facies*: Flat face, broad forehead, hypertelorism, short nose, low set ears, wide mouth, and hypoplastic teeth **(Fig. 5.70)**. For example, William's syndrome, mental retardation, and supravalvular AS.
- *Potter's facies*: Prominent epicanthic fold, hypertelorism, and low set ears. For example, Potter's syndrome (pulmonary hypoplasia and renal agenesis).
- *Down syndrome*: Prominent epicanthic fold, small ears, short stature, single palmar crease, VSD, and mental retardation **(Fig. 5.71)**.

Neurologic Facies

Parkinson's disease: Masked facies, immobile, fixed, and expressionless face with infrequent blinking of the eyes. Normal rate of blinking is about 20/minute. In Parkinsonism, the rate

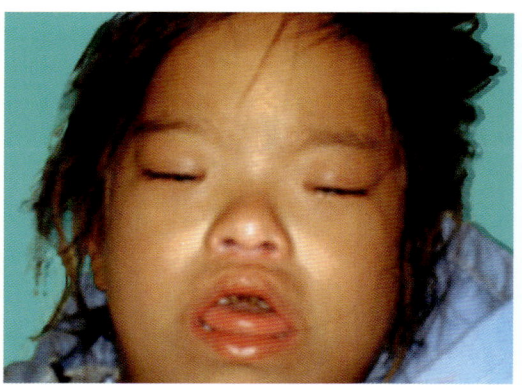

FIG. 5.70: Elfin facies.

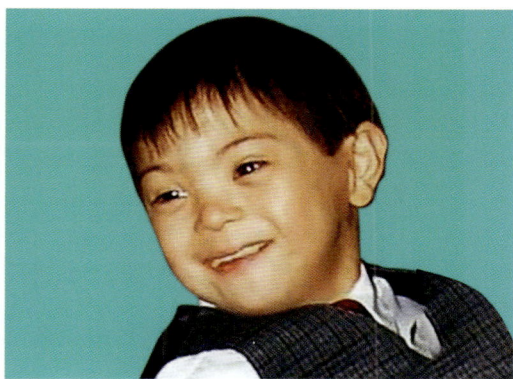

FIG. 5.71: Down's facies.

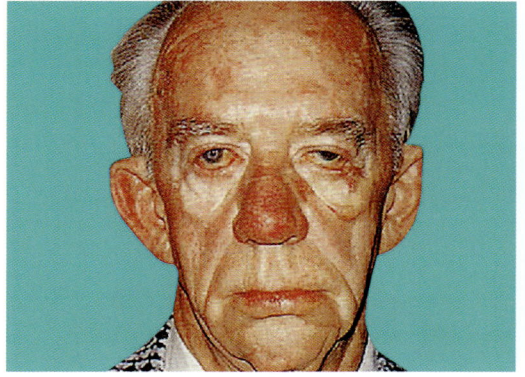

FIG. 5.72: Masked facies.

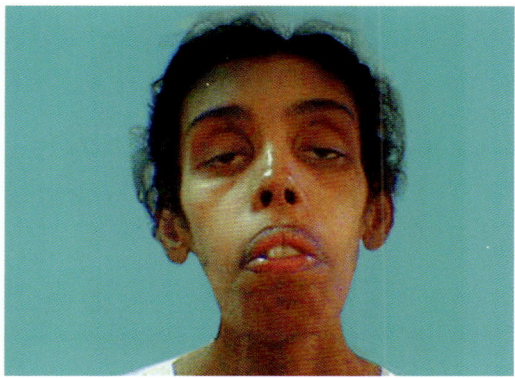

FIG. 5.73: Hatchet facies.

of blinking is reduced to <10/min. On closing the eyes, fluttering of the eyelids is seen (blepharoclonus). In postencephalitic parkinsonism, oculogyric crisis (tonic upward deviation of the eyes) may be seen. A jaw tremor may also be seen **(Fig. 5.72)**.

Myotonic Facies

Hatchet facies: Hollowing of temples and jaws, eyes are hooded, lower lip droops, global weakness of face leads to sagging of lower face, accompanied by wasting of neck muscles giving a swan neck appearance **(Fig. 5.73)**.

Myasthenic Facies

Snarling facies (sagging of corner of face, drooping of eyelids, and weakness of facial muscles) **(Fig. 5.74)**.

Cardiovascular Facies

- *Aortic facies*: Pale and shallow face
- *Mitral facies*: Acrocyanotic face (rosy cheeks, while rest of the face has bluish tinge)
- *Marfanoid facies*: Long face, long thin nose, and hypotelorism **(Fig. 5.75)**

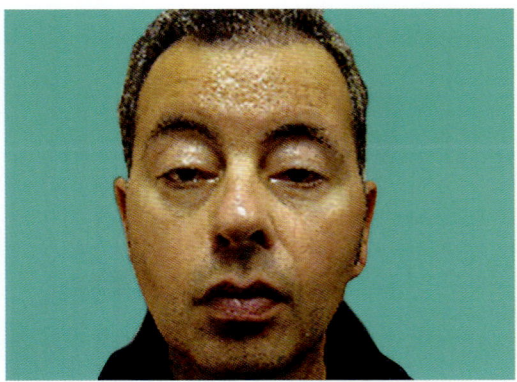

FIG. 5.74: Myotonic facies.

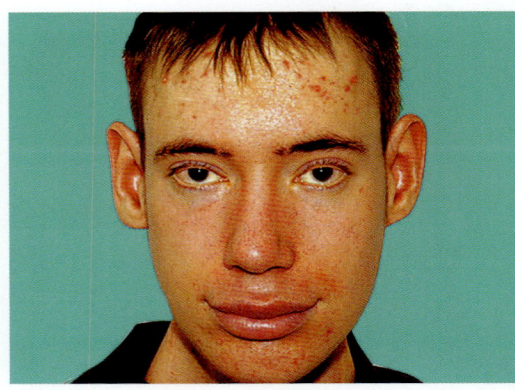

FIG. 5.75: Marfanoid facies.

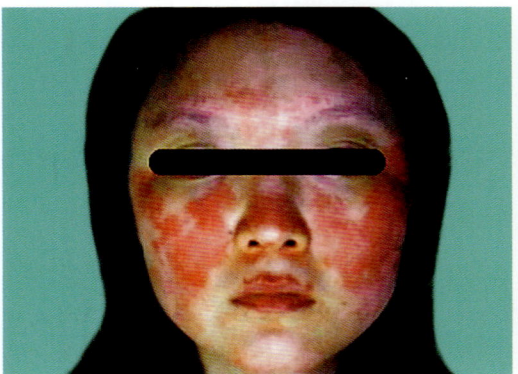

FIG. 5.76: Butterfly rash over cheeks.

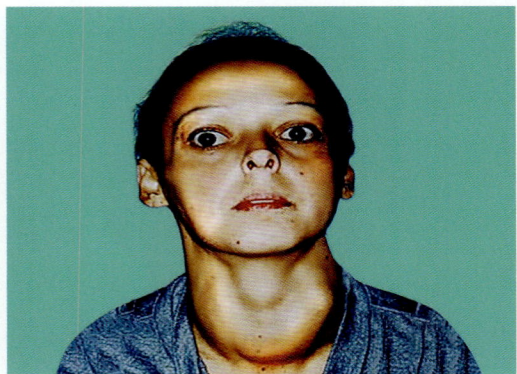

FIG. 5.77: Graves' facies.

Rheumatologic Facies

- *Systemic lupus erythematosus*: Butterfly rash over cheeks **(Fig. 5.76)**
- *Scleroderma*: Tight skin, loss of wrinkle, sharp nose, and tight mouth opening
- *Face in Sjögren's syndrome*: There is enlargement of the lacrimal gland on both sides along with enlargement of the parotid and submandibular glands on both sides.

Endocrine or Metabolic Facies

- *Renal facies*: Puffiness of face, periorbital edema, and coarse hair (mouse facies)
- *Graves' facies*: Anxious look, exophthalmos, and lid lag **(Fig. 5.77)**
- *Acromegaly*: Coarse face, prominent mandible, large nose, and lips (gorilla-like facies) **(Fig. 5.78)**
- *Cushing facies*: Moon facies, increased hair, plethora, and acne **(Fig. 5.79)**
- *Myxedematous facies*: Puffiness of face, coarse hair, and dry and rough skin (Torpid facies)
- *Cretinism*: Face is pale and has a stupid and dull look. Nose is broad and flattened. Lips are thick and separated by a large and fissured protruding tongue. Hair on eyebrows, eyelashes, and scalp are scanty. The presence of prominent medial epicanthal folds and low set ears **(Fig. 5.80)**.

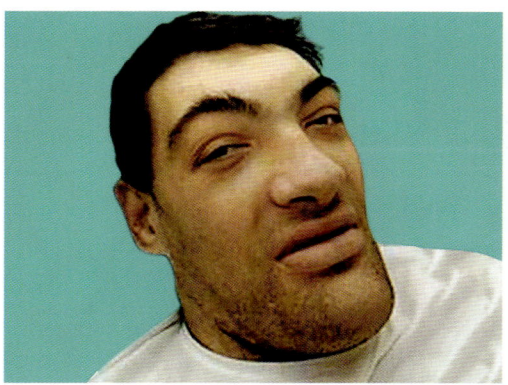

FIG. 5.78: Acromegaly facies.

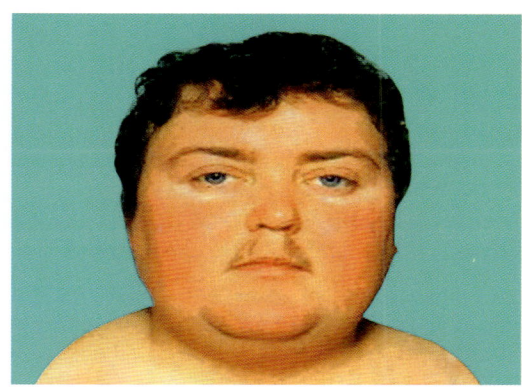

FIG. 5.79: Cushing facies.

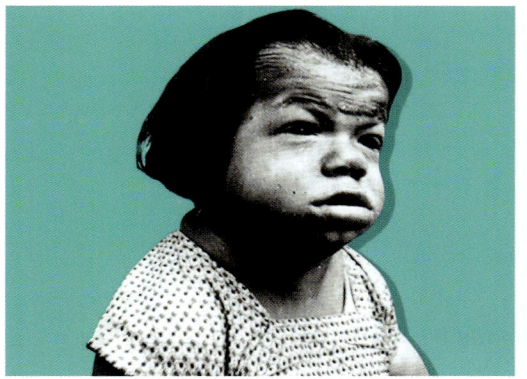

FIG. 5.80: Cretin facies.

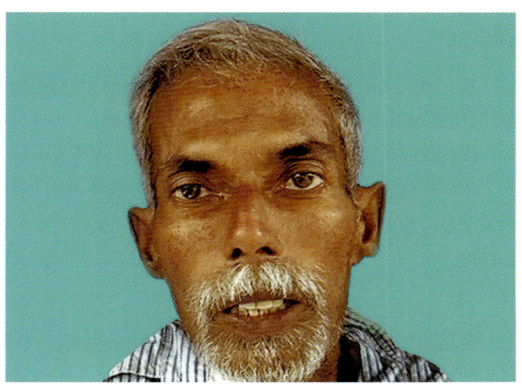

FIG. 5.81: Hepatic facies.

Other Facies

- *Frog facies*: Intranasal tumor
- *Marshall Hall's facies*: Hydrocephalus
- *Lions facies*: Paget's disease
- *Hepatic facies*: Sunken eyes, pinch up noses, temporal hallow, malar prominence, and muddy complexion are found in CLD **(Fig. 5.81)**.
- *Leonine facies*: In lepromatous leprosy, thickening of the skin and ear lobes with a flattened nasal bridge and loss of hair over the lateral aspect of eyebrows and eyelashes (madarosis) can be seen.
- *Thalassemic facies*: Frontal bossing, depressed nasal bridge, zygomatic prominence, and malocclusion of teeth **(Fig. 5.82)**
- *Raccoon eyes*: Bruising around eyes found in amyloidosis or head injury
- *Face in pneumonia*: In lobar pneumonia, the alae nasi are overactive, eyes are bright and shiny, and herpetic lesions may be present over the angles of the mouth.
- *Face in COPD*: Anxious look with bluish discoloration of lips, tip of the nose, ear lobes, and breathing out through pursed lips
- *Tabetic facies*: Partial ptosis with wrinkling of forehead and unequal, small and irregular pupils

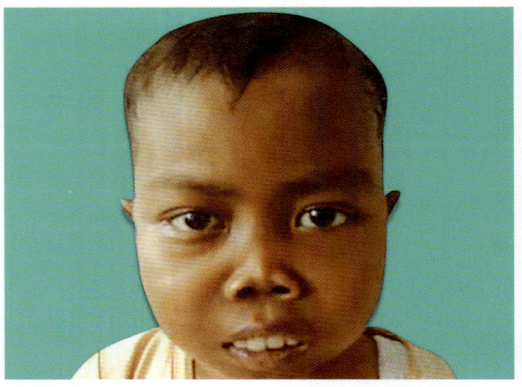

FIG. 5.82: Thalassemic facies.

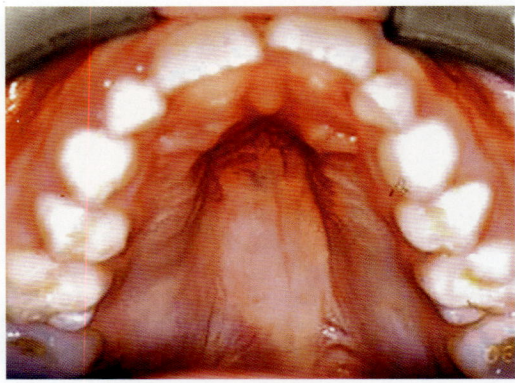

FIG. 5.83: High-arched palate.

Nose

- Saddle-shaped nose—congenital syphilis
- Parrot-beaked nose—scleroderma
- Nasal flare—acute exacerbation of COPD
- Collapsed nasal bridge—Wegner's bridge

Lips

- Cyanosis
- Angular stomatitis (usually caused due to Vitamin B2 deficiency)
- Herpes labialis
- Pigmentation—Peutz–Jeghers syndrome
- Pursed lip breathing—acute exacerbation of COPD

Palate

Hard palate: In healthy person, it is whitish in color, firm texture, and irregular transverse ridges.

Soft palate: Light pink, smooth and movable upwardly, and uvula seen in midline. On uttering "Ah" it moves upward equally.

High-arched palate: The palate is usually high arched and narrow, e.g., Marfan syndrome, Turner syndrome, and Noonan's syndrome **(Fig. 5.83)**.

■ HAND EXAMINATION

Hand

- *Cold extremities*: Peripheral circulatory failure and peripheral vascular disease, e.g., Raynaud's disease **(Fig. 5.84)**
- *Jaundice*

- *Hyperpigmentation* **(Fig. 5.85)**:
  - Causes: Arsenic intoxication and Addison's disease
- *Sweating*: Anxiety and thyrotoxicosis
- *Cherry-red color*: Carbon monoxide (CO) poisoning
- *Palmar erythema*: Alcoholic CLD **(Fig. 5.86)**
- *Dupuytren's contracture* (painless flexion contracture of ring and little fingers due to thickening, fibrosis, and shortening of ulnar side of palmar fascia) **(Fig. 5.87)**.
  - Causes:
    - Trauma
    - Alcoholic cirrhosis
    - Phenytoin therapy
    - Peyronie's disease
    - Idiopathic
- *Simian crease*: Single in Down's syndrome **(Fig. 5.88)**
- *Triple hand*-thickened, velvety texture of hand, and other sign of visceral malignancy
- *Arachnodactyly (long slender fingers)*: Marfan syndrome
- *Polydactyly*: ASD and single atrium

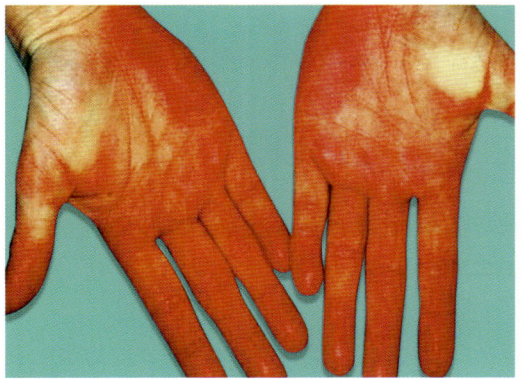

FIG. 5.84: Cold extremities.

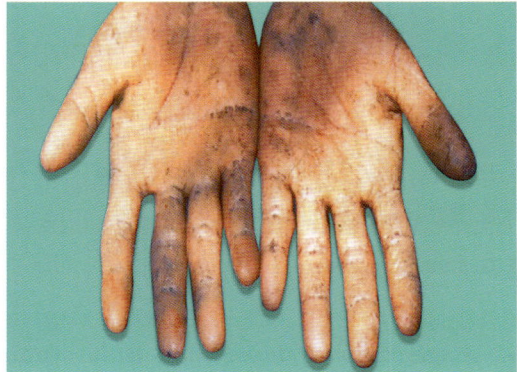

FIG. 5.85: Arsenic hyperpigmentation.

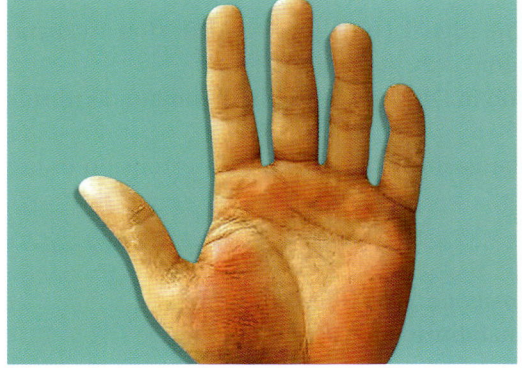

FIG. 5.86: Palmar erythema.

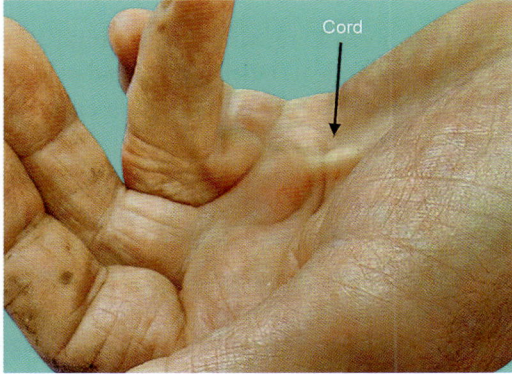

FIG. 5.87: Dupuytren's contracture.

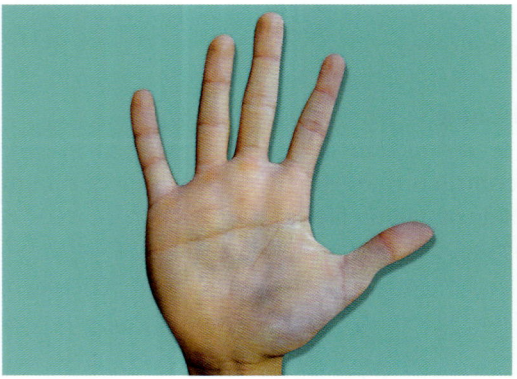

FIG. 5.88: Simian crease.

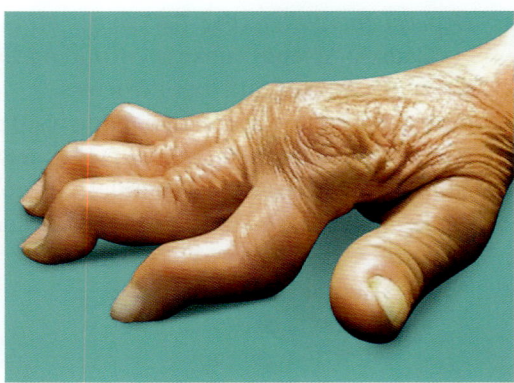

FIG. 5.89: Swan neck.

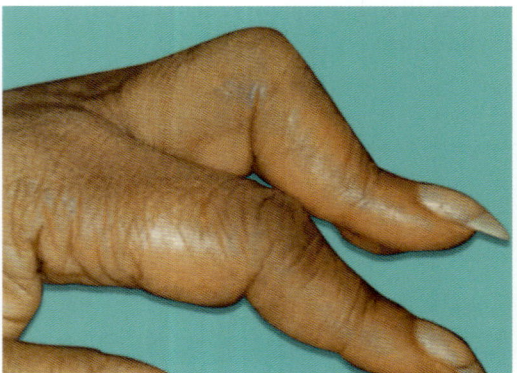

FIG. 5.90: Boutonniere.

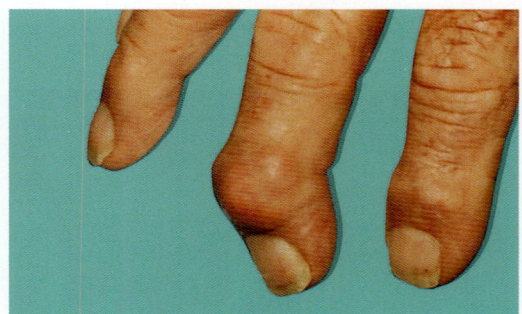

FIG. 5.91: Heberden's node.

- *Fingerization of thumb*: Holt–Oram syndrome
- *Hypermobility of wrist joint*: Ehler–Danlos syndrome

Deformity

- *Swan neck*: Extension in proximal interphalangeal (PIP) joint and flexion in distal interphalangeal (DIP) joint, found in rheumatoid arthritis **(Fig. 5.89)**
- *Boutonniere*: Flexion in PIP joint and extension in DIP joint found in rheumatoid arthritis **(Fig. 5.90)**
- *Z-shaped thumb*: Flexion of metacarpophalangeal (MCP) thumb with extension of the other joint
- *Ulnar deviation*: Rheumatoid arthritis
- *Wrist subluxation*: Rheumatoid arthritis
- *Heberden's node*: Swells at DIP joint. Seen in osteoarthritis **(Fig. 5.91)**.
- *Ape hand*: Median nerve damage leading to inability to oppose thumb
- *Claw hand*: Ulnar nerve damage

- *Movement*: Passive or active movement of joints
  - Active—make a fist:
    - Wrist extension and flexion
    - Flexion, extension at MCP, and IP joints
    - Pincer grip: Thumb and index finger should touch each other.
    - Prayer sign: Patient is instructed to put his hands together as if doing prayer. This test may be used to look for limited joint mobilities of hand.
  - Passive—of all joints
  - Sensorimotor function:
    - Basic purpose is to test sensory and motor function of radial, ulnar, and median nerve along with interossei group of muscles.
    - Loss of sensation in peripheral neuropathy
- *Sensation*: Loss of sensation in peripheral neuropathy
- *Temperature and tenderness*: Inflammation and fracture

Allan's Test

It is a test for arterial flow to hand. Fist both hands, elevate hands, and occlude both radial arteries simultaneously. Now suddenly release pressure over radial artery. Color will change from pale to rubor quickly. If it fails, it indicates an arterial occlusive disease of arm.

Tinel's Sign

- Test for carpal tunnel syndrome
- Tingling sensation over hand after tapping over median nerve

Capillary Refill Time

Press nail bed capillary and release. Normal change of color from pale to rubor is less than 3 seconds. If more than 5 seconds, it indicates dehydration and decreased peripheral perfusion.

Hand Examination in Different Systemic Diseases

Gastrointestinal System

- *Palmar erythema*: Thenar or hypothenar eminences in CLD
- *Dupuytren's contracture*: Thickening and fibrous contracture of palmar fascia, especially on fourth and fifth metacarpals. It can lead to fixed deformity from fifth to third finger in CLD, alcoholic person.
- Pallor
- Clubbing
- *Hepatic flap*:
  - Hand dorsiflexion at wrist
  - Fingers outstretched and separated
  - Hold 15 seconds
  - Jerky intermittent movement at wrist and MCP joints.

Cardiovascular System

- Temperature
- Sweating
- Nail
- Clubbing
- Janeway lesion [(nontender maculopapular lesions in thenar eminence in subacute bacterial endocarditis (SBE)] **(Fig. 5.92)**
- Cyanosis
- Osler's node (tender papule in pulp of fingers, e.g., SBE) **(Figs. 5.93A and B)**
- Splinter hemorrhages (linear longitudinal hemorrhages under nail, e.g., SBE, trauma, scurvy, and psoriasis) **(Fig. 5.94)**
- *Thumb sign (in Marfan's syndrome)*: If the patient clenches fingers around flexed thumb, normally thumb should not cross ulnar side. In Marfan's syndrome, the thumb crosses ulnar side.
- *Wrist sign (in Marfan's syndrome)*: Normally wrist cannot be encircled by thumb and little finger. In case of Marfan's syndrome, it can be done very easily **(Fig. 5.95)**.
- Xanthomata: Raised yellow lesion caused by build-up lipids beneath skin at extensor tendon **(Fig. 5.96)**

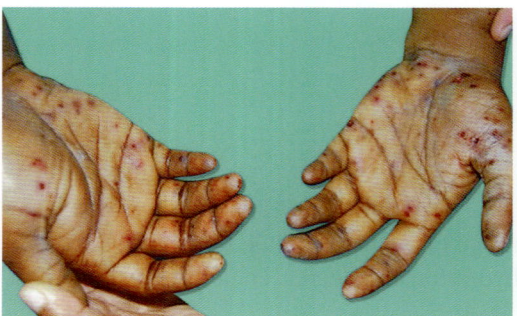

FIG. 5.92: Janeway lesion.

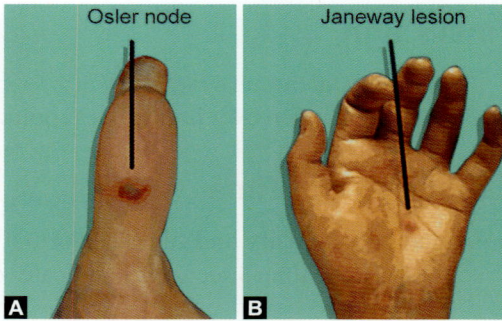

FIGS. 5.93A AND B: Osler's node.

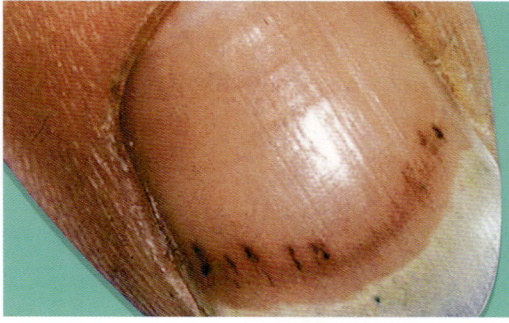

FIG. 5.94: Splinter hemorrhages.

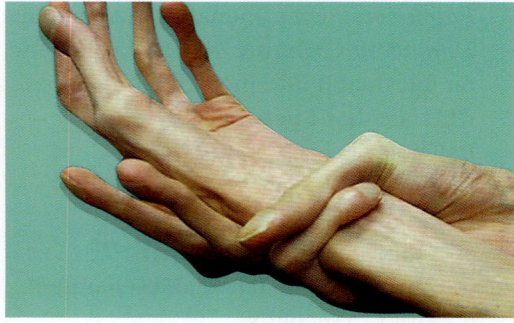

FIG. 5.95: Wrist sign in Marfan's syndrome.

CHAPTER 5: General Examination

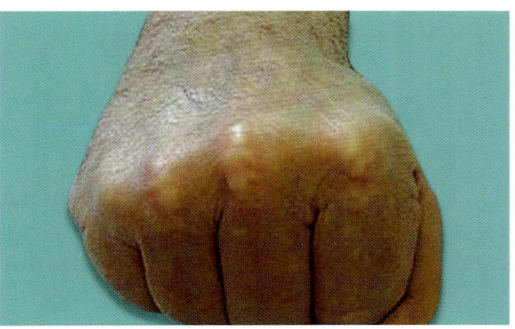

FIG. 5.96: Xanthomata.

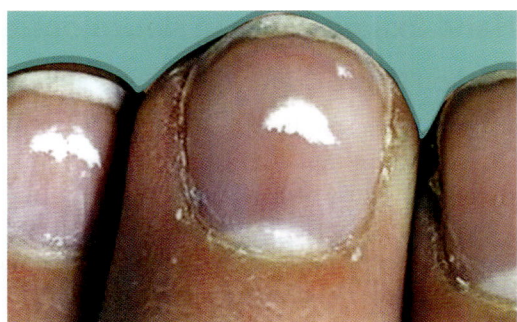

FIG. 5.97: Leukonychia.

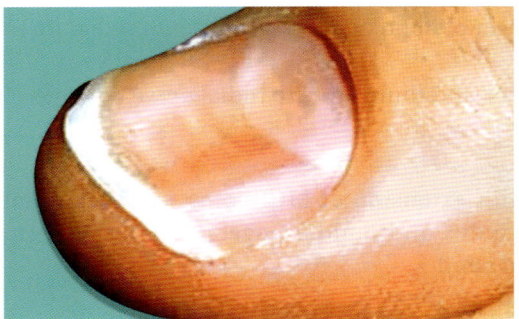

FIG. 5.98: Koilonychia.

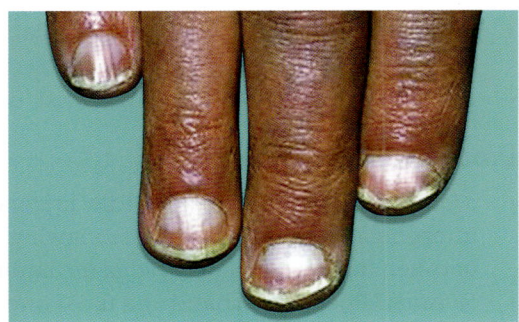

FIG. 5.99: Half-and-half nail.

Respiratory System
- Temperature—warm extremity
- Cyanosis
- Clubbing
- Pulse—full bounding pulse
- *Tremor*:
  - Fine tremor—salbutamol
  - Flapping—respiratory failure
- Nicotine staining

Renal System
- Dry hand
- Flapping tremor—uremia
- Leukonychia—hypoalbuminemia in nephrotic syndrome **(Fig. 5.97)**
- Koilonychia—iron deficiency anemia—abnormal thin nails, lost convexity, and flat and brittle nail **(Fig. 5.98)**
- AV fistula
- Bruising
- Half-and-half nail (distal brown transverse band)—CKD **(Fig. 5.99)**

Hand Examination in Neurological Disorder

Median Nerve Damage
- *Motor*: Loss of flexion at wrist, loss of flexion of radial half of digits and thumb, loss of opposition, and abduction of thumb
- *Sensory*: Loss of sensation in lateral three and half of digits including nail bed and thenar eminence
- *Ape hand deformity*: Hyperextension of index and thumb along with adducted thumb due to median nerve damage

Radial Nerve Damage
- *Motor*: Loss of extension of wrist, fingers, and thumb
- *Sensory*: Loss of sensation in dorsoradial aspect of hand and dorsal aspect of radial three and half digits
- *Wrist drop*: Inability to extend the wrist, fingers, and thumb due to radial nerve damage

Ulnar Nerve Damage
- *Motor*: Clawing of ring and little fingers with extension at MCP joints and flexion at interphalangeal joints and less clawing of index and middle fingers with loss of grip between fingers along with radial deviation of hand
- *Sensory*: Ulnar side of hand and ulnar one and half digits
- *Claw hand deformity*.

Charcot–Marie–Tooth Disease
Thenar flattening with preserved hypothenar muscle bulk.

Motor Neuron Disease
Wasting of predominantly thenar muscles. Abductor pollicis brevis first to be affected followed by first dorsal interosseous muscle. Muscle wasting gradually progresses to other areas.

Dystonia
Repetitive involuntary movement followed by abnormal posturing of neck/face/hand muscles.

Parkinsonism
- Flexion of MCP joints with hyperextension of IP joints with ulnar deviation
- Micrographia with rest tremor (pill rolling/drum beating) may be present.

Striatal hand: Flexion of MCP joints with hyperextension of IP joints with adduction of all the fingers and opposition of thumb to index finger is seen in parkinsonism.

Tremor: Involuntary rhythmic contraction of muscles.
- *Rest tremor*: Occurs with the body part in complete repose, e.g., parkinsonism
- *Action tremor*:
  - Postural tremor: It occurs with maintenance of a posture.

- Intention tremor (kinetic tremor): It occurs with moving a body part to and from a target, e.g., diseases of the cerebellar outflow, multiple sclerosis, trauma, and tumor.

Chorea

Brief semidirected irregular purposeless movements.

Athetosis

Slow involuntary convoluted writhing movements.

Hand in Rheumatological Disorder

- Color—inflammation, erythema
- Scars
- Rashes—sign of vasculitis
- Sclerodactyly—long tapered fingers [CREST (calcinosis, Raynaud phenomenon esophageal dysmotility, sclerodactyly, and telangiectasia) syndrome]
- Thin skin—steroid intake
- Soft tissue wasting or growth
- Nail pitting—psoriasis
- Temperature—warm in inflammation
- Deformities in:
  - *Rheumatoid arthritis*:
    - Z thumb, swan neck deformity
    - Boutonniere deformity, ulnar
    - Deviation of fingers, radial
    - Deviation of wrist
  - *Osteoarthritis*:
    - Heberden's node (distal interphalangeal joint)
    - Bouchard's node (PIP joint)
    - Tender joints
    - Crepitation in joints

■ HAIR

- *Hair loss*:
  - Alopecia:
    - Localized
      » Scarring—infection, SLE, and lichen planus
      » Nonscarring—hair pulling and fungal infection
    - Generalized—age related, cytotoxic drug-induced, and hypothyroidism
  - Secondary hair loss—old age and cirrhosis of liver
- *Abnormal hair growth* **(Fig. 5.100)**:
  - Hirsutism—occurs in female. Male pattern of hair growth especially on face, genitalia, body, and on abdomen. It may be idiopathic or androgen secreting tumor.

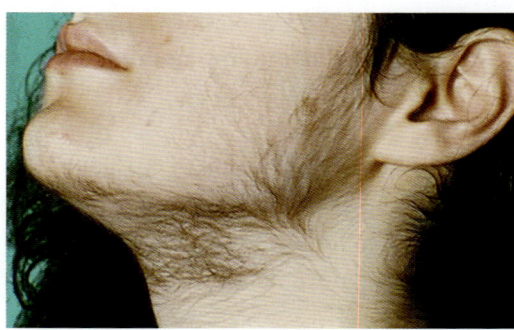

FIG. 5.100: Abnormal hair growth.

■ CONCLUSION

General examination is the mirror of systemic examination. A careful general examination usually gives positive and negative clues for the diagnosis of respiratory examination. General examination, particularly the vitals, is important for the management of patients.

SUGGESTED READINGS

1. Loscalzo J, Fauci A, Kasper D, Hauser S, Longo D, Jameson JL. Harrison's Principles of Internal Medicine. 21st Edition. McGraw Hill; New York. 2022. p 2131.
2. Dover AR, Innes JA, Fairhurst K. Macleod's Clinical Examination. 15th Edition. Elsevier; UK. 2023.

CHAPTER 6

Evaluation of Respiratory System

Supriya Sarkar

■ INTRODUCTION

The first step for the diagnosis of a clinical puzzle is the "clinical data collection." The first step includes: (1) Detailed and comprehensive history taking, (2) meticulous clinical examination, and (3) judiciously selected investigations. Questionnaire is the most important for the diagnosis of respiratory diseases, and the rest can only supplement the first one. Faulty or incomplete data collection will be a disaster.

Proper history taking will assist in selecting proper investigation and subsequently that will help in establishing a complete diagnosis. History should be taken at least thrice. The first one should be taken before clinical examination to have the preliminary idea of disease. The second one should be taken after completion of clinical examination. For example, when clinical examination suggests the left-sided pleural effusion, specific history for that condition should be taken. The third one should be taken after the completion of investigations. When a high-resolution computed tomography (HRCT) scan of the thorax suggests interstitial lung disease, history should be taken to identify the cause of that condition.

Uncomplicated tuberculosis or a lesion surrounded by normal lung parenchyma may not have any physical sign. On the other hand, a combination of signs may indicate pleural effusion or interstitial lung fibrosis. Sometimes, an asymptomatic subject may come with abnormal chest radiology. Next and most important step is "clinical data analysis" that needs knowledge, experience, and clinical sense.

The examination of the respiratory system is divided into two parts: (1) Examination of upper respiratory tract and (2) examination of lower respiratory tract.

■ UPPER RESPIRATORY TRACT

The examination of the respiratory system must start with examination of upper respiratory tract. All components of upper respiratory tract including oral cavity should be carefully examined separately. Although the oral cavity is not a component of upper respiratory tract, it is unequivocally important for the diagnosis of respiratory diseases. For example, poor oral hygiene may lead to aspiration pneumonia and lung abscess.

Nose and Sinuses

First inspect the nose for any deformity, enlargement or depression of nasal bridge (saddle nose). The deformity of the nose may be found in fracture; and inflamed enlarged nose may be found in rhinophyma. The destruction of nasal septum may be found in congenital syphilis. The deviation of nasal septum is more common than expected, and it increases the risk of nasal obstruction and infection. The patency of each nostril should be examined by closing that nostril by pressing finger and asking patient to close mouth and exhale through other nostril. Direct examination of nasal cavity and inferior turbinate is done preferably with the aid of a nasal speculum. Nasal polyp (pearly gray smooth surfaced) or bleeding points must be looked for. Paranasal sinuses can be palpated for tenderness as: (1) Frontal sinus by pressing upward beneath the medial side of supraorbital ridge; (2) maxillary sinus by pressing against the anterior wall of malar prominence below the inferior orbital margin; and (3) ethmoidal sinus by pressing medially against the medial wall of the orbit. Any discharge from sinuses or postnasal discharge should be looked for.

Oral Cavity

The examination of oral cavity includes lips, teeth, gums, tongue, floor of mouth, cheeks, palate, tonsils, and oropharynx. Those structures are carefully inspected for signs of inflammation, infection, deformity, ulcer formation, and white patch (candidiasis). The pigmentation of oral cavity may suggest Addison's disease. Teeth are examined for tobacco staining, caries, discoloration, etc. Gums are examined for gum bleeding, gum hypertrophy, gingivitis, etc. The presence of halitosis should be noted. The tongue is examined for pallor, cyanosis, ulceration, leukoplakia, and movement.

Larynx

The examination of the larynx is done by direct or indirect laryngoscopy usually done by ear, nose, and throat (ENT) specialists. Indirect evidence of laryngeal disease should be carefully looked for, for example, hoarseness of voice may indicate laryngeal palsy, vocal cord nodule, or laryngeal inflammation. Similarly, edema of lips, tongue, around eyes, and front of neck along with dyspnea and choking of voice may indicate laryngeal edema that may indicate a life-threatening condition, angioedema.

■ EXAMINATION OF LOWER RESPIRATORY SYSTEM

The examination of thorax has four components: (1) inspection, (2) palpation, (3) percussion, and (4) auscultation.

Inspection

Inspection part is important as some findings are appreciable only during inspection. For example, important signs of volume loss or gain (flattening or bulging) are only assessed by inspection. Some findings such as the movement of upper part of the chest are better observed by inspection. Inspection of front and lateral aspect of thorax is done with patient on supine or semirecumbent position with the chest and upper abdomen properly exposed, with proper illumination and with arms sufficiently abducted to make axillary areas clearly visible. For the examination of the back, patients are made to stand or sit upright with arms folded across the chest. For better understanding, findings of inspection may be grouped into eight subheadings. Thoracic movement is assessed during inspection and palpation. It is preferable to club them to have a complete assessment.

Respiration

It includes respiratory rate, depth, type, symmetry, and special character.
- *Respiratory rate*: The number of breaths in a full 1 minute should be counted by observing chest wall movement after diverting patients' attention by palpating pulse. Never put palm on patients' thorax or abdomen, as unlike heart rate, respiratory rate may be altered by patient voluntarily. The normal respiratory rate is 10–14 breaths/min, with an approximate 1:3 ratio of inspiration to expiration. Increased respiratory rate is called tachypnea and may be found in all pathologies of the respiratory system.
- *Respiratory depth*: It is very difficult to assess depth of respiration unless it is gross. Increased depth of inspiration (air hunger) can be seen in metabolic acidosis (ketoacidosis and uremia) and massive pulmonary embolism. It should not be confused with dyspnea in obstructive airway diseases.
- *Type of respiration*: In adult female, respiration is thoracoabdominal whereas it is abdominothoracic in male and children of any sex. Predominantly thoracic respiration may be found in bilateral diaphragmatic palsy, peritonitis, ascites, abdominal tumor, pregnancy, and even in gaseous distension of bowel. Exclusive abdominal respiration is found in ankylosing spondylitis, intercostal muscle paralysis, or persons with pleural pain.

Special character:
- "Periodic or Cheyne–Stokes breathing" is a cyclical variation of rate and depth of respiration and is characterized by periods of apnea that are interspersed between cycles of progressively increasing and decreasing respiratory rates. It occurs mainly in left ventricular failure due to long circulatory time delaying chemostimulators to reach respiratory centers.
- "Kussmaul breathing" is a rapid and deep breathing caused by acidotic stimulation of the respiratory centers. It can indicate metabolic acidosis such as diabetic ketoacidosis and uremia.
- "Biot breathing" is an irregular breathing pattern alternating between tachypnea, bradypnea, and apnea. It is probably an indicator of impending respiratory failure.

Shape of Chest and Deformity

Normal shape is elliptical with anteroposterior diameter and transverse diameter ratio 5:7; in flat chest, the ratio may be as low as 1:2; and in barrel chest, it is more than 1:1. Anteroposterior diameter may be increased in kyphosis. Flattening and bulging of whole or part of hemithorax indicate volume loss or volume gain, respectively. Flattening or bulging is assessed in respect to normal hemithorax. For unilateral disease, hemithorax with decreased movement is considered as abnormal.

Barrel chest: Ribs lose their typical 45° downward angle and become more horizontal, leading to an increase of the anteroposterior diameter of the chest. The ratio between anteroposterior diameter and transverse diameter is more than 1:1, and subcostal angle is more than 90° **(Fig. 6.1)**. Barrel chest is found in hyperinflation of lung such as emphysema and sometimes in asthma.

Pectus carinatum (pigeon chest): It is characterized by a localized prominence of sternum with adjacent costal cartilages, and it is often accompanied by indrawing of the ribs forming symmetrical horizontal grooves. It is usually a sequel of chronic respiratory illness or recurrent infection in childhood, or it may be a feature of rickets in undernourished subjects.

Pectus excavatum (funnel chest): It is characterized by either depression of lower part of sternum or whole length of sternum along with attached ribs. It is usually asymptomatic, but severe form can displace heart toward left and can cause palpitation. It is often congenital but may be acquired in shoemakers (cobbler's chest).

Thoracic kyphoscoliosis: It varies from minor variation of spinal curvature to gross deformity **(Fig. 6.2)**. Scoliosis itself can cause displacement of mediastinum with shifting of trachea and apical impulse. Gross deformity can decrease lung volumes and capacities, causing increasing work of breathing, hypoxia, hypercapnia, and even cor pulmonale.

Chest wall bulging/flattening: Bulging in comparison to normal hemithorax indicates volume gain as in case of pleural effusion, pneumothorax, or sometimes by a large mass lesion. Flattening of chest indicates volume loss and found in lung fibrosis, collapse, or fibrothorax. The degree of flattening depends on the duration of illness; as a result, it is less in collapse than fibrosis. Flattening and bulging are more marked in pleural diseases than lung parenchymal diseases.

Signs of thoracic operation: These include the scars from incision and signs of volume loss in lobectomy or pneumonectomy. Deformity is more marked in thoracoplasty, where ribs are cut at both ends and pushed into thorax to close a cavity or to obliterate a space.

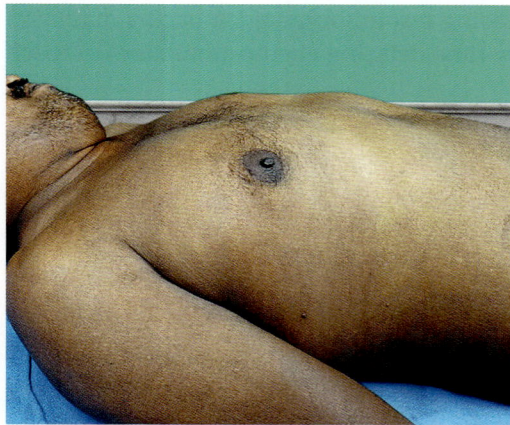

FIG. 6.1: Barrel chest.

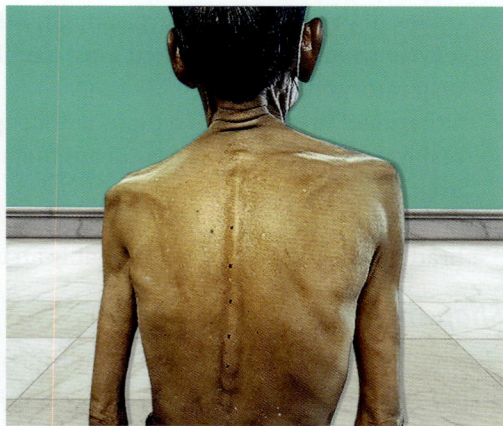

FIG. 6.2: Thoracic kyphoscoliosis and dropping of shoulder.

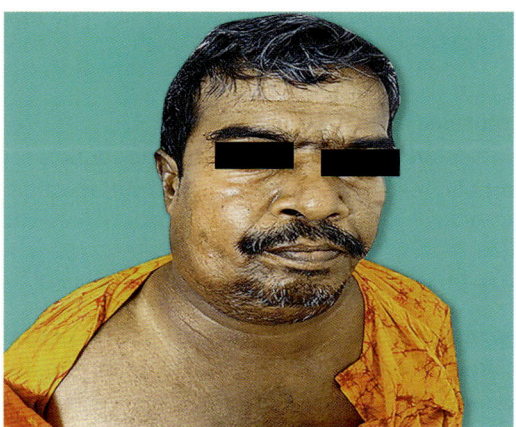

FIG. 6.3: Superior vena cava syndrome.

Cutaneous and Subcutaneous Lesions over Chest Wall

Skin lesions should be inspected and palpated carefully as they sometimes give important clue to diagnosis such as superior vena cava (SVC) obstruction. SVC obstruction causes swelling with congestion of the face and upper chest wall **(Fig. 6.3)**. On the other hand, swelling with paleness of face (puffy face) is found mainly in renal diseases. We should look for cutaneous and subcutaneous lesions, subcutaneous emphysema, vascular abnormalities, direction of venous flow, and other lesions such as gynecomastia.

Partial ptosis of the eye (due to paralysis of Müller's muscle) may be observed as a part of Horner's syndrome also called Bernard–Horner syndrome or oculosympathetic palsy. Pseudoptosis should be differentiated from true ptosis (due to paralysis of third cranial nerve) by: (1) Correction of ptosis when patient is asked to look upward, and (2) absence of other manifestations of third nerve palsy. Components of Horner's syndrome include miosis (constricted pupil), partial ptosis, enophthalmos (depressed eye ball), and anhidrosis (decreased sweating).

Pulsation

Pulsation may be seen at precordium, epigastrium, and rarely in other areas of the thorax. Pulsation in the precordium is usually noted as cardiac pulsation. Whereas, apical pulsation is the pulsation seen over apex of heart and that should be confirmed by palpation. Pulsation over the epigastrium usually indicates right ventricular enlargement commonly seen in cor pulmonale. Rarely, epigastric expansile pulsation may be observed due to aneurysm of descending aorta. A vascular tumor or increased vascularity over a tumor is sometimes visible.

Signs of Dyspnea

Although dyspnea is a symptom, there are many physical signs suggestive of dyspnea. Sometimes, a patient may complain of dyspnea without sign then the possibility of malingering or psychological dyspnea should be considered. On the other hand, there may be signs of dyspnea though patient denies any complain particularly in case of chronic dyspnea

where the patient may be habituated with dyspnea or adjust it by lifestyle modification. Signs of dyspnea include:
- Increased respiratory rate
- The use of accessory muscles of respiration*
- Suprasternal, supraclavicular, intercostal, or epigastric suction
- Paradoxical movement of chest wall or anterior abdominal wall
- Pursed lip breathing

Examination from Back

It is important to recognize volume changes in hemithorax. Loss of hemithorax volume is found in pleural fibrosis, lung parenchymal fibrosis, long standing lung collapse, or following lung resection (pneumonectomy or lobectomy). Increased hemithorax volume is usually not clinically appreciable from the back. As mentioned earlier, changes are more in pleural diseases than parenchymal diseases.
- *Dropping of shoulder*: Downward displacement of shoulder in comparison to normal side indicates volume loss of the affected hemithorax or spinal deformity **(Fig. 6.2)**.
- *Winging of scapula*: Lateral rotation of scapula due to volume loss of ipsilateral hemithorax that should be confirmed during palpation by measuring spinoscapular distance.
- *Examination of spine for thoracic kyphosis and scoliosis*: Kyphosis (increased anterior concavity of dorsal spine) is difficult to appreciate clinically, unless gross. Scoliosis (lateral bending of spine) can be easily demonstrated by marking spinous processes of dorsal spines with skin marking pencil. Scoliosis may be postural, congenital, idiopathic, or may result from neuromuscular diseases or skeletal diseases such as caries spine and trauma. In volume loss of hemithorax, scoliosis is found with concavity toward the same side.
- Any other abnormality in the back should be noted.

Thoracic Movement

It is a combined inspiratory and palpatory finding as movement of upper part of thorax that moves upward (pump handle movement) is better visible than palpable. On the other hand, movement of lower part of thorax is due to upward and outward movements of lower ribs (bucket handle movement) and is better palpable than visible. Ideally movement should be inspected from the foot end of bed with patient lying supine and window light coming from the head end of the patient. Movement should be looked for tangentially, keeping examiner's eyes at the level of thorax. Bilateral movement is assessed by chest wall expansion, and unilateral movement is assessed by comparing movement of the diseased side with that of normal side. Asymmetry of thoracic apical movement can be observed by looking downward standing behind the patient while the patient is sitting on a tool.

Accessory muscles of respiration: Accessory muscles of inspiration are mainly neck muscles (sternocleidomastoids act by lifting sternum upward; and anterior, middle, and posterior scalene muscles act by lifting first two ribs). Muscles those fix shoulder girdles and back muscles act indirectly by making a fulcrum upon which neck muscles can act. Accessory muscles of expiration are mainly abdominal muscles (rectus abdominis and obliques) act by pushing the diaphragm upward. Internal intercostal muscles depress ribs and thereby assist forced expiration.

Specific Inspiratory Signs

- *Hoover's sign*: Indrawing of lower chest wall due to contraction of low flat diaphragm, and that may be found in hyperinflated lungs in emphysema.
- *Sternomastoid sign (trail sign)*: Shifting of trachea causes prominence of sternomastoid of that side.
- *Tietze's syndrome*: Inflammation of the costochondral joints of the upper part of chest causes swelling and tenderness of upper costochondral joints.

Palpation

Superficial Palpation

It should include temperature, tenderness, examination to detect the venous flow, and examination of swelling. Apart from routine examination of chest wall swelling, cough impulse and pulsation of the swelling must be examined.

Examination of Trachea

Upper 4–5 cm of trachea can be felt in the neck between cricoid cartilage and suprasternal notch. Thyroid enlargement can cause displacement of trachea. In chronic obstructive pulmonary disease (COPD), trachea may be dragged into thorax during inspiration.

Tracheal position: We should remember certain facts before examining trachea: (1) Trachea is a movable structure—so examine it gently, (2) lowest palpable part of trachea better reflects mediastinal position, and (3) trachea moves with movement of head. For examination of trachea; first fix head with left hand, then palpate trachea from above downward up to suprasternal angle, then gently push finger between trachea and sternomastoid muscles on both sides to feel the gaps. Trachea shifting is indicated by ipsilateral reduction of gap **(Fig. 6.4)**. Normal tracheal position is central (slight right anatomical shift at the level of bifurcation is not clinically appreciable). Shifting of trachea indicates upper mediastinal shifting. Ipsilateral shifting of trachea occurs in fibrosis or collapse involving upper lobe of

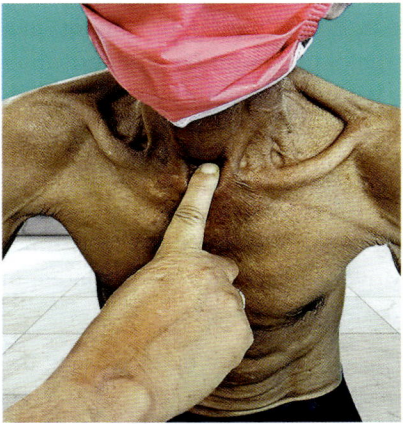

FIG. 6.4: Examination of trachea.

lung, whereas contralateral shifting occurs in case of pleural diseases (pneumothorax and pleural effusion) and due to mass lesion of thyroid, lung, lymph node, mediastinal mass, etc.

Tracheal movement: Trachea moves downward during inspiration normally, but that is not clinically appreciable. In obstructive airway disease, the movement gets prominence. Finger is placed just below cricoid cartilage, the distance between suprasternal notch and cricoid cartilage will decrease during inspiration.

Tracheal tug/Oliver's sign: The sign is an extreme downward movement of trachea during systole that is found in aneurysm of arch of aorta as arch of aorta encircles left main stem bronchus.

Apical Impulse

Apical impulse should be palpated in anatomical position (standing or sitting). Apical impulse is defined as the most downward, most outward, and definite cardiac impulse palpable over precordium. Normal position of apical impulse is 1 cm medial to left midclavicular line at the fifth intercostal space. Shifting of the position of apical impulse indicates shifting of lower mediastinum or cardiomegaly. Ipsilateral shifting of apical impulse occurs in volume loss (fibrosis or collapse) of lower lobe, whereas contralateral shifting occurs in pleural diseases. In addition, leftward shifting of apical impulse may occur in cardiomegaly, and rarely in pectus excavatum and congenital absence of pericardium.

Apical impulse may not be palpable in obese patients, in emphysema, pericardiac effusion, left-sided pleural effusion, and apical impulse positioned behind the ribs or sternum. In dextrocardia, apical impulse is on the right side and that can be differentiated from rightward shifting of heart by normal position of trachea and the presence of cardiac dullness in right parasternal line.

Shifting of trachea along with apical impulse suggests shifting of total mediastinal due to whole lung volume loss (ipsilateral) and pleural diseases (contralateral).

Movement of Chest

To elicit movement inequality, we compare movement of both sides considering the fact that disease-side will move less. For palpating movement, palm should be placed over the area firmly not too lightly so that you cannot feel the movement or too tightly so that chest wall movement is hampered. If you place your fingers instead of palm, you will not get the feeling of movement. Another area of concern is the taking of skin ridge. That is not absolutely necessary, and it is necessary only to demonstrate movement.

Movement at the infraclavicular areas: This is done in supine position, head resting on pillow, head and trunk in straight line, shoulders are relaxed and in symmetric position, and see the movement tangentially. Movement can also be palpated, but that is less effective. Some physicians avoid that maneuver.

Movement at the lower anterior chest: This is done placing the palms over costal margins, thumb fingers looking to the xiphoid process, a loose fold of skin between two thumbs may be taken, and patient is asked to take deep breath **(Fig. 6.5)**. The movement of both sides is assessed by feeling the movement of two sides and observing the movement of thumbs.

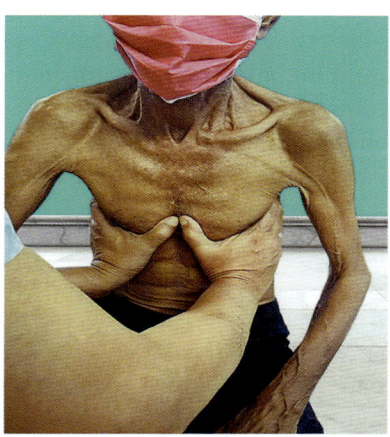 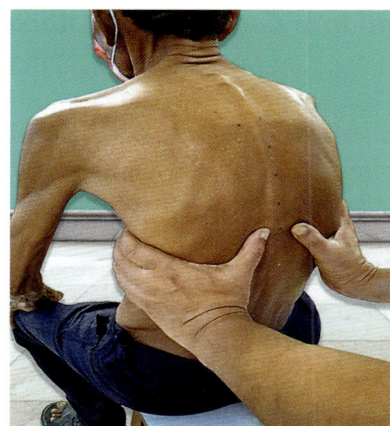

FIG. 6.5: Examination of lower anterior chest wall movement.

FIG. 6.6: Examination of lower chest wall movement from back.

Movement at the infrascapular areas: Here inspection is seldom helpful. The movement of these areas is assessed by asking the patient to sit erect and take deep breath; palms are placed below scapula and tips of both thumbs are brought together in the region of 10th thoracic spine **(Fig. 6.6)**.

Movement of the apex of lungs: This is better seen from the back and looking from above, and patient is sitting erect and symmetrically. Palpation of movement of apex was done by placing palms firmly over the middle third of trapezius with fingers directing anteriorly toward clavicles and feeling the upward movement of trapezius.

Chest Wall Expansion

Expansion of thorax is measured at lower two-thirds of chest by recording the maximum difference between full inspiration and full expiration. Expansion should be above 5 cm. Decreased chest wall expansion is found in COPD, asthma, diffuse parenchymal lung diseases, and ankylosis spondylitis.

Vocal Fremitus

It is a crude test and has no added advantage over vocal resonance. It is assessed by placing the ulnar side of palm over the intercostal space; asking the patient to utter "one-one-one"; feeling the vibration; and comparing it with the corresponding part of the opposite side. Ulnar surface of palm is preferred, as it is said to be more sensitive, and can be better placed over the intercostal areas. Similarly, vibrations from low-pitched rhonchi arising from large bronchus and pleural rub of chronic pleurisy may be palpable.

Crowding of Ribs

The interspace between the ribs of one side is compared with other side by insinuating fingers in the intercostal spaces. Rib crowding is found in pleural fibrosis and less commonly in lung parenchymal fibrosis. Overriding of ribs, where one rib rides over other ribs, is found exclusively in pleural fibrosis.

Palpation of Cardiovascular Abnormalities

Superficial pulsations other than apical impulse should be palpated for confirmation as well as to elicit the expansile nature of pulsation. Venus flow should be noted, and any bruit should be palpated. Palpable pulmonary component of second heart sound indicates pulmonary hypertension. Similarly, left parasternal heave by the side of sternum is a sign of right ventricular enlargement.

Measurements

- *Anteroposterior diameter and transverse diameter*: Normal chest is elliptical with ratio between anteroposterior and transverse diameters 5:7 **(Figs. 6.7A and B)**.
- *Subcostal angle*: It is the angle between two costal margins, and it should be less than 90°.
- *Chest wall expansion*: It is normally more than 5 cm. It is reduced in diseases of chest wall, neuromuscular diseases involving thorax, pleural, lung parenchymal, or airway diseases.
- *Hemithorax expansion*: Decrease movement of one hemithorax can be documented by measuring chest wall expansion of each hemithorax separately (from tip of the spine in back to mid-sternum in front) and comparing them with other side.

Percussion

During percussion, three things should be noted: (1) Sound/note, (2) feeling of resistance, and (3) tenderness. Percussion is done by hammering with the right middle finger (at 90° angle and movement coming from right wrist joint) over the second phalanx of left middle finger firmly placed over the area to be percussed. Left index and ring fingers must not touch chest wall as it will decrease vibration of chest wall producing sound. Normal percussion note over chest is resonant as lungs mainly contain air. Lung note loses its resonance in pleural diseases other than pneumothorax and in consolidation, fibrosis, collapse, etc. Percussion note over consolidation is usually impaired to dull; it is dull over solid organs (heart, liver, and spleen), and it is stony dull (dull + sense of resistance) over pleural effusion. On the other

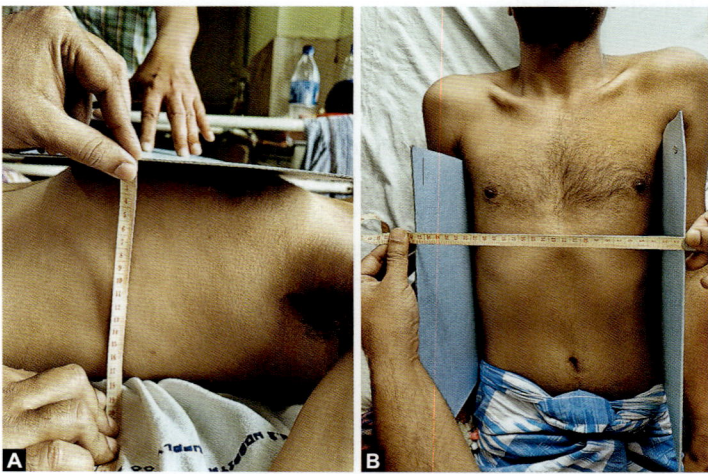

FIGS. 6.7A AND B: Examination of anteroposterior and transverse diameter of thorax.

hand, it is hyperresonant in the presence of excess air such as pneumothorax, emphysema, large cyst, and superficial cavity. Bilateral hyperresonant note is indirectly assessed by the absence of normal dullness over the liver and heart. Tympanitic note is found over a hollow organ such as fundus of stomach, distended guts, and over pneumothorax.

Percussion through Midclavicular Line

Midclavicular line is a vertical line from midpoint between middle of sternal notch and acromion process **(Fig. 6.8)**. Percussion along midclavicular lines is done in patient lying in supine and symmetrical position or patient in sitting position.

Percussion through Midaxillary Line

Midaxillary line is a vertical line drawn from axilla at the midpoint between anterior and posterior axillary folds. Percussion along midaxillary line is done with patient in sitting position and raising both hands straight over the side of the head.

Percussion of Back

Patient's position is sitting with arms crossed over the chest directing toward opposite shoulder.
- *Percussion in suprascapular area*: This is done by placing fingers vertically in the suprascapular areas, and percussion is done from medial to laterally.
  - *Percussion in interscapular area*: Here percussion is done by placing fingers horizontally from above downward.
  - *Percussion through scapular line*: Scapular line is a vertical line from the tip of angle of scapula. In these lines, percussion is done placing fingers obliquely directing medially and upward.

Percussion in Kronig's Isthmus

Kronig's isthmus is a place bounded medially by neck muscles, anteriorly by clavicle, laterally by acromion process, and posteriorly by trapezius. Percussion of Kronig's isthmus should be done from the back placing pleximeter fingers over middle-third of trapezius extending to

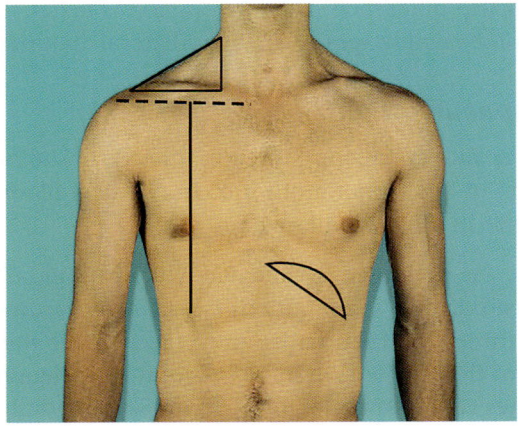

FIG. 6.8: Midclavicular line, Kronig's isthmus, and Traube's space.

supraclavicular fossa (**Fig. 6.8**). The area represents the apex of lungs. Dullness over the area is found in any lesion of apex of lungs such as tuberculosis, Pancoast tumor, and apical cap.

Percussion for Liver Dullness

It is a deep percussion over right midclavicular line to find out the upper border of liver dullness. It is not effective in presence of fluid in right pleural space.

Percussion of Traube's Space

Traube's space is a crescent-shaped tympanitic area over the left lower chest anteriorly, bounded medially by left border of liver, above by left dome of diaphragm, and below by costal margin. The surface marking of Traube's space is left sixth rib above with convexity upward up to the ninth rib in midaxillary line and bounded inferiorly by left costal margin (**Fig. 6.8**). The normal tympanitic node is obliterated in left-sided pleural effusion, pericardial effusion, hepatomegaly, splenomegaly, and tumor over fundus of stomach.

Cardiac Percussion

Cardiac percussion to delineate the cardiac boundary is not done as there is a risk of dislodgement of thrombi. For pulmonary medicine, deep percussion over left parasternal line is done to notice the presence or absence of cardiac dullness in the fourth and fifth spaces. Left parasternal line is resonance in emphysema and shifting of heart to right.

Right Parasternal Percussion

It is usually resonant. Dullness may be found in anterior mediastinal mass or sometimes in fourth and fifth space in rightward shifting of heart or dextrocardia.

Tidal Percussion

This is a crude method to demonstrate diaphragmatic movement. It is done by deep percussion over back in the scapular line to delineate the lowest border of lung resonance. Then the difference between the resonance at full inspiration and forceful expiration is noted. It is usually one intercostal space difference. Tidal percussion is negative in severe emphysema. Paradoxical movement of the diaphragm occurs in unilateral diaphragmatic palsy.

Percussion for Hydropneumothorax

Horizontal fluid level: The line connecting the upper levels of dullness anteriorly, laterally, and in back is horizontal in hydropneumothorax. In classical pleural effusion, the highest point of that line should be in the midaxillary line.

Shifting dullness: At first, the dullness is delineated while patient is in sitting position. Then keeping the finger placed at that area, patient is asked to lie down in lateral decubitus posture. Then wait for three normal breaths and percuss over the area. A resonant note indicates replacement of fluid by air. Then ask patient to sit again and percuss over the area. A dull note indicates replacement of air by fluid. Shifting dullness is classically found in hydropneumothorax. Rarely, it may be found over a large superficial cavity with fluid, hydropneumopericardium, and herniation of gut. Delayed shifting dullness may be found in pleural effusion, and when detected it indicates free fluid and healthy underlying lung.

Mediastinal Percussion

Mediastinal percussion is done over sternum. Manubrium sterni is usually resonant and if it is dull, it indicates anterior mediastinal mass. Body of sternum is usually dull, and it may be resonant in emphysema, tension pneumothorax, and mediastinal emphysema.

Auscultation

Auscultation is done over areas of thorax and comparing them with other side. Areas are infraclavicular, mammary, and inframammary anteriorly; axillary and infra-axillary laterally; and suprascapular, interscapular, and infrascapular in the back. During auscultation, the patient must be instructed how to breathe, how to pronounce notes, and how to whisper; followed by observing patients taking breathe. Then to perform auscultation with stethoscope.

In auscultation, the following points should be noted: Breath sound, vocal resonance, added sound, and special sound. Three characters of breath sound must be noted: (1) Frequency/pitch (waves/sec) measured as hertz (Hz); (2) amplitude/loudness (height of wave), measured as decibel (dB); and (3) timber/quality (that differentiates sounds of equal pitch and loudness).

Auscultation should be done in quite atmosphere. Patient should sit on a tool after removing clothes over the chest. Patient should be instructed properly before auscultation. Hear more than one full breath, preferably three, comparing normal with abnormal side.

Breath Sound

Breath sound is produced in the large airways by turbulent airflow. As it passes through lungs and chest wall (a low-pass filter), there is a sharp drop of frequency and amplitude.

Vesicular breath sound: This is characterized by rustling in character, no gap between inspiration and expiration, and the duration of expiratory phase is less than that of inspiratory phase. Breath sound increases its intensity during inspiration and quickly fades away during expiration. Vesicular breath sounds are of four types:
1. *Normal vesicular*: The breath sound heard over normal lungs. Puerile breath sound is normal breath sound that is clearly audible and found in children, thin-built persons, and hyperinflated lungs.
2. *Diminished vesicular breath sound*: Breath sound is normal but low in amplitude, and it is usually found in pleural diseases and hyperinflation of lung (emphysema).
3. *Vesicular with prolong expiration*: It is found in obstructive airway diseases.
4. *Harsh vesicular breath sound (bronchovesicular)*: When the inspiratory part of breath sound is of bronchial character and expiratory part is of vesicular character. It is found in compensatory emphysema/hyperinflation.

Bronchial breath sound: Bronchial breath sound is blowing in character with a gap between the end of inspiration and start of expiration. In bronchial breath sound, the expiratory part of sound is as long as and as loud as inspiratory sound, and inspiratory and expiratory sounds are equal in pitch and intensity. Bronchial breath sound is found when the sound bypasses

the low-pass filter. Bronchial breath sound may be heard over C-7 to T-3 spine, in normal persons. Bronchial breath sounds are of three types:
1. *High-pitched bronchial (tubular) breath sound*: This is typically found in consolidation. It may be found in upper border of pleural effusion, peripheral lung collapse with patent bronchus, pulmonary fibrosis, and mediastinal tumor close to a large patent bronchus. Transmitted sound may be heard in case of tracheal shifting in collapsed lung. Tracheal sound is a very loud sound with equal duration of inspiration and expiration.
2. *Low-pitched bronchial (cavernous) breath sound*: This is typically found over a superficial cavity with patent bronchus.
3. *Amphoric breath sound*: It is a low-pitch sound with a metallic character typically found in pneumothorax with bronchopleural fistula and rarely may be found over a large superficial cavity with a communicating bronchus. The sound may be observed by blowing an empty jar with a pipe.

Vocal Resonance

Vocal resonance is the sound produced in the vocal cord transmitted and heard over chest wall. Voice sounds are faintly audible due to low-pitch filtering effect of lungs and chest wall. It may be distinctly audible when lung is consolidated.
- Normal vocal resonance
- *Decreased and absent vocal resonance*: Mainly found in pleural diseases and emphysema
- *Increased vocal resonance*: Usually found over consolidation, transmitted sound due to shifting of trachea, upper border of pleural effusion, etc.
   - Bronchophony: It is the voice sound that is distinct with more intensity and clarity.
   - Egophony: This is a nasal intonation and beating quality of vocal resonance typically found over upper border of pleural effusion and consolidation. Egophony came from the Greek ward "ego" meaning goat.
   - Whispered pectoriloquy: When whispered sound is audible distinctly without any alteration and individual syllables can be clearly recognized. It is found over consolidation.

Added Sound

Rhonchi: It is a dry, continuous/uninterrupted, and musical sound that lasts more than 250 ms. Rhonchus is a Latinized version of Greek rhonchus, meaning wheeze. Its use should be restricted to musical sound produced by narrowed bronchi. It has been suggested that rhonchi should be replaced by wheeze. Wheeze is high pitch with frequency of 400 Hz or more and may be heard without stethoscope. Rhonchi can be classified as:
- *High pitched (sibilant)*: Rhonchi with frequency more than 400 Hz is found in obstruction in smaller airways.
- *Low pitched (sonorous)*: Rhonchi with frequency less than 200 Hz is found in obstruction in large airways.

Rhonchi/wheeze is recently classified as:
- Monophonic wheezing consists of a single musical note starting and ending at different times. It can be:
   - Fixed monophonic: Wheeze has a constant frequency and a long duration; it is found in intrabronchial tumor, foreign body, bronchostenosis, and mucus accumulation.

- Random monophonic: Wheeze has a varying frequency and duration presenting in both phases of respiration. It is seen in asthma.
- Polyphonic wheezing consists of multiple musical notes starting and ending at the same time and is typically produced by the dynamic compression of the large, more central airways. Polyphonic wheeze is confined to the expiration only. It is found in COPD.

Crepitation: Crepitation is derived from Latin word crepitare, meaning crackle or rattle. It is unambiguously used for nonmusical, short, and explosive crackling sound that lasts <20 ms. It is also described as moist, nonmusical, leathery sound mainly audible during inspiration. Some prefer to use crackles over crepitation. Fine crackles are produced within small airways, medium crackles are caused by air bubbling through mucus in small bronchi, and coarse crackles arise from large bronchi or the bronchiectatic segments.

- Fine crackles are due to opening up of closed airways. Fine crepitation is softer, shorter in duration, and higher in pitch than coarse crackles. Fine crackles are heard on mid to late inspiration and occasionally on expiration, unaffected by cough, gravity dependent, and not transmitted to mouth. Late inspiratory crepitation previously called Velcro crepitation (sounds such as opening of Velcro straps) is typically found in diffuse parenchymal lung diseases (interstitial lung diseases). It is also seen in pulmonary edema and pneumonia.
- Coarse crackles are heard on early inspiration and throughout expiration, affected by cough and transmitted to mouth. It is caused by bubbling of air through secretions. It is found in bronchiectasis, chronic bronchitis, fibrosis, and cavities.

Pleural rub: It is a friction sound, biphasic occurring at the end of inspiration and just after starting of expiration. The main difference between pleural rub and coarse crepitation is that it does not change in quality or quantity after coughing.

Succussion splash: It is a splashing sound heard over the chest directly or by stethoscope at the air-fluid level with sudden sharp movement of thorax. This sign should not be elicited as it may push fluid from pleural space to lung in the presence of bronchopleural fistula.
- *d'Espine sign*: It is described as bronchial breath sound and whispering pectoriloques heard over the spinous processes below T3 vertebrae in adult.
- *Reverse d'Espine sign*: It is also described as anterior d'Espine sign. It is described as bronchial breath sound and bronchophony heard over supracardiac area due to large anterior mediastinal mass/lymphadenopathy between trachea and sternum.

Special Signs

Stridor: It is a loud high-pitched musical sound produced by the turbulent flow in the upper airways. It is louder over the neck than over chest wall. Stridor is mainly inspiratory sound. It is heard without stethoscope and may be heard from a distance. Stridor is inspiratory when it is associated with extrathoracic lesions. Stridor may be heard over expiration in intrathoracic lesions.

Coin test: It was described as a sign for tension pneumothorax. To elicit the sign, place a metallic coin flat against the chest wall just below the mid-clavicle, strike the coin with the edge of another metal coin with the help of an assistant or by patient himself, and place the diaphragm of stethoscope at the opposite corresponding point in the posterior wall of chest of the affected side. Coin test is positive if high-pitched metallic and bell-like sounds are heard.

Scratch sign: The test is done with patient in either sitting or supine position, place the diaphragm of stethoscope at the midpoint over the sternum, scratch with finger or a blunt object over lateral wall of both sides of chest at equidistant points, and sounds of two sides are compared. A positive sign consists of a considerably louder and harder sound on the side of pneumothorax.

Hamman's sign: The sign was described by Louis Hamman in 1939. The presence of free air between heart and chest wall produces crunching sounds that are synchronous with cardiac cycle and best heard over the precordium. The sign is found in pneumomediastinum and left-sided pneumothorax.

Subcutaneous crepitation: Subcutaneous emphysema produces an unusual cracking sensation under the skin when pressed with fingers due to the presence of air in the subcutaneous tissue.

Forced expiratory time: It is a simple, inexpensive, and sensitive test to detect airflow obstruction at bedside. Forced expiratory time (FET) is defined as the time taken for an individual to complete forceful exhalation after maximum inspiration. More than 6-second FET indicates obstructive airway diseases.

■ CONCLUSION

Examination of respiratory system should be aimed to determine the underline pathology. Examination should be aimed to pin-point the anatomical structure involved such as pleural diseases, lung parenchymal diseases, airway diseases, and mediastinal diseases, or diseases involving a combination of structures. Examination should be aimed to detect exact pathology such as consolidation, lung fibrosis, collapse, interstitial pneumonia/fibrosis, pleural effusion, and pneumothorax or a combination of pathologies. A properly taken history can only determine the etiology. A combination of examination findings may suggest pleural effusion, but without proper history, the diagnosis will remain inconclusive. A detailed history taking and meticulous clinical examination will give a provisional diagnosis, and that should be confirmed by investigations.

SUGGESTED READINGS

1. Kasper DL, Hauser SL, Jameson JL, Gauci AS, Longo DL, Loscalzo J. Harrison's Principles of Internal Medicine. 19th edition. McGraw-Hill Education, New York, 2017. pp. 1661-2.
2. Munro JF, Campbell IW. Macleod's Clinical Examination. 7th edition. ELBS. Reprinted 1987. pp. 1-16, 153-91.

CHAPTER 7

Basic Investigations: Indications and Interpretations

Subir Kumar Dey, Sukanta Kumar Dey, AG Ghoshal, Shyam Krishnan, Udas Chandra Ghosh, Sekhar Chakraborty, Indranil Halder, Subhra Mitra, Jaydip Deb, Sumit Roy Tapadar

A. EXAMINATION OF SPUTUM

Subir Kumar Dey, Sukanta Kumar Dey

■ INTRODUCTION

When there is an inflammation of the lungs and airways, pus cells and other inflammatory products produced reach the tracheobronchial tree as sputum (phlegm/mucus). Sputum is not the same as saliva, and it has some lung cells in it. Easy differentiation can be made by microscopic examination of alveolar macrophages.

The respiratory tract of a normal adult produces about 100 mL mucus per day. The condition in which the mucus volume exceeds 100 mL per day is defined as bronchorrhea, usually occurring in infective exacerbations, bronchiectasis, asthma, chronic bronchitis, alveolar cell carcinoma, acute organophosphorus poisoning, and ingestion of neurotoxins from eating neurotoxic fishes. When excess sputum is formed, the normal process of removal may be ineffective and causes accumulation. Mucous membrane is stimulated, and this mucus is coughed out. Sometimes cough is also provoked by postural changes as in bronchiectasis. Sputum is basically a representative sample of the lungs and lower respiratory tract.

■ SPUTUM ANALYSIS

Sputum analysis is the simplest, cost-effective, and noninvasive investigation, which helps in the diagnosis of many diseases, though at times, it is the most controversial clinical sample to be collected due to the difficulty in obtaining expectorated sputum sample of adequate quality, which can lead to a low yield of bacterial culture. Up to 50% of patients have nonproductive cough, and 50% of the productive cough samples are contaminated with upper respiratory tract secretions, despite the possibility that some pathogens may be a part of the commensal flora. In those unable to expectorate sputum, nebulization with hypertonic saline is fruitful. A more significant microbiological sample of sputum can be obtained by bronchoscopic techniques. When sputum cannot be coughed up, it is induced. Induced sputum (IS) can be obtained by inhalation of hypertonic saline 3–5% usually used via nebulization (though other agents such as distilled water, glucose solution, and surfactant active agents such as TYLOXAPOL, tegemist, and β2-agonist can be used). An ultrasonic nebulizer delivers about 5–7 mL of hypertonic solution for about 10 minutes. Sometimes preinduction nebulization with a β2-agonist is helpful. It was first used by Bickerman et al. in 1958 in the cytology of lung cancer. Later on IS was used for diagnosis of many diseases. Various studies over past decades have favored superior yield of sputum induction over fiberoptic bronchoscopy (FOB). This has been very helpful in resource poor or rural settings, especially among young women, mostly having dry cough, scanty sputum and may have minimal disease. It is a boon in Revised National Tuberculosis Control Program (RNTCP) where demonstration of acid-fast bacilli (AFB) is an essential requirement.

A good and adequate sample has <10 squamous epithelial buccal cells and >25 polymorphonuclear neutrophils per low power field. Alternatively, a leukocyte-to-epithelial cell ratio >5 denotes adequate sputum sample and signifies minimal oropharyngeal contamination. Increased number of epithelial cells and decreased number of neutrophils suggest contamination. An easy differentiation can be made by microscopic observation of alveolar macrophages. Differentiation from gastric contents can be made by testing for pH.

■ HOW TO OBTAIN A SPUTUM SAMPLE?

No special preparation is required. Only if samples for AFB are taken, it is advisable to see that patients are not on antibiotics such as fluoroquinolones, which have an antitubercular action. Usually, a morning sample is obtained in disposable wide mouth container—sterile or nonsterile—depending on test required after a bout of deep cough failing which it is induced.

■ MICROSCOPIC FEATURES OF SPUTUM

- Volume (mL/24 hours)—discussed earlier
- *Appearance*:
  - Serous
  - Mucoid
  - Mucopurulent
  - Purulent: It may contain a variable amount of pus mixed with mucus often looking like a ripe lemon. Purulent sputum is usually yellow, but if it is stagnant, as may happen when the patient has had a long sleep or in diseased states such as bronchiectasis, it may appear greenish owing to the liberation of the green enzyme verdoperoxidase from the cells as they are broken down.
    - Blood-stained sputum: Hemorrhage in the alveoli may cause streaking of sputum with fresh blood. Hemoptysis is massive when there is bleeding from the

bronchial artery, which is at systemic pressure. Common causes are tuberculosis, bronchiectasis and carcinoma. In many cases, no explanation is found for casual slight blood streaking of sputum.
- Rusty sputum: An acute hemorrhagic exudate in the alveoli, as in pneumonia, may result in round particles of altered blood, which is called rusty sputum.
- Blackish sputum (melanoptysis): It results from expectoration of the contents of necrotic progressive massive fibrosis (PMF). Such sputum may even be jet black in case of coalminers suffering from pneumoconiosis.
- Anchovy sauce-like sputum is the characteristic feature of ruptured amoebic liver abscess.
- Dentistry: A search for anaerobic infections is very much rewarding wherever possible.
- Others: Plugs or casts of bronchi looking like worms as found in asthma or allergic bronchopulmonary aspergillosis (ABPA) and jelly-like expectoration may be found in ruptured hydatid cyst.
- *Consistency*: Viscosity (mm^2) can be determined by using a thromboelastograph modified by Morgagnie and Grassi and spinnability (mm) measured by Seafan thread meter.
- *Odor*:
  - Very offensive smell may be found in anaerobic lung infection, e.g., lung abscess.
  - Gram-negative organisms may impart a distinctive odor to sputum, similar to that of *Escherichia coli*.
  - These odors may be used as a guide to initial antibiotic treatment while awaiting bacteriological results.

The most important elements which may be identified are: bacteria or pus cells, eosinophils, malignant cells, ova and fungi (pneumonia due to *Pneumocystis jirovecii*), asbestos bodies, or lung flukes (*Paragonimus westermani*).

The presence of eosinophils suggests an allergic process such as in asthma, pulmonary eosinophilia, ABPA, and intermittently in chronic bronchitis. We may also find hooklets scolices of *Echinococcus granulosus* when the hydatid cyst ruptures into the bronchus.

CLINICAL APPLICATION OF SPUTUM IN THE DIAGNOSIS OF PULMONARY DISEASES

- *Pulmonary tuberculosis*:
  - By examining a sputum smear under microscope by Ziehl–Neelsen method, we can see acid and alcohol fast bacilli (AAFB) commonly known as AFB. The probability of finding AFB in sputum depends on the number of tubercle bacilli in the sputum (If the count is 10,000 bacilli per mL, then we may find one acid-fast bacteria).
  - GeneXpert, launched by Cepheid, California, US, uses the rapid molecular beacons based Xpert MTB/RIF assay (*Mycobacterium tuberculosis*/Rifampicin) utilizing the commercially available cartridge-based nucleic acid amplification test (CBNAAT) technology. The test detects *M. tuberculosis* and rifampicin resistance directly after minimal decontamination by sodium hydroxide (NaOH) and centrifugation of the specimen of untreated sputum/tissue/body fluids. The overall sensitivity is 92.2%

(98.2% for smear positive and 72.5% for smear negative TB) and specificity is 99.2%. The test has much better accuracy than the microscopy or culture methods and takes 1 hour and 45 minutes.
- *Asthma*: In many cases, diagnosis is not possible by pulmonary function test (PFT) alone, especially in asthma and chronic obstructive pulmonary disease (COPD) overlap. An increased eosinophil count above the upper limit of 3% of nonsquamous cells is used as a diagnostic tool. Also, increased levels of eosinophil allow the forecast of glucocorticoid use. It can be used for assessing drug activity, response to treatment, and also to decide on the minimal dose of inhaled corticosteroid.
- *Lung cancer*: The presence of malignant cells in sputum is more in case of central lesions and in bronchoalveolar cell carcinoma, where there is profuse expectoration.
- *Pneumonia*: A simple Gram-stain of sputum can give the idea of the infective organism within hours before chemotherapy is initiated as culture takes some time. Antigen testing in sputum can help in the diagnosis of pneumonia (newly developed antigen detection kit RAPIRUN). GeneXpert technology can also detect methicillin-resistant *Staphylococcus aureus* (MRSA) and antimicrobial resistance [*mecA* gene and staphylococcal cassette chromosome mec (SCCmec)].
- *COPD*: Sputum analysis has given evidence of the increased number of macrophages, neutrophils, and eosinophils in COPD. Changes in various mediators have been found in sputum supernatant of COPD patients [IL-8, LTB-4, and tumor necrosis factor-alpha (TNF-α)].
- *Interstitial lung diseases*: IS has been used to study interstitial lung disease (ILD), more specifically pneumoconiosis, sarcoidosis, and nongranulomatous etiology in ILD.
- *Opportunistic infection (OI) in immunocompromised host*: In human immunodeficiency virus (HIV)/acquired immunodeficiency syndrome (AIDS), *P. jirovecii (carinii)* cysts can be diagnosed when sputum smear is stained with Grocott methenamine silver stain which will be taken up by the cell wall.
- *Lung fluke*: The presence of ova of *P. westermani* in sputum is diagnostic of lung fluke and can be better seen by adding 1% sulfuric acid.
- *Others*: Cough due to gastroesophageal reflux disease (GERD) has shown increased macrophages laden with lipid in IS.

Sputum will always remain an important diagnostic tool because of the ease and simplicity in obtaining a sample.

SPUTUM EXAMINATION IN REVISED NATIONAL TUBERCULOSIS CONTROL PROGRAM

As per recent guidelines of RNTCP, sputum should be examined for all cases of presumptive pulmonary TB cases. Presumptive TB cases are patients with cough for >2 weeks, unexplained fever for >2 weeks, hemoptysis, unexplained weight loss, and abnormal chest X-ray (CXR). CXR and sputum smear examination for AFB should be done simultaneously. CBNAAT should be done in smear negative but X-ray positive cases, people living with HIV infections, pediatric patients, and in smear and CXR negative cases with strong clinical suspicion for TB.

Sputum smear microscopy as before, as the primary tool for diagnosing tool.

Using rapid molecular diagnostics nucleic acid amplification (NAAT)—CBNAAT/TrueNat upfront wherever possible for early diagnosis of TB and all notified new patients for testing resistance to rifampicin.

For upfront NAAT, one specimen is tested using NAAT and if TB is detected the other sample is used for further cascade testing by line probe assay (LPA) and liquid culture.

■ CONCLUSION

Sputum being the mirror for many diseases of the Lung, non-invasive be used more and more.

SUGGESTED READINGS

1. Jauregin W, Comerana JM. Activated terapentua de la acebrofillena en la enfermedad obstructive clonica o arm bronghial. Orient Med. 1987;36(1336):29-30.
2. Bickerman HA, Sproul EE, Barach AL. An aerosol method of producing bronchial secretion in human subjects: a clinical technic for the detection of lung cancer. Dis Chest. 1958;33(4):347-62.
3. Long MH, Johansson E, Lonnroth K, Eriksson B, Winkvist A, Diwan VK. Longer delays in tuberculosis diagnosis among women in Vietnam. Int J Tuberc Lung Dis. 1999;3(5):388-93.
4. Gupta KB, Garg S. Sputum induction—a useful tool in diagnosis of respiratory diseases. Lung India. 2006; 23:82-6.
5. Iredate MJ, Wanklyn SA, Phillips IP, Krausz T, Ind PW. Non-invasive assessment of bronchial inflammation in asthma: no correlation between eosinophilia of induced sputum and responsiveness to inhaled hypertonic saline. Clin Exp Allergy. 1994;24(10):940-5.
6. Popov TA, Pizzichini MM, Pizzichini E, Kolendowicz R, Punthakee Z, Dolovich J, et al. Some technical factors influencing the induction of sputum for cell analysis. Eur Respir J. 1995;8(4):559-65.
7. Chalmers JD, Pletz MW, Aliberti S. Community-acquired Pneumonia. Lausanne: European Respiratory Monograph; 2014. pp. 26-9.
8. Seaton A, Seaton D, Leitch AG. Crofton and Douglas Respiratory Disease, 5th edition. London: Blackwell publisher; 2008. pp. 104-5.
9. Fukushima K, Nakamura S, Inoue Y, Higashiyama Y, Ohmichi M, Ishida T, et al. Utility of a sputum antigen detection test in Pneumococcal pneumonia and lower respiratory infectious disease in adults. Intern Med. 2015;54(22):2843-50.
10. Tadolini M, Centis R, D'Ambrosio L, et al. Clinical diagnosis of TB and role of GeneXpert. Breathe. 2012;9:104.

CHAPTER 7: Basic Investigations: Indications and Interpretations

B1. INTERPRETING THE CHEST X-RAY

AG Ghoshal, Shyam Krishnan

"Every chest X-ray has a story"

■ INTRODUCTION

Medical imaging continues to play an ever-important role in diagnoses and patient management. Throughout the years, chest X-ray (CXR) has remained the day-to-day workhorse for health professionals.

Chest X-ray uses a very small dose (≈0.2 mSv) of ionizing radiation to produce pictures of the inside of the chest. X-rays are a type of electromagnetic radiation. The term X-ray is shorthand for X-radiation, so named simply because it was an unknown form of radiation when discovered. X-rays were discovered by Wilhelm Röntgen, which is why X-rays are sometimes called Röntgen rays in other parts of the world. Röntgen was the recipient of the first Nobel Prize in Physics for his discovery.

The CXR often represents the first imaging step, not only in diseases that focus on the cardiovascular and respiratory systems, but in systemic illness too. A CXR as an investigation has its own limitations and biases.

In a CXR, one can recognize *air, water, and bone density*. About 99% of the lung is air, while the pulmonary vasculature and interstitial space constitute just 1% of the lung.

Traditionally, the X-ray film was exposed, developed, coded, and placed in an envelope or packet, and stored for review. However, with the advent of digital radiography and the picture archiving and communication system (PACS), the images can be viewed remotely and manipulated via a workstation by clinicians in different locations, almost as soon as they are acquired.

■ TECHNICAL ASPECTS

- *Focus film distance*: 1.85 m (6 ft)
- kVp 60–80
- Centering at T5
- Full inspiration (right)—anterior end of sixth rib; posterior end of 10th rib.

For a standard CXR, the following aspects must be considered:
- Orientation
- Position
- Rotation
- Penetration
- Lung volume
- Artifacts

Orientation

To ensure that the orientation is correct, we place a *side marker* for the right or left side.

Position/Projection

The erect position is optimal for chest radiography. All posterior-anterior (PA) films will be obtained with the patient in standing position, and most anterior-posterior (AP) films with the patient in either standing or sitting position. All supine films are obtained AP and reserved for sick patients receiving intensive therapy. Again, all films other than those taken PA erect should be labeled with the position. Positioning has a significant influence on the appearance of air, fluid, and blood vessels within the chest.

Rotation

In the case of rotation, one side of the radiograph becomes darker than the other. This phenomenon is known as *increased transradiancy*. Therefore, one side becomes more transradiant (darker) than the other. The diagnostic error here is that the reviewer may misinterpret this difference in transradiancy as pathology **(Fig. 7B1.1)**.

Penetration

With the correct exposure factors, the end plates of the lower thoracic vertebral bodies should be just visible through the cardiac shadow. An underpenetrated film looks diffusely opaque (too white), structures behind the heart are obscured, and left lower lobe pathology may be easily missed. An overpenetrated film looks diffusely lucent, the lungs appear darker than usual, and the vascular markings and lung detail are poorly seen.

Lung Volumes

Full inspiration is required to detect intrapulmonary abnormalities. The diaphragm should be seen at the level of the 8th–10th posterior ribs or the right sixth anterior rib with good inspiration. Poor inspiration may cause increased opacification of the lungs because of atelectasis, most commonly affecting the base of each lung.

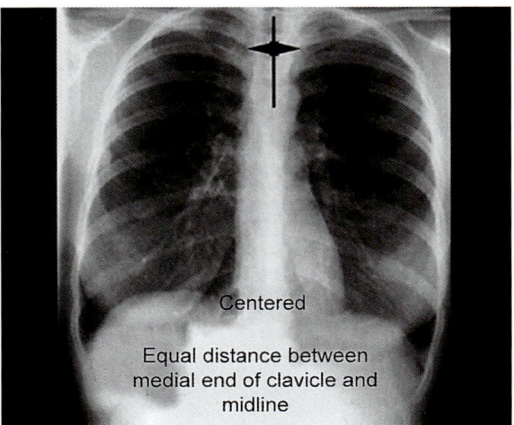

FIG. 7B1.1: Chest radiograph image showing an equal distance between medial end of clavicle and midline.

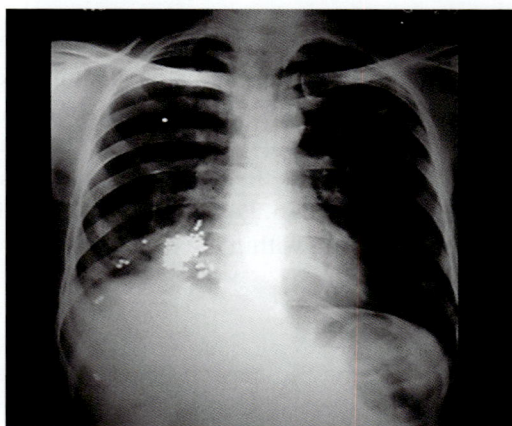

FIG. 7B1.2: Gun pellets lodged in the subcutaneous tissue overlying the right lower lobe.

Artifacts

Common artifacts include electrocardiogram (ECG) stickers, the patient's ornaments and clothing, hospital bedding, skin folds, etc. The presence of an opacity with a very well-defined margin, or one that is projected over both the lungs and adjacent soft tissues, should prompt a visual examination of the chest wall **(Fig. 7B1.2)**.

Discarding or Repeating Images

If the image is not of the best quality but the clinical question can still be answered, a CXR need not be repeated. If you are not sure if a repeat image will be of use, then discuss the case with a radiographer or radiologist. Do not immediately discard a CXR because it is not perfect. Even suboptimal images demonstrate life-threatening abnormalities, which may require your immediate attention.

Errors

There are interobserver errors as well as intraobserver errors. These errors tend to crop up due to two main factors:
1. Quality of the film
2. Familiarity with the disease

■ TECHNIQUE FOR RADIOGRAPH VIEWING

- Directed search through a systematic pattern
- Free global search

Systematic Review

- Airways
- Bones

- Cardiac silhouette
- Diaphragm
- Edges
- Fields
- Gas
- Hilum
- Instrumentation—lines and tube

Airways
- *Ensure trachea is visible and in midline*:
    - Trachea gets pushed away from abnormality, e.g., pleural effusion or tension pneumothorax.
    - Trachea gets pulled toward abnormality, e.g., atelectasis.
    - Trachea normally narrows at the vocal cords.
    - View the carina, angle should be between 60 and 100°.
    - Beware of things that may increase this angle, e.g., left atrial enlargement, lymph node enlargement, and left upper lobe atelectasis.
    - Follow out both main stem bronchi.
- *Check for a widened mediastinum*:
    - Mass lesions (e.g., tumor and lymph nodes)
    - Inflammation (e.g., mediastinitis and granulomatous inflammation)
    - Trauma and dissection (e.g., hematoma and aneurysm of the major mediastinal vessels)

Bones
- Check for fractures, dislocation, subluxation, and osteoblastic or osteolytic lesions in clavicles, ribs, and thoracic.
- Spine and humerus including osteoarthritic changes
- At this time, also check the soft tissues for subcutaneous air, foreign bodies, and surgical clips.
- Caution with nipple shadows, which may mimic intrapulmonary nodules:
    - Compare side-to-side, if on both sides the "nodules" in question are in the same position, then they are likely to be due to nipple shadows.

Cardiac Silhouette
- *Check heart size and heart borders*:
    - Cardiothoracic ratio: Cardiac size is measured by drawing vertical parallel lines down the most lateral points on each side of the heart and measuring between them. Thoracic width is measured by drawing vertical parallel lines down the inner aspect of the widest points of the rib cage and measuring between them **(Fig. 7B1.3)**.
    - The cardiothoracic ratio is frequently expressed as a percentage. A value of greater than 1:2 (50%) is considered abnormal.
    - Assessment of heart size is measured in the PA view, and that cardiac size is not exaggerated by factors such as patient rotation.

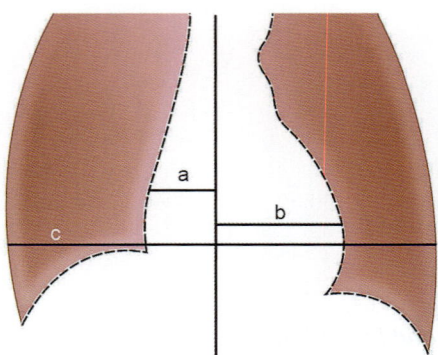

FIG. 7B1.3: Cardiothoracic ratio = [a+b/c]. Values >1:2 is considered abnormal.

- *Check aorta*: Widening, tortuosity, and calcification
- *Check heart valves*: Calcification and valve replacements
- *Check superior vena cava (SVC), inferior vena cava (IVC), and azygos vein*: Widening and tortuosity

Diaphragm

- *Right hemidiaphragm*:
    - Should be higher than the left
    - If much higher, think of effusion, lobar collapse, and diaphragmatic paralysis.
    - If you cannot see parts of the diaphragm, consider infiltrate or effusion.
    - Normally the angle made by the diaphragm with the chest wall is an acute angle; if there is a pleural effusion, the costophrenic angle will be blunted.
    - The diaphragm is normally rounded in contour, but there will be flattening if the lungs are hyperinflated.
- If film is taken in erect or upright position, you may see free air under the diaphragm if intra-abdominal perforation is present.

Edges

Borders of heart and mediastinum—*"Silhouette Sign"*: When two adjoining surfaces are of different densities, due to their differential absorption of the X-rays, they appear distinct. But when the adjoining surfaces are of similar densities, due to similar X-ray absorption they merge with each other with loss of the outline (Silhouette) demarcating them. The Silhouette sign describes the loss of a normal lung or soft tissue interface or "silhouette", caused by any pathology which either replaces or displaces normal air-filled lung. This sign is commonly applied to the heart, mediastinum, chest wall, and diaphragm.

Fields

- *Check for infiltrates*:
    - Identify the location of infiltrates by use of known radiological phenomena, e.g., loss of heart borders or of the contour of the diaphragm.

- Remember that right middle lobe abuts the heart, but the right lower lobe does not.
  - The lingula abuts the left side of the heart.
- *Identify the pattern of infiltration*:
  - Interstitial pattern (reticular) versus alveolar (patchy or nodular) pattern
  - Lobar collapse
  - Look for air bronchograms, tram tracking, nodules, and Kerley B lines.
  - Pay attention to the apices.
- Shadowing, opacification, increased density, and increased whiteness are all acceptable terms.
- *Lesion descriptors* may lead you toward a diagnosis. Be descriptive rather than jumping to a diagnosis.

Lesion descriptors:
- *Tissue involved*: Lung, heart, aorta, bone, etc.
- *Size*: Large/small/varied
- *Side*: Right or left; unilateral or bilateral
- *Number*: Single or multiple
- *Distribution*: Focal or widespread
- *Position*: Anterior/posterior/lung zone, etc.
- *Shape*: Round/crescentic, etc.
- *Edge*: Smooth/irregular/spiculated
- *Pattern*: Nodular/reticular (net-like)
- *Density*: Air/fat/soft tissue/calcium/metal

Gas

- Check the correct position of the gastric bubble.
- Look for free air.
- Look for bowel loops between diaphragm and liver.
- Beware of hiatus hernia.

Hilum

The hilar point on either side of the heart represents the intersection of the pulmonary arteries and veins. The left hilar point normally lies higher than the right. Aside from this, the hila should always be equal in size and density **(Fig. 7B1.4)**.
- Check the position and size bilaterally.
- Enlarged lymph nodes
- Calcified nodules
- Mass lesions
- Pulmonary arteries, if greater than 1.5 cm, think about possible causes of enlargement.

Instrumentation—Lines and Tubes

- Check for tubes, pacemaker, wires, lines, foreign bodies, etc.
- *Central lines* should pass to the lower SVC and should not enter the right atrium.

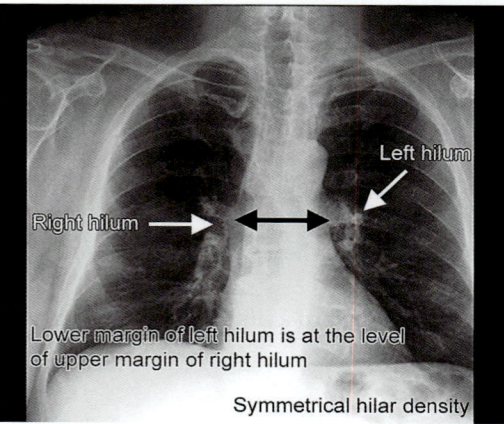

FIG. 7B1.4: Chest radiograph showing left and right hilar points.

- *Pulmonary artery catheters* should not be wedged into small branches.
- *Endotracheal tubes* should have the tip at least 2.5 cm above the carina, optimally midway between the carina and thoracic inlet.
- *Gastric tubes* should pass below the diaphragm and into the stomach.
- *Chest drains*: Check the position. The tip of the tube should lie in an effective position and not be misplaced or displaced into lung tissue.

■ COMMON RADIOLOGICAL SIGNS

Some common radiological signs encountered **(Fig. 7B1.5)** in daily practice are described here.

Consolidation

Consolidation is the result of filling of the alveoli by any cause, e.g., fluid (e.g., pulmonary edema), pus, blood (e.g., pulmonary hemorrhage), and tumor (especially bronchioloalveolar cell carcinoma). Clinical correlation is therefore essential to make the diagnosis. Lobar consolidation usually obeys the anatomical fissures; consolidation is limited to the affected lobe **(Fig. 7B1.6)**.

Atelectasis

It refers to collapse of the lung resulting in loss of aeration of the lung tissue. Collapse results mostly from an intrabronchial mass or mucus plug or clot obstructing the bronchus. It may also result from an extrinsic compression obliterating the bronchial lumen **(Fig. 7B1.7)**.

Pleural Effusions

Abnormal collection of pleural fluid in the pleural space is called pleural effusion. Over 150 mL pleural fluid is required for it to appear on an "erect" CXR, lower volumes >75 mL

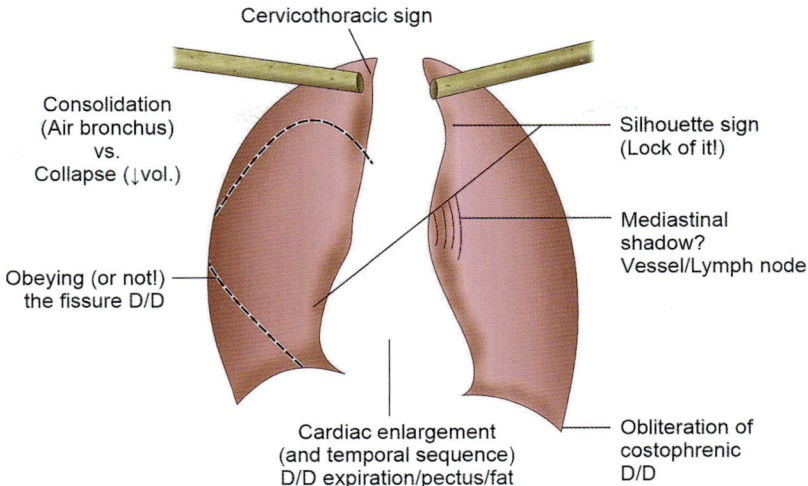

FIG. 7B1.5: Radiological signs encountered in daily practice.

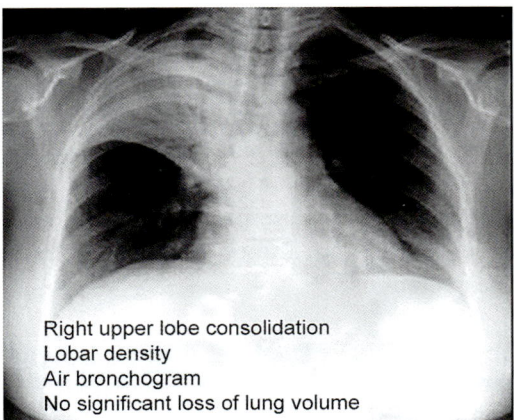

Right upper lobe consolidation
Lobar density
Air bronchogram
No significant loss of lung volume

FIG. 7B1.6: Chest radiograph showing right upper lobe consolidation.

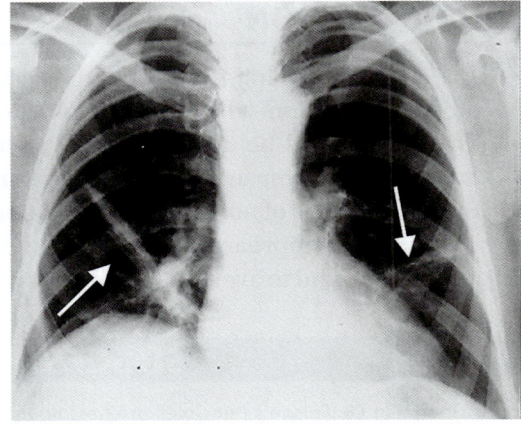

FIG. 7B1.7: Chest radiograph demonstrating the collapse of right middle lobe collapse and left lingular collapse.

can be detected in a decubitus film. It initially appears as a blunting of the respective costophrenic angle, but as the volume increases, it eventually appears as an area of increased density with a meniscus rising up the lateral chest wall **(Fig. 7B1.8)**.

Pneumothorax

The presence of air in the pleural space is called pneumothorax. It is classified as *simple* and *tension* pneumothorax based on the clinical features and amount of air in the pleural space **(Fig. 7B1.9)**.

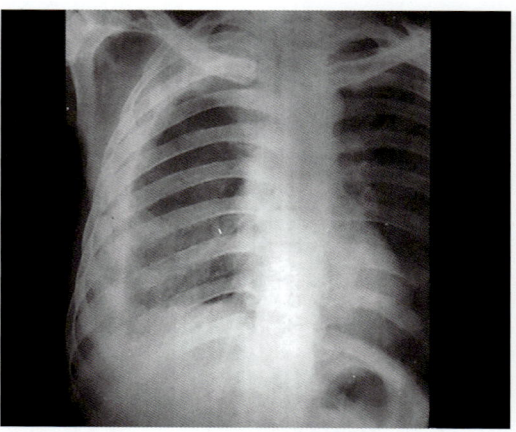
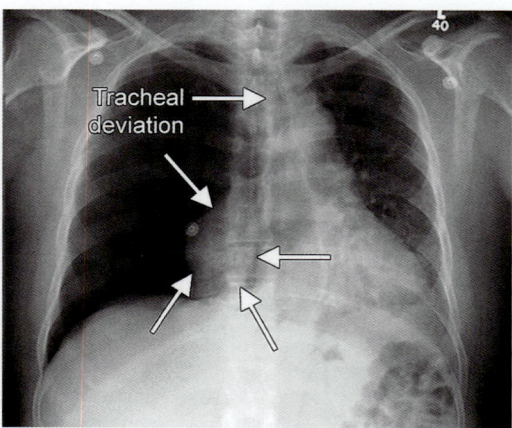

FIG. 7B1.8: Chest radiograph showing right-sided costophrenic angle with a right-sided peripheral vertical column of increased density suggestive of a lamellar effusion.

FIG. 7B1.9: Chest X-ray film of tension pneumothorax showing right-sided hyperlucency accompanied with leftward shift of the trachea and the white arrows showing the collapsed lung border.

■ CONCLUSION

- The chest radiograph is an affordable, accessible, and effective diagnostic tool. Like any other investigation, it has share of limitations as it is prone to errors and biases.
- The CXR should be used to answer specific clinical questions and should always be interpreted keeping the clinical history in mind.
- Basic knowledge of normal thoracic anatomy is essential when interpreting the CXR.
- A systematic approach to CXR review is necessary to gain the optimum diagnostic information and to avoid potential errors in interpretation.

SUGGESTED READINGS

1. Goodman LR. Felson's Principles of Chest Roentgenology: A Programmed Text. Elsevier Health Sciences; 2014. p. 424.
2. Sperber M (Ed). Radiologic Diagnosis of Chest Disease. Springer Science & Business Media; 2012. p. 602.
3. McLoud T. Thoracic Radiology: The Requisites. Elsevier Health Sciences; 2010. p. 1865.
4. Boyars M. Chest Roentgenography for Pulmonary Evaluation. In: Walker HK, Hall WD, Hurst JW (Eds). Clinical Methods: The History, Physical, and Laboratory Examinations, 3rd edition. Boston: Butterworths; 1990.

B2. ROLE OF CHEST X-RAY (LATERAL VIEW) IN RESPIRATORY SYSTEM

Udas Chandra Ghosh

■ INTRODUCTION

Chest X-ray (CXR) or film is the most frequently requested radiological investigation in clinical medicine. Plain posteroanterior (PA) film is commonly asked for, but lateral film should not be undertaken routinely.

A high kVp (120–170 kVp) or normal kVp technique with or without grid may be required for lateral film. For sharpness, the side of interest (right or left) is nearest to the film. The patient's arms are folded and extended above the head or displaced back if the anterior mediastinum is of interest.

Figures 7B2.1A to C show the lateral view of both sides of chest showing lobes and different segments (including middle lobe).

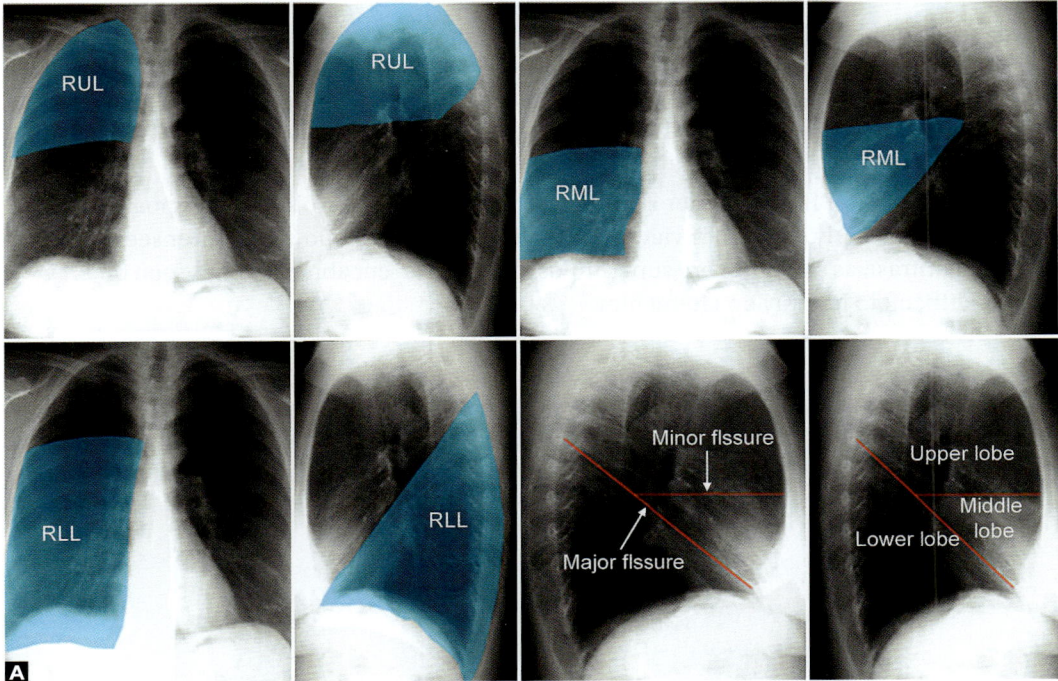

FIGS. 7B2.1A TO C: *Continued.*

Continued

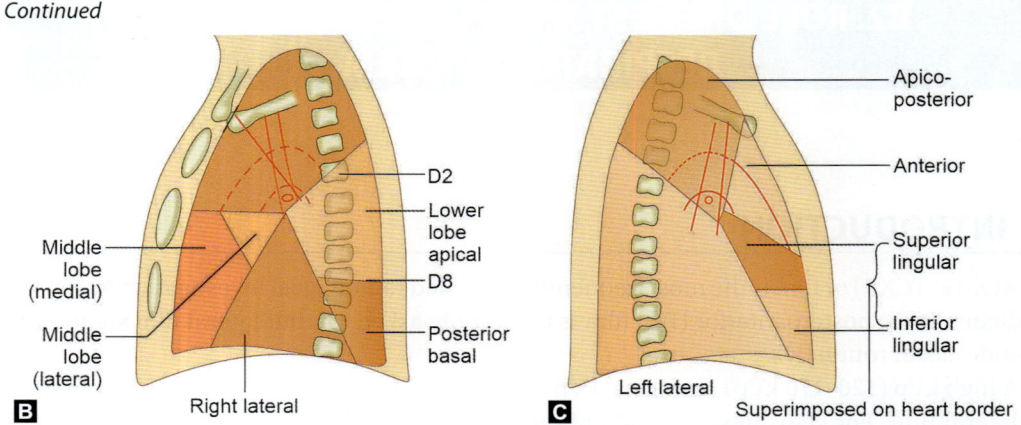

FIGS. 7B2.1A TO C: Lateral view of both sides of chest showing lobes and different segments (including middle lobe).
(RLL: right lower lobe; RML: right middle lobe; RUL: right upper lobe)

■ IMPORTANCE OF LATERAL VIEW

Lesions obscured on the PA film are often clearly demonstrated on the lateral view. As the left side of the chest is more obscured than right side in PA film, left side is positioned adjacent to the film but when there is a specific lesion, that side is positioned adjacent to the film. Anterior mediastinal masses are merged with mediastinal shadow which is cleared on lateral view **(Fig. 7B2.2)**.

Encysted pleural fluid is better seen in lateral view, and consolidation in posterior basal segment is not clearly seen in PA view due to overlying heart shadow but better seen in lateral view. By contrast, as two lungs are superimposed, the clear-cut abnormalities seen on PA view may be difficult to identify on lateral film.

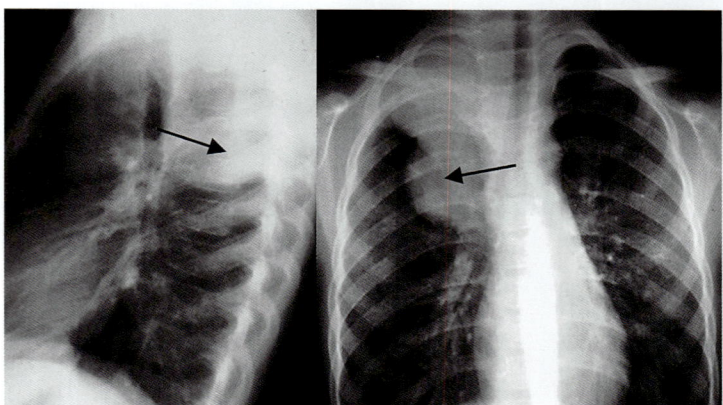

FIG. 7B2.2: Posterior mediastinal mass.

Other Views [Oblique, Apical, Apical Lordotic, Decubitus (Supine and Lateral) and Expiratory and Inspiratory]

The different plain films, e.g., *oblique, apical, apical lordotic, decubitus* (supine and lateral) and **expiratory and inspiratory** films may assist in the diagnosis of the complex problems of the respiratory system before proceeding to the expensive and invasive procedure.

The retrocardiac area, the posterior costophrenic angles, and the chest wall with pleural plaques are clearly demonstrated in *oblique* views. When the patient is unable to stand, or in portable radiographs, AP film is taken where the ribs and the posterior chest wall are well shown. In PA film, scapulae overlie the upper lungs and clavicles are projected more cranially over the apices, and the disk spaces of cervical spines are more clearly seen. In portable AP view, the shorter film-focus distance (FFD) results in apparent enlargement of the heart.

For good visualization of the apex, apical view or apical lordotic view on PA film is useful. To differentiate the subpulmonary effusion from any other cause of elevated diaphragm and or lower lobe consolidation, supine and decubitus position of PA view is helpful where the free fluid is displaced in subpulmonary effusion. The lateral decubitus film helps to differentiate the small amount of pleural fluid from thickened pleura.

Paired inspiratory and expiratory films demonstrate air trapping and diaphragm movement. Small pneumothorax and interstitial shadow are more apparent on the expiratory film. However, these paired films accurately diagnose small pneumothorax which is more prominent in expiratory film. These paired films are very important in children with a possible diagnosis of inhaled foreign body.

■ CLINICAL IMPORTANCE

Lateral view is helpful to diagnose middle lobe syndrome; the minor and major fissures are parallel to each other (arrows), and the atelectic lobe can be seen as a band of opacity between the fissures projecting over the cardiac silhouette **(Figs. 7B2.3A and B)**.

Lateral view is also helpful to diagnose pneumothorax and pneumomediastinum **(Figs. 7B2.4A to C)**.

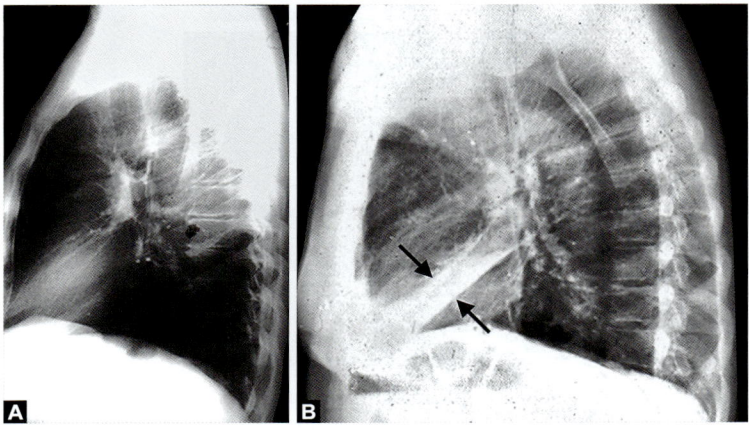

FIGS. 7B2.3A AND B: (A) Normal lung; (B) Right middle lobe atelectasis.

Lateral view of X-ray differentiates pleural effusion from large cystic lesion and encysted pleural effusion **(Figs. 7B2.5 to 7B2.7)**.

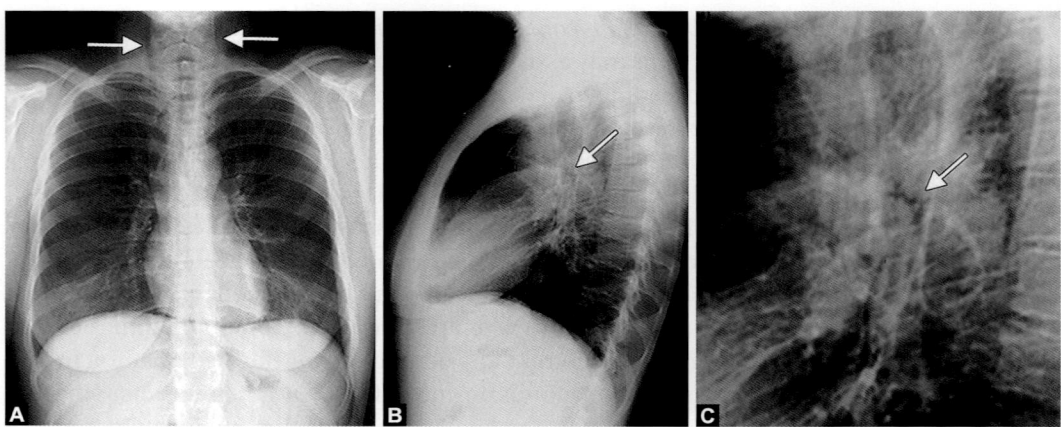

FIGS. 7B2.4A TO C: (A) Linear lucencies overlying the upper chest and neck (arrows)—pneumomediastinum; (B) "Ring around the artery" sign (arrow), a finding seen in pneumomediastinum; (C) A magnified view of the "ring around the artery" sign (arrow).

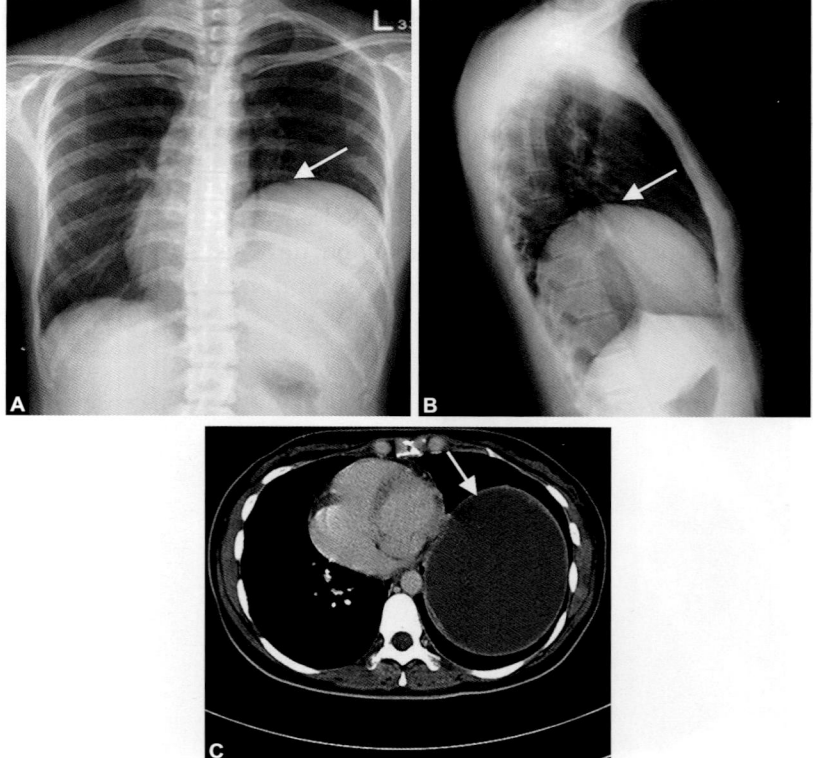

FIGS. 7B2.5A TO C: (A and B) Chest X-ray posteroanterior and lateral: Left lower lung mass mimicking elevated left side diaphragm (arrows); (C) CT scan: A huge encapsulated cystic tumor (arrow) at left lower lung field and right displacement of the heart.

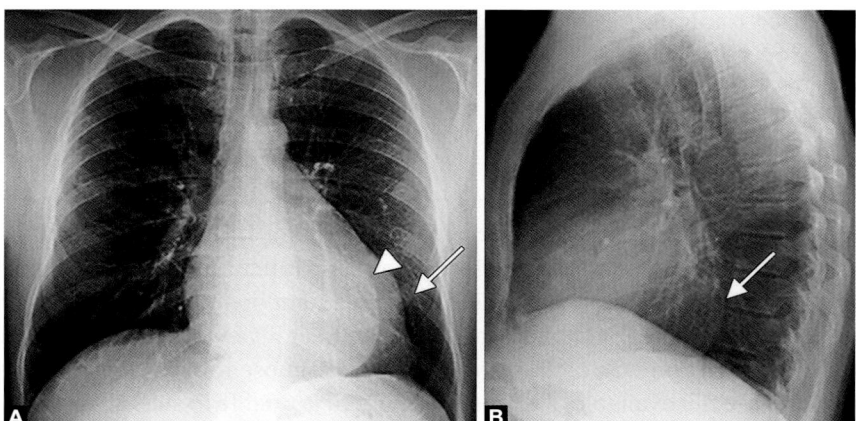

FIGS. 7B2.6A AND B: (A) Chest X-ray posteroanterior view shows the border of the left ventricle (arrowhead) surrounded by a lower density border of a pericardial lipoma (arrow); (B) A lateral view shows the posteriorly positioned low-density lipoma of the pericardium (arrow).

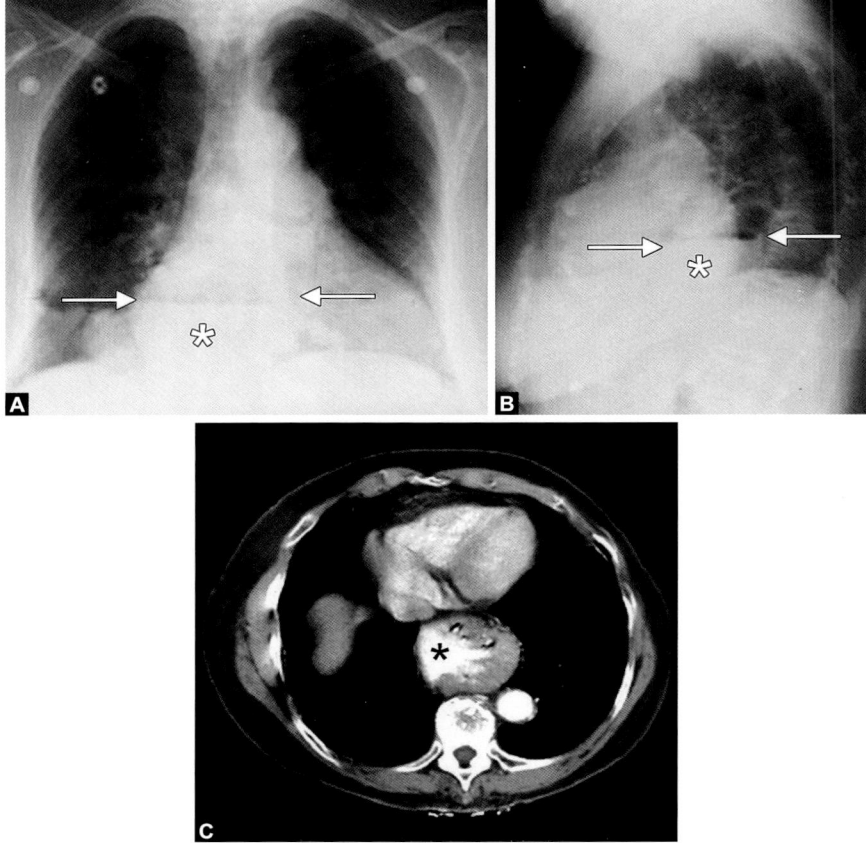

FIGS. 7B2.7A TO C: (A) Chest X-ray (anteroposterior) shows a hiatus hernia (asterisk) with an air-fluid level (arrows); (B) A lateral chest X-ray confirms a hiatus hernia (asterisk) and an air-fluid level in the hernia (arrows); (C) A CT scan shows contrast in the hiatus hernia (asterisk).

So, apart from traditional PA views, lateral view, and other views are helpful to diagnose the disease processes, where CT scan facilities are not available and when the patient is unable to stand.

■ CONCLUSION

The lateral films should not be undertaken routinely. The lateral CXR is less frequently requested and more difficult to interpret. Nevertheless it contains much information on the thoracic cage, pleura, lungs, pericardium, heart, mediastinum and upper abdomen. Lesions obscured on the PA film are often clearly demonstrated on the lateral view. So, apart from traditional PA views, lateral view, and other views are helpful to diagnose the disease processes, where CT scan facilities are not available and when the patient is unable to stand.

SUGGESTED READINGS

1. David Sutton, Textbook of Radiology and Imaging, Seventh edition, Volume 1, pp. 13-15.
2. Harrison's Principles of Internal Medicine, 21st edition, Volume 2, 2024 pp. 2142-43.

C. ARTERIAL BLOOD GAS ANALYSIS—A STEP-WISE APPROACH

Sekhar Chakraborty

■ INTRODUCTION

Any critically ill patient should be examined in intensive care unit (ICU) or in emergency with a proper arterial blood gas (ABG) analysis to arrive at a correct diagnosis and to offer appropriate management. Therefore, all intensivists and critical care physicians should be conversant with the ABG analysis at bed side.

■ APPLICATIONS OF ARTERIAL BLOOD GAS

- To assess acid–base imbalance in critical illness
- To document respiratory failure and assess its severity
- To monitor patients on ventilators and assist in weaning
- To assess response to therapeutic interventions and mechanical ventilation
- To assess preoperative patients

■ STEP-WISE APPROACH TO ANALYZE ARTERIAL BLOOD GAS

Step 1: To collect an arterial blood sample
Step 2: To take focused history and to do clinical examination
Step 3: To validate ABG report
Step 4: To assess oxygenation
Step 5: To look at pH-acidemia or alkalemia
Step 6: To assess primary acid–base disorder
Step 7: To assess whether the disorder is acute or chronic if the primary disorder is respiratory
Step 8: To assess the degree of compensation
Step 9: To mind the gaps
Step 10: To look for mixed acid–base disturbances

Step 1: To Collect an Arterial Blood Sample

- Arterial blood gas sample should be collected at room air.
- Radial artery is preferred, but it can be collected from arteria dorsalis pedis, femoral, and brachial arteries.
- A 22-gauge needle and 2-mL syringe are preferred.
- Syringe must be occupied >50% by blood.
- Syringe should be preheparinized with 0.5 mL of heparin (1:1,000) and emptied immediately.
- Avoid air bubbles.
- Cool the sample immediately.

Table 7C.1: Berlin criteria for acute respiratory distress syndrome (ARDS) severity.

PaO_2/FiO_2 ratio	Inference
200–300 mm Hg	Mild ARDS
100–200 mm Hg	Moderate ARDS
<100 mm Hg	Severe ARDS

Table 7C.2: Normal values of arterial blood gas.

	Normal range	For calculation
pH	7.34–7.45	7.4
pCO_2	35–45	40
HCO_3	22–26	24
PO_2	>80	>95

Table 7C.3: List of primary acid–base disorders.

Disorder	pH	pCO_2 or HCO_3^-
Respiratory acidosis	pH low ↓	pCO_2 high ↑
Metabolic acidosis	pH low ↓	HCO_3^- low ↓
Respiratory alkalosis	pH high ↑	pCO_2 low ↓
Metabolic alkalosis	pH high ↑	HCO_3^- high ↑

In Case of Accidental Collection of Venous Sample

- Absence of flash of blood on puncturing the vessel
- Absence of pulsation during filling of syringe
- Absence of auto filling

Potential Errors While Collecting the Sample

- Air contamination—spurious high pO_2
- Froth in sample—discard it immediately
- Duration between collection and examination is more—blood cells consume oxygen and produce CO_2, hence lower the pH
- Excess anticoagulant-drop in pCO_2 and pO_2; pH usually remains unchanged.

Step 2: To Take Focused History and to do Clinical Examination

- History of pulmonary, renal, or any metabolic disorder
- History of vomiting (primary acid–base problem could be metabolic alkalosis due to loss of hydrochloric acid)
- History of diarrhea (primary problem could be metabolic acidosis due to loss of bicarbonate ions through stool)
- Duration of illness—acute or chronic

- History of drug intake or poisoning
- History of dyselectrolytemia

Step 3: To Validate Arterial Blood Gas Report

- If there is discrepancy between clinical condition and ABG values of the patient, check the validity of the report.
  - Calculate H⁺ ion concentration:
    - $[H^+] = 24 \times pCO_2/HCO_3^-$ Calculate $[H^+]$ from pH in ABG
    - $[H^+] = 80$ – last two digits of pH after decimal in ABG
  - Match the H⁺ ion concentration by two methods—A and B
    - If it is matched—ABG is valid.
    - If not matched—recheck the ABG.

Step 4: To Assess Oxygenation

- Look at oxygenation (PaO_2 and SaO_2)
- Look at PaO_2/FiO_2 ratio
  - Normally the ratio is 1:400 to 1:500.
  - If the ratio is <1:400—consider ventilation–perfusion (V/Q) mismatch or diffusion defect or intracardiac shunt.
  - It the ratio is <1:300—consider acute respiratory distress syndrome (ARDS) **(Table 7C.1)**.
- Look for A–a gradient (PAO_2-PaO_2). Here PAO_2 is partial pressure of oxygen in alveoli, and PaO_2 is partial pressure of oxygen in arterial blood.
- In room air, $PAO_2 = 150 - PaCO_2/0.8$
- PaO_2 is obtained from ABG.
- If the A–a gradient is >20 mm Hg at any age, it is abnormal.

Step 5: Look at pH—Acidemia or Alkalemia?

- If the pH is low—acidemia
- If the pH is high—alkalemia
- If the pH is normal—normal acid-base status or mixed acid-base disorder
  - An acidemia can result from—low HCO_3^- or high CO_2
  - An alkalemia can result from—high HCO_3^- or low CO_2

Step 6: To Assess Primary Acid–Base Disorder

- It is imperative at this point to know the normal values of ABG **(Table 7C.2)**.
- Look at CO_2 and HCO_3^- to determine whether the primary problem is metabolic or respiratory **(Table 7C.3)**.

Metabolic Acidosis

- *Primary decrease in HCO_3^-*: It is due to either the loss of bicarbonate or utilization of bicarbonate.

- The next step is to calculate anion gap (AG):
  - AG = $Na^+ - (Cl^- + HCO_3^-)$
  - Normal AG = 12 ± 2 mEq/L
  - HAG (high anion gap) = presence of unmeasured anions.
  - NAG (normal anion gap) = bicarbonate losses are compensated by cation loss.
- *Correct AG if there is hypoalbuminemia*:
  - For 1 g drop of albumin (below 4 g%), add 2–3 to calculated AG.

The causes of HAG and NAG metabolic acidosis can be memorized as the following mnemonics:
- *HAGMA are MUDPILERS*:
  - HAGMA = High anion gap metabolic acidosis
  - MUDPILERS:
    M = Methanol
    U = Uremia (chronic)
    D = Diabetic ketoacidosis
    P = Paraldehyde
    I = INH, iron
    L = Lactate
    E = Ethanol, ethylene glycol
    R = Rhabdomyolysis
    S = Salicylate
- *NAGMA are HARD-UP*:
  - NAGMA = Nonanion gap metabolic acidosis
  - HARD-UP:
    H = Hyperalimentation
    A = Acetazolamide
    R = Renal tubular acidosis
    D = Diarrhea
    U = Uremia (acute)
    P = Postventilation hypocapnia
- In case of non-AG metabolic acidosis, urinary AG is calculated.
  - Urinary AG = $UNa^+ + UK^+ - UCl^-$
- Urinary AG is usually negative or it may remain negative in case of diarrhea (nonrenal loss of bicarbonate).
- Urinary AG becomes positive in RTA (renal tubular acidosis).

Metabolic Alkalosis

- Due to increase of bicarbonate either by gain of HCO_3^- or extracellular volume contraction
- *Two types*:
  1. Saline responsive—> 20 mEq/L urinary chloride
  2. Saline nonresponsive—< 20 mEq/L urinary chloride

Respiratory Acidosis

- Due to primary rise in pCO_2
- Cause is alveolar hypoventilation.

Respiratory Alkalosis
- Due to primary fall in pCO_2
- Cause is alveolar hyperventilation.

Step 7: To Assess Whether the Disorder is Acute or Chronic if the Primary Disorder is Respiratory

- Consider history of the patient.
- Calculate the change in pH from 7.4 (normal pH).
  - In case of acute respiratory disorder (acidosis or alkalosis):
    - Change in pH = 0.008 × ($PaCO_2$ – 40)
    - Expected pH = 7.4 ± change in pH
  - In case of chronic respiratory disorder (acidosis or alkalosis):
    - Change in pH = 0.003 × ($PaCO_2$ – 40)
    - Expected pH = 7.4 ± change in pH
  - Compare pH on ABG with expected pH:
    - If the pH on ABG is close to A—acute disorder
    - If the pH on ABG is close to B—chronic disorder

Step 8: To Assess the Degree of Compensation

Compensatory responses and mechanisms for the primary acid–base disorders are listed in **Table 7C.4**.

Table 7C.4: List of compensatory mechanisms for primary acid–base disorders.

Primary disorder	Initial chemical change	Compensatory response	Compensatory mechanism	Expected level of compensation
Metabolic acidosis	↓ HCO_3^-	↓ pCO_2	Hyperventilation	pCO_2 = (1.5 × [HCO_3^-]) + 8 + 2 pCO_2 = last two digits of pH
Metabolic alkalosis	↑ HCO_3^-	↑ pCO_2	Hypoventilation	pCO_2 = (0.7 × [HCO_3^-]) + 21 + 2 pCO_2 = last two digits of pH
Respiratory alkalosis	↑ pCO_2	↑ HCO_3^-		
Acute			Buffering–rule of 1	↑ [HCO_3^-] = 1 mEq/L for every 10 mm Hg delta pCO_2
Chronic			Generation of new HCO_3^- —rule of 3	↑ [HCO_3^-] = 3 mEq/L for every 10 mm Hg delta pCO_2
Respiratory alkalosis	↓ pCO_2	↓ HCO_3		↓ [HCO_3^-] = 2 mEq/L for every 10 mm Hg delta pCO_2
Acute			Buffering–rule of 2	
Chronic			Decreased reabsorption of HCO_3^- —rule of 4	↓ [HCO_3^-] = 4 mEq/L for every 10 mm Hg delta pCO_2

Step 9: To Mind the Gaps

- Calculate AG and adjust AG in case of metabolic acidosis.
- Calculate delta gap = delta AG – delta HCO_3^-
  - Delta AG = calculated AG – 12
  - Delta CO_3 = 24 – patient's HCO_3^-
  - Normally delta gap is zero if there is only acidosis
  - Raised or decreased delta gap = mixed disorder
- Osmolar gap = calculated plasma osmolality–measured osmolality
  - Normally the gap is < 20 mOsmol/Kg H_2O
  - If it is raised—unaccounted anions

Step 10: Look for Mixed Acid–Base Disturbances

Mixed acid–base disturbances are suspected when there is:
- Absence of compensation
- Overcompensation
- Long-standing pulmonary or renal disease
- Respiratory assistance required

■ CASE VIGNETTE 1

A 50-year-old male has undergone gastrectomy and discharged. He returned after 2 weeks with nausea, vomiting, and altered mental status. He was readmitted to the ICU. His temperature was 39°C, BP was 86/50 mm Hg, and pulse rate was 130 beats/min. He is drowsy and minimally responsive lungs: clear, respiratory rate: increased, no rub, no edema, and abdomen is diffusely tender.

His ABG is ......

pH	7.24	Na^+	132
pCO_2	24	K^+	8.2
HCO_3^-	12	Cl^-	95
pO_2	68	HCO_3^-	12

- pH: 7.24 (low), acidosis
- pCO_2: 24 (low), respiratory alkalosis
- HCO_3^-: 12 (low), metabolic acidosis
- Anion gap: 132 – (95 + 12) = 25
- Winter's equation (expected pCO_2): (12 × 1.5 = 18) + 8 = 26 (observed = 24)
- Delta change HCO_3^-: (25 – 12 = 13) + 12 (observed) = 25 (a normal HCO_3^-)
- What is the acid base disorder?
- *Answer*:
  - Anion gap metabolic acidosis
  - Compensatory respiratory alkalosis

CHAPTER 7: Basic Investigations: Indications and Interpretations

CASE VIGNETTE 2

A 24-year-old female presented with lethargy and shortness of breath for last 3–4 days. She had upper abdominal pain and vomiting 1 week ago. Examination revealed: Temperature: 37°C; BP: 100/60 mm Hg; Pulse: 129/min; Respiratory rate: 30; Lungs: clear; Abdomen: normal, no edema; Skin: poor turgor, and dry mucous membranes.

pH	7.10	Na^+	140
pCO_2	15	K^+	6.5
HCO_3^-	5	Cl^-	100
pO_2	110	HCO_3^-	5

- pH: 7.1 (low), acidosis
- pCO_2: 15 (low), respiratory alkalosis
- HCO_3^-: 5 (low), metabolic acidosis
- Anion gap: 140 − (100 + 5) = 35
- Winter's equation (expected pCO_2): (5 × 1.5 = 7.5) + 8 = 15.5 (observed = 15)
- Delta changes HCO_3^-: (35 − 12 = 23) + 5 (observed) = 28 (an elevated HCO_3^-)
- What is the acid base disorder ?
- *Answer*:
  - Anion gap metabolic acidosis
  - Compensatory respiratory alkalosis
  - Metabolic alkalosis

CASE VIGNETTE 3

A 55-year-old man collapsed in a bar and was brought to the emergency room (ER). He was unresponsive, BP was not obtainable, pulse was found to be 140 beats/min, and he had peritoneal signs.

pH	6.86	Na^+	139
pCO_2	81	K^+	3.9
HCO_3^-	14	Cl^-	84
pO_2	55	HCO_3^-	16

He was intubated, started on pressors, and treated with HCO_3^-.

pH	7.04	Na^+	148
pCO_2	34	K^+	4.5
HCO_3^-	9	Cl^-	93
pO_2	110	HCO_3^-	10

On admission:
- pH: 6.85 (low), acidosis
- pCO_2: 81 (high), respiratory acidosis
- HCO_3^-: 16 (low), metabolic acidosis

- Anion gap: 139 − (84 + 16) = 39
- Winter's equation (expected pCO_2): (16 × 1.5 = 24) + 8 = 32 (lower than observed, 81)
- Delta change HCO_3^-: (39−12 = 27) + 16 (observed) = 43
- What is the acid base disorder ?
- Answer:
  - Anion gap metabolic acidosis
  - Respiratory acidosis
  - Metabolic alkalosis

After Intubation

- pH: 7.04 (low), acidosis
- pCO_2: 34 (low), respiratory alkalosis
- HCO_3^-: 10 (low), metabolic acidosis
- Anion gap: 148 − (93 + 10) = 45 (increasing)
- Winter's equation (expected pCO_2): (10 × 1.5 = 15) + 8 = 23 (lower than observed, 34)
- Delta change HCO_3^-: (45 − 12 + 33) + 10 (observed) = 43
- What is the acid base disorder ?
- Answer:
  - Anion gap metabolic acidosis (lactate was 24)
  - Respiratory alkalosis
  - Metabolic alkalosis

■ CASE VIGNETTE 4

A 20-year-old female attempted suicide by taking pills from mother's medicine box. She was brought to the ER. She was found alert, but agitated. BP: 140/60 mm Hg; Pulse: 126 beats/min; Temperature: 37°C, Respiratory rate: 32 breaths/min. Neurological examination was noncontributory.

pH	7.56	Na^+	140
pCO_2	15	K^+	4.5
HCO_3^-	13	Cl^-	107
pO_2	88	HCO_3^-	13

- pH: 7.56 (high), alkalosis
- pCO_2: 15 (low), respiratory alkalosis
- HCO_3^-: 13 (low), metabolic acidosis
- Anion gap: 140 (107 − 13) = 20
- Winter's equation (expected pCO_2): (13 × 1.5 = 19.5) + 8 = 27.5 (higher than observed, 15)
- Delta change HCO_3^-: (20 − 12 = 8) + 13 (observed) = 21 (only minimally reduced HCO_3^-)
- What is the acid base disorder ?
- Answer:
  - Salicylate poisoning
  - Anion gap metabolic acidosis
  - Primary respiratory alkalosis

CHAPTER 7: Basic Investigations: Indications and Interpretations

■ CASE VIGNETTE 5

A 34-year-old male of 60 kg body weight, brought to accident and emergency in a semicomatose state. He has a long history of alcohol abuse.

pH	7.16	Na⁺	140
pCO_2	23	K⁺	5.8
HCO_3^-	8	Cl⁻	103
pO_2	65	HCO_3^-	8

What is the acid–base disorder in this patient?
- *Answer*:
  - Metabolic acidosis with respiratory compensation

■ CASE VIGNETTE 6

- A 55-year-old woman presented with complaints of lethargy, thirst, muscle weakness, and generalized body pains. Previous emergency department visits with hypokalemia.
- Her serum potassium level was 2.6 mmol/L.
- *Other electrolytes*:
  - Sodium: 138 mmol/L
  - Chloride: 116 mmol/L
  - HCO_3^-: 17 mmol/L
  - BUN (blood urea nitrogen)/creatinine: Normal
  - Glucose: 75 mg/dL
- Urine analysis: pH 5.4, 2 + glucose
- Urine anion gap: –20
- ABG:
  - pH: 7.25
  - pCO_2: 28
  - pO^2: 100
  - Total bicarbonate: 15.1 mmol/L
  - Base excess: 13.7 mmol/L

What is the acid–base disorder in this patient?
- *Answer*:
  - Metabolic acidosis with respiratory compensation with type 2 RTA. (With negative urine AG, pH < 5.5 and low serum K)

SUGGESTED READINGS

1. Ghosh AK. Diagnosing acid-base disorders. J Assoc Physicians India. 2006;54:720-4.
2. Fencl V, Jabor A, Kazda A, J Figge. Diagnosis of metabolic acid-base disturbances in critically ill patients. Am J Resp Crit Care Med. 2000;162(6):2246-51.
3. Gluck SL. Acid–base. Lancet. 1998;352(9126):474-9.
4. Haber RJ. A practical approach to acid-base disorders. West J Med. 1991;155(2):146-51.

D. INTERPRETATION OF THE SPIROMETRY

Indranil Halder

■ INTRODUCTION

Interpretation of the spirometry result begins with a review and comment on test quality. Quality review of the spirometry curves (flow/volume and time/volume) should be done, and relying only on numerical results for clinical decision should not be done.

The standard of the forced vital capacity (FVC) should be checked. A minimum of three acceptable FVC maneuvers must be obtained. Repeatability criteria should be checked and met when there is no >100 mL ideally (and certainly no >150 mL in the occasional highly variable patient) between each blow. Encourage maximum effort at the start of each blow by verbally encouraging patient to continue to exhale to achieve maximal effort. The patient is to be observed so as to ensure that each FVC is performed to the best by ensuring that:
- The patient breathes into maximal inspiration.
- The mouthpiece is not obstructed with their teeth or tongue.
- There are no leaks from the mouthpiece.

The flow/volume curve is to be observed as each FVC maneuver is being performed to identify if there is any:
- Slow starts
- Early stops
- Variability in flow within maneuver

Ensure the patient exhales fully and that this is demonstrated in the graph showing a time/volume plateau.

No more than 8 FVC maneuvers are to be performed in one session. If the patient is unable to achieve these standards, it is to be recorded why this has not been possible, and arrangement for a further appointment to repeat the test is to be made if appropriate.

■ SELECTING THE BEST VALUE FOR CLINICAL USE

The best values are selected from three technically acceptable results selected from up to eight efforts, where the repeatability criteria are met.

■ CALCULATING THE REFERENCE

Value for Clinical Use

Predicted values and normal ranges can be obtained from reference tables. They are calculated from the patient's height in meters, age in years, and sex, and this is used to calculate the mean predicted values for forced expiratory volume in 1 second (FEV_1), FVC, and vital capacity (VC). Predicted values should be obtained from studies of "normal" or "healthy" subjects with the same anthropometric data (e.g., sex, age, and height) and, where relevant, ethnic characteristics of the patient being tested. The actual best measurement and the mean predicted value are used to calculate the % predicted value. The lower limit of normal (LLN) or range is calculated from the mean predicted value and the residual standard deviation.

Manufacturers usually provide software that allows the users to easily select among a panel of reference equations. They should also allow easy insertion of new equations. The reference values used should be documented on every spirometry report.

■ REPORTING THE SPIROMETRY RESULTS

The results should be reported with graphs of time/volume and flow/volume superimposing all efforts and a clear table of results showing at least the following values for FEV_1, FVC, FEV_1/FVC, peak expiratory flow (PEF), and VC. The actual, the mean predicted values, the % predicted value, and LLN range should also be displayed. A comparison of test results is done with reference values based on healthy subjects; comparison is also done with a known disease or abnormal physiological patterns (i.e., obstruction and restriction). A comparison with self is done for evaluating change in an individual patient.

A final step in the lung function report is to answer the clinical question that prompted the test. Poor preparatory steps increase the risk of misclassification, i.e., a falsely negative or falsely positive interpretation for a lung function abnormality. Patients whose results are near the thresholds of abnormality are at a greater risk of misclassification.

■ TYPES OF VENTILATORY DEFECTS

Spirometric tests can show the following patterns: Normal, obstructive, restrictive, and mixed abnormalities **(Fig. 7D.1)**.

Spirometry interpretations should be clear, concise, and informative. A mere statement of which values are normal or low is not helpful. Tests are not to be interpreted in the absence of any clinical information. Whenever possible, ask the physicians who are responsible for ordering tests to state the clinical question to be answered, and also, before testing, ask patients why they were sent for testing. Similarly, recording respiratory symptoms, such as cough, phlegm, wheezing, and dyspnea, as well as smoking status, and recent bronchodilator use could be helpful in this regard.

The interpretation will be most meaningful if the interpreter can address relevant clinical diagnoses, and for this the chest radiograph appearance and the most recent hemoglobin value may be helpful. Neuromuscular disease or upper airway obstruction (UAO) where relevant should also be suspected.

The FVC, FEV_1, and FEV_1/FVC ratio are the basic parameters used to properly interpret lung function.

Obstructive Abnormalities

A reduction in maximum expiratory airflow relative to the maximum volume that can be expelled from the lung (the VC, measured as a forced maneuver) reflects an obstructive

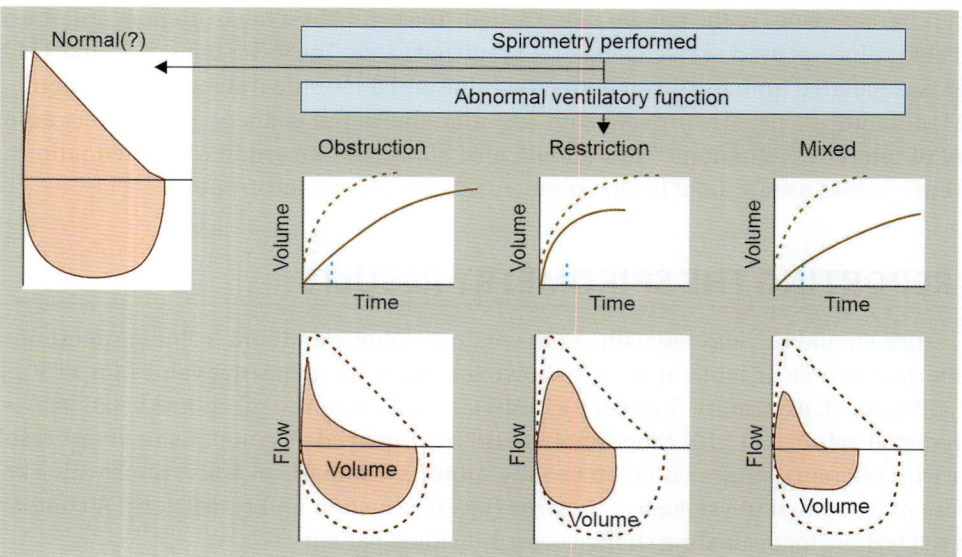

FIG. 7D.1: Volume-time and flow-volume curves under different ventilator defects.

ventilatory defect due to narrowed airways. In practice, the presence of airway obstruction is suggested by a reduced FEV_1/FVC ratio, and the expiratory flow volume curve will appear concave. Examples of obstructive lung abnormalities may be seen in patients of asthma and chronic obstructive pulmonary disease (COPD). Several organizations, e.g., Global Initiative for Chronic Obstructive Lung Disease (GOLD), have sought to simplify the diagnosis of airflow limitation by replacing the LLN with a fixed cut-off of 0.70. However, since the FEV_1/FVC ratio is dependent on age, height, and sex, this leads to overdiagnosis of obstructive lung disease in elderly subjects, and underdiagnosis in young subjects. Therefore, the presence of obstructive lung disease is better to be based on an FEV_1/FVC ratio below the LLN.

Special attention must be paid when FEV_1 and FVC are concomitantly decreased and the FEV_1/FVC ratio is normal or almost normal. This pattern most frequently reflects failure of the patient to inhale or exhale completely. It may also occur when the flow is so slow that the subject cannot exhale long enough to empty the lungs to residual volume (RV). In this circumstance, the flow/volume curve should appear concave toward the end of the maneuver. Total lung capacity (TLC) will be normal, and forced expiratory flow (FEF) will be low. Measurement of slow VC (inspiratory or expiratory) may then give a more correct estimate of the FEV_1/VC ratio.

When this pattern is observed in a patient performing a maximal, sustained effort, it may be useful to repeat spirometry after treatment with an inhaled bronchodilator. Significant improvement in the FEV_1, FVC or both would suggest the presence of reversible airflow obstruction.

Restrictive Abnormalities

Interstitial lung disease or extrinsic disorders such as kyphoscoliosis and ankylosing spondylitis as well as obesity may cause a restrictive lung defect. This is characterized by a normal or increased FEV_1/FVC ratio and a low FVC, and the expiratory flow volume curve will appear convex. However, the results of pulmonary function tests are highly dependent on patient cooperation. Premature termination of the FVC maneuver or failure to take a maximal inhalation can result in a high FEV_1/FVC ratio. Indeed the most common cause of a restrictive picture is poor technique. A true restrictive ventilatory defect may also occur concurrently with airway obstruction if the FVC and FEV_1/FVC are both below their LLN. This represents a mixed ventilatory defect, i.e., restriction and airway obstruction. This diagnosis cannot be made on the basis of spirometry alone. If there is clinical evidence for restrictive lung disease, referral to a pulmonary function laboratory with facilities to measure TLC and gas transfer is recommended.

Mixed Abnormalities

A mixed ventilatory defect is characterized by the coexistence of obstruction and restriction, and is defined physiologically when both FEV_1/FVC and FVC are below the LLN. Since FVC may be equally reduced in both obstruction and restriction, the presence of a restrictive component in an obstructed patient cannot be inferred from simple measurements of FEV_1 and FVC.

The maximal voluntary ventilation (MVV) is not generally included in the set of lung function parameters necessary for diagnosis or follow-up of the pulmonary abnormalities because of its good correlation with FEV_1. However, it may be of some help in clinical practice. For example, a disproportionate decrease in MVV relative to FEV_1 may be seen in neuromuscular disorders.

■ SEVERITY CLASSIFICATION

For general purposes, severity of obstructive lung function impairment is based on $FEV_1\%$ predicted **(Table 7D.1)**.

The FEV_1 may sometimes fail to properly identify the severity of a defect, especially at the very severe stages of the diseases. $FEV_1\%$ prediction correlates poorly with symptoms and may not, by itself, accurately predict clinical severity or prognosis for individual patients.

Severity grading based on degree of airflow obstruction is arbitrary, and correlates poorly with respiratory symptoms and quality of life. Additional measures of disease impact (for example, dyspnea score, exacerbation rate, and validated measure of health status) are required for a comprehensive assessment of COPD severity.

Table 7D.1: Severity of airway obstruction forced expiratory volume in 1 second (FEV_1) as a percentage of the predicted/reference value.		
Degree of severity	**GOLD stage**	**$FEV_1\%$ predicted**
Mild	I	>80
Moderate	II	50–79
Severe	III	30–49
Very severe	IV	<30

BRONCHODILATOR RESPONSE

There is no consensus about the drug, dose, or mode of administering a bronchodilator in the laboratory. Short-acting β2-agonists, such as salbutamol, are recommended. Four separate doses of 100 mg should be used when given by metered dose inhaler using a spacer. Tests should be repeated after a 15-minute delay. The first step in interpreting any bronchodilator test is to determine if any change greater than random variation has occurred.

Percent change from baseline and absolute changes in FEV_1 and/or FVC in an individual subject is used to identify a positive bronchodilator response.

An increase in FEV_1 and/or FVC >12% of control and >200 mL constitutes a positive bronchodilator response. In the absence of a significant increase in FEV_1 and/or FVC, an improvement in lung function parameters within the tidal breathing range, such as increased partial flows and decrease of lung hyperinflation, may explain a decrease in dyspnea. The lack of a bronchodilator response in the laboratory does not preclude a clinical response to bronchodilator therapy.

The interpretation of spirometry may be summarized and simplified in the **Flowchart 7D.1**.

CENTRAL AND UPPER AIRWAY OBSTRUCTION

Special attention should be paid by the technicians to obtain maximal and repeatable PEFs and forced inspiratory maneuvers if there is a clinical or spirometric reason to suspect a UAO. This may be confirmed by imaging and/or endoscopic techniques.

When patient's effort is good, the pattern of a repeatable plateau of forced inspiratory flow, with or without a forced expiratory plateau, suggests a variable extrathoracic central or UAO. Conversely, the pattern of a repeatable plateau of FEF, along with the lack of a forced inspiratory plateau, suggests a variable, intrathoracic central or UAO. The pattern of a

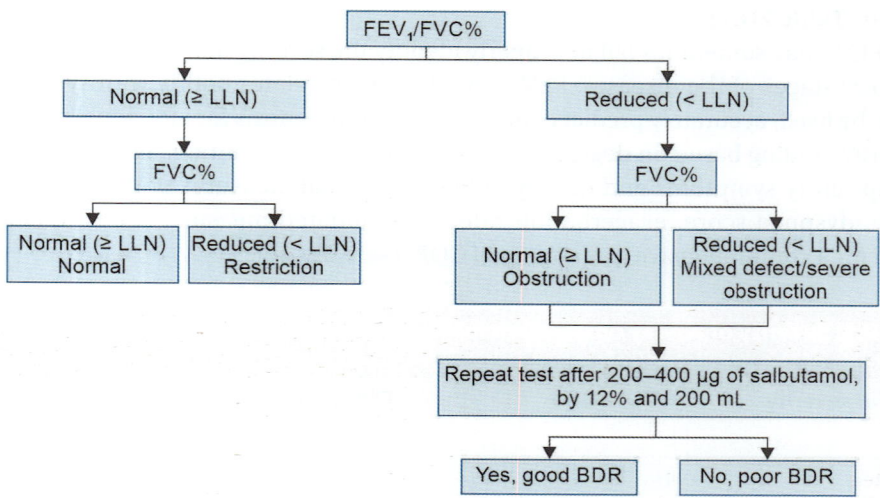

FLOWCHART 7D.1: Interpretation of spirometric data.
(BDR: bronchodilator response; FEV_1/FVC: forced expiratory volume in 1 second/forced vital capacity; LLN: lower limit of normal)

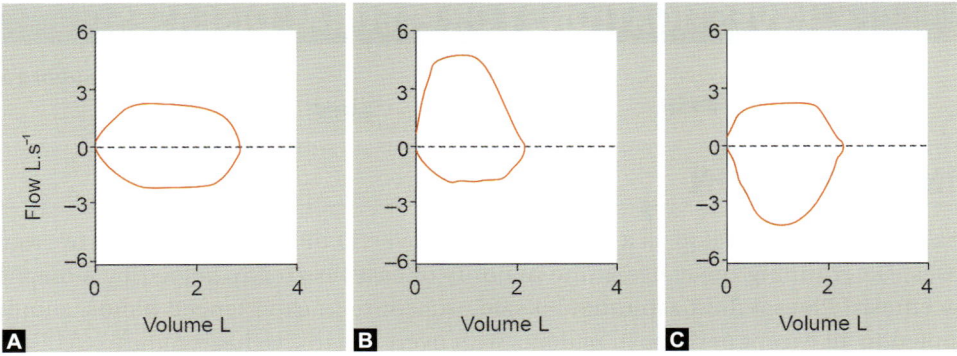

FIGS. 7D.2A TO C: Idealized examples of (A) fixed, (B) variable extrathoracic, and (C) variable intrathoracic airway obstruction.

repeatable plateau at a similar flow in both forced inspiratory and expiratory flows suggests a fixed central or UAO.

The effects of anatomical or functional lesions on maximum flows depend on the site of the obstruction, kind of lesion (variable or fixed), and the extent of anatomical obstruction **(Figs. 7D.2A to C)**.

■ CONCLUSION

Spirometry is an important tool for the approach of respiratory disease. It divides respiratory diseases into obstructive, restrictive, and mixed respiratory disease. It can assess the severity of diseases. It can also assess the reversibility, thereby the response to treatment.

SUGGESTED READINGS

1. Global Initiative for Chronic Obstructive Lung Disease (GOLD). Global Strategy for the Diagnosis, Management, and Prevention of COPD-2016. [online] Available from http://goldcopd.org/ global-strategy-diagnosis-management-prevention-copd-2016/ [Last accessed October, 2024].
2. Laszlo G. Standardisation of lung function testing: helpful guidance from the ATS/ERS Task Force. Thorax. 2006;61(9):744-6.
3. Pellegrino R, Viegi G, Brusasco V, Crapo RO, Burgos F, Casaburi RE, et al. Interpretative strategies for lung function tests. Eur Respir J. 2005;26:948-68.

E. INVESTIGATIONS FOR PLEURAL DISEASES

Subhra Mitra

■ INTRODUCTION

Pleural effusion can develop as a complication of over 50 different pulmonary or systemic diseases. Determining the cause in the majority of cases is greatly helped by a diagnostic thoracentesis. Pleural fluid aspiration, a safe procedure in experienced hands, should be attempted in all except perhaps in patients with overt congestive heart failure (CHF) where the response to antifailure treatment may be awaited.

Complications of thoracentesis include pneumothorax (2–6%) and hemothorax (1%) with about half of the pneumothoraxes requiring intercostal tube drainage (ICTD). Ultrasound guidance helps in small or multiloculated effusion or when procedure risk is high as in patients with chronic obstructive pulmonary disease (COPD) with bullae.

■ THORACENTESIS

Exudate versus Transudate

Pleural fluid analysis is needed to distinguish exudates from transudates. Exudates have a pleural fluid protein level of >3 g/dL. However, to enhance the diagnostic accuracy further, Light's criteria is used according to which an exudative effusion is positive for any of the following: (1) Pleural fluid protein/serum protein ratio greater than 0.5, (2) pleural fluid lactate dehydrogenase (LDH)/serum LDH ratio greater than 0.6, and (3) pleural fluid LDH level greater than two-thirds of the normal upper limit for serum. Transudative effusion meets none of the above criteria. Transudates usually result from imbalances in hydrostatic and oncotic pressure with pleura essentially remaining normal and therapy is directed toward CHF, cirrhosis, or nephrotic syndrome, the common causes. Very low pleural fluid protein (<0.5 g/dL) suggests urinothorax, an effusion secondary to peritoneal dialysis, or misplaced central intravascular line (transudates of extravascular origin).

Light's criteria may misclassify a transudative effusion as exudative in up to 25% of cases, particularly if the patient is on diuretics. If a patient of CHF or cirrhosis has pleural fluid which meets the exudative criteria, then the difference between the protein concentration of the serum and pleural fluid is calculated. If the measured difference exceeds 3.1 g/dL, it is likely that the patient has a transudative effusion. Alternatively, if the pleural fluid N-terminal pro-B-type natriuretic peptide (NT-proBNP) is raised (1,300 pg/mL), the patient most likely suffers from CHF. Overall, when the laboratory values are near the cut-off levels then clinical judgment has to be relied upon in evaluation of these patients.

Exudative pleural effusion usually complicates lung or pleural inflammation, infection, and malignancy. A minority of effusions have an extravascular origin of pleural fluid as in chylothorax, esophageal rupture, pancreaticopleural fistula or Meigs's syndrome with ascites (peritoneal fluid moves into low pressure pleural space through diaphragmatic defects).

Gross Appearance

Pale-yellow color seems to suggest transudate, sometimes exudate. If grossly bloody pleural fluid hematocrit is obtained. If pleural fluid hematocrit is >50% of that of the peripheral blood, the patient has hemothorax and that calls for ICTD. If pleural fluid hematocrit is <1%, the blood in the pleural fluid is nonsignificant. However, pleural fluid hematocrit in the range of 1–50% signifies a malignant pleural effusion, trauma, or pulmonary embolism (PE) as a cause of pleural effusion. Turbid or pus-like aspirate suggests pleural space infection. However, chylous or pseudochylous effusions have a similar appearance. Centrifugation helps in differentiation. Turbidity clears if it is due to infection and turbidity persists in the two latter entities. A raised pleural fluid triglyceride (>110 mg/dL) supports the diagnosis of chylothorax. An intermediate level of triglyceride (50–110 mg/dL) requires chylomicron analysis. In pseudochylothorax effusions, the triglyceride level is not raised, cholesterol crystals may be present together with elevated levels of cholesterol (>250 mg/dL).

Brown or chocolate sauce aspirate hints at amoebic liver abscess with hepatopleural fistula or a long-standing bloody effusion.

A foul odor on aspiration suggests bacterial infection possibly with anaerobes whereas the rarely occurring smell of urine points toward urinothorax.

Pleural Fluid Differential: Total Count (TC) and Differential Count (DC)

Transudates usually have a white blood cell (WBC) count <1,000/µL while counts above 10,000/µL are common in pleural space infection but are also found in pancreatitis, PE, and connective tissue diseases (CTD).

Lymphocytosis (>50% small lymphocytes) alerts the physician to malignancy, lymphoma, or tuberculosis as the likely causes suggesting the need for a needle biopsy of the pleura. Lymphocytosis is also seen in chronic rheumatoid pleurisy, sarcoidosis, and post-coronary artery bypass graft (post-CABG)-related effusion.

Eosinophilia (≥10% eosinophil on DC) is common in pneumothorax or hemothorax but is also found in malignancy (lymphoma), PE, benign asbestos pleural effusion, and drug reactions (nitrofurantoin). Sometimes pleural fluid eosinophilia in a patient with hemothorax may lead to peripheral blood eosinophilia.

Pleural Fluid Lactate Dehydrogenase

This reflects the degree of inflammation in the pleural space, so if the level increases on serial thoracentesis, a more aggressive diagnosis/therapeutic approach is suggested.

Pleural Fluid Glucose

A low-pleural fluid glucose (<60 mg/dL) narrows the possibilities to parapneumonic effusion, malignant effusion, tuberculous effusion, and rheumatoid effusion.

Pleural Fluid pH

This is most useful in determining the need for ICTD in parapneumonic effusion (pH < 7.2), but as an accurate measurement it is difficult (requires the same care as measurement of arterial pH). We can use pleural fluid glucose measurement instead for determining the need for drainage (<40 mg/dL), since this provides a similar information.

In the context of need for drainage of a parapneumonic effusion, the indications are presence of frank pus, pleural fluid Gram-stain, culture positivity or low pleural fluid glucose (<40 mg/dL), pH < 7.20, and LDH > 1,000 IU/L.

Adenosine Deaminase

In a lymphocytic pleural effusion, measurement of adenosine deaminase (ADA) helps in the differential diagnosis between a malignant effusion and a tuberculous effusion, when the initial cytology is negative. A high ADA is suggestive of a tubercular etiology whereas a low ADA (<40 U/L) virtually rules out the diagnosis of tuberculosis. ADA may be raised in neutrophilic effusions and parapneumonic effusions and in some effusions due to lymphoma.

Pleural Fluid Amylase

A greater reading than the upper limit of normal for serum amylase or a pleural fluid to serum amylase ratio >1.0 narrows the differential diagnosis of the effusion to acute pancreatitis, chronic pancreatic pleural effusion, esophageal rupture, or malignancy. A correct diagnosis of chronic pancreatic pleural effusion will never be made unless a high pleural fluid amylase (>1,000 U/L) is measured or a contrast-enhanced computed tomography (CECT) scan shows the sinus tract and mediastinal pseudocyst connecting the pancreatic pseudocyst and pleural space (usually left), because these patients often appear chronically ill without any abdominal symptoms.

Pleural Fluid Cytology and Other Tests for Malignancy

Cytological study of the pleural fluid establishes the diagnosis in 40–87% malignant pleural fluid effusions. Positive cytology is more common with adenocarcinoma than with squamous cell carcinoma. The yield is higher if slides are examined together with cell block preparations and repeat samples (three) are examined which provide a higher percentage of fresher cells.

If lymphoma is suspected, fluid can be sent for flow cytometry or immunohistochemistry. Immunohistochemical tests on cell blocks of pleural fluid or pleural biopsy specimens can help in confirming a diagnosis and specifying a tumor type.

Estimation of tumor markers (CA 15-3, CA 19-9, CA 125, etc.) has not been very promising. A low value of pleural fluid mesothelin can be useful in ruling out a diagnosis of mesothelioma.

Fluorescent in situ hybridization (FISH) with specific probes visualizes prespecified chromosomal aberration in cytologic smears to confirm an aberrant mesothelial cell as truly malignant and to complement cytology in diagnosis of malignant effusions.

Immunologic Tests

A positive pleural fluid antinuclear antibody (ANA) (>1:40), though not diagnostic, is a sensitive tool for detecting lupus pleuritis in patients with a known diagnosis of lupus. However, ANA titer lacks specificity (positive also in malignancy and parapneumonic effusion) and perhaps a negative titer is more useful for ruling out a diagnosis of lupus pleuritis in patients with a known diagnosis of lupus with effusion of unknown etiology. In a patient with rheumatoid arthritis with pleural effusion, a pleural fluid rheumatoid factor ≥1:320 and more than and equal to serum titer favor rheumatoid pleuritis as the cause of the effusion.

Microbiological Tests

Pleural fluid from undiagnosed exudative pleural effusion should be cultured for bacteria (both aerobically and anaerobically), mycobacteria (BACTEC 960 liquid culture system), and fungi. Gram-stain and acid-fast bacillus (AFB) smear should be done. Culture of pleural fluid from chest tube drainage is discouraged.

Molecular Techniques in Tuberculous Pleural Effusions

Nucleic acid amplification (NAA) techniques have high specificity but overall low sensitivity. False positive results may occur due to deoxyribonucleic acid (DNA) contamination or presence of dead bacilli.

Xpert MTB/RIF (*Mycobacterium tuberculosis*/resistance to rifampin) also has a poor sensitivity at 46%, but specificity is higher at 99% compared to culture. While a positive Xpert result in pleural fluid can be treated as TB, a negative result does not exclude the disease. The test is not advised by World Health Organization (WHO) in their recommendations on the use of Xpert MTB/RIF in 2013. Therefore, pleural fluid ADA, culture, and pleural biopsy remain important tools in the diagnosis of tuberculous pleural effusion.

■ IMAGING STUDY

Ultrasound

Ultrasound detects pleural effusion as a relative echo-free space demarcated by the usual anatomic boundaries, the visceral pleura and lung, chest wall and parietal pleura, and the diaphragm. Ultrasound obviates the need for lateral decubitus chest radiograph for detection of a "possible" small effusion. In critically ill patients, ultrasound identifies the effusion in a supine position. The anechoic or heterogeneously echoic character of the pleural fluid helps in differentiation between transudates and exudates. An ultrasound detects septations or loculated nature of pleural collections where this diagnostic tool is sometimes superior to chest computed tomography (CT) scan. Thoracocentesis can be performed and ICTD/ pigtail drainage catheter placements can be done under ultrasound guidance when effusion is small or loculated.

Ultrasound detects hypoechoic thickening on the pleural surface and guides needle biopsy in malignant effusion. Additionally ultrasound easily discovers liver abscess, peripancreatic collections, and ovarian tumors, which are important abdominal causes of pleural effusion.

Chest X-ray

About 150–200 mL of pleural fluid is required for detection in a posteroanterior or lateral chest X-ray (CXR). A large effusion causes mediastinal shift to opposite side but when no shift is detected, lung collapse or a fixed mediastinum or mesothelioma is likely. CXR often gives a clue to the cause of effusion in the form of cardiomegaly, a lung or pleura based mass lesion, lung collapse, and rib erosion. Free fluid collection in a subpulmonic location simulates a raised dome, whereas fluid between fissures mimics a lung mass or a "phantom tumor", often occurring in a CHF patient and "disappearing" with diuretic therapy. In parapneumonic effusions, "D" shaped loculations sometimes develop usually between the chest wall (base of the D) and the lung, better visualized on a lateral film and ultrasound.

Computed Tomography

Computed tomography scan of thorax with contrast enhancement is often performed in patients with undiagnosed pleural effusion where malignancy is suspected as well as in complicated parapneumonic effusion and empyema. CECT scans help in distinguishing parenchymal abnormality and pleural fluid (will not enhance with contrast). CT may also demonstrate a lung mass, a lobar collapse, an enhancing breast nodule, an anterior mediastinal mass, or extensive mediastinal adenopathy, suggesting a malignant effusion **(Figs. 7E.1 and 7E.2)**.

Computed tomography can differentiate between benign and malignant pleural thickening **(Fig. 7E.3)**. Malignancy is suspected if parietal pleural thickening is >1 cm and/or any of the following is present—circumferential pleural thickening, nodular pleural thickening, and mediastinal pleural thickening. CT-guided needle aspiration or cutting needle biopsy is possible.

Computed tomography is also useful in differentiating a parenchymal lung abscess located near the chest wall from encysted empyema with bronchopleural fistula.

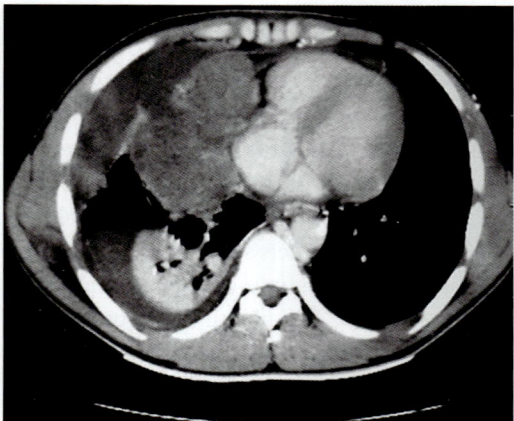

FIG. 7E.1: Contrast-enhanced computed tomography (CECT) of thorax showing anterior mediastinal mass with pleural effusion. Patient's blood biomarker levels were (Beta human chorionic gonadotropin—2252 m IU/mL; alpha-fetoprotein—81,454 ng/mL) and USG-guided biopsy was suggestive of nonseminomatous germ cell tumor.

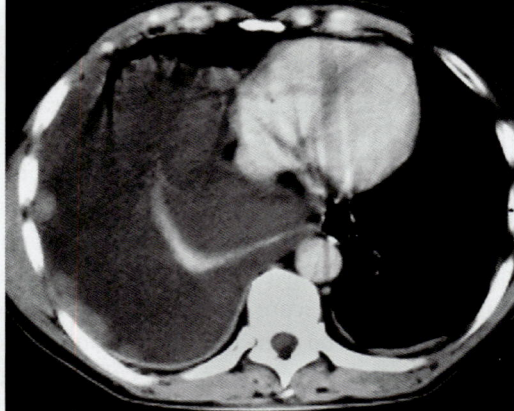

FIG. 7E.2: Contrast-enhanced computed tomography (CECT) of thorax showing large volume pleural effusion with pleural enhancement and pleural nodules (a highly specific but less sensitive finding, found in only 17% cases) suggestive of pleural metastasis.

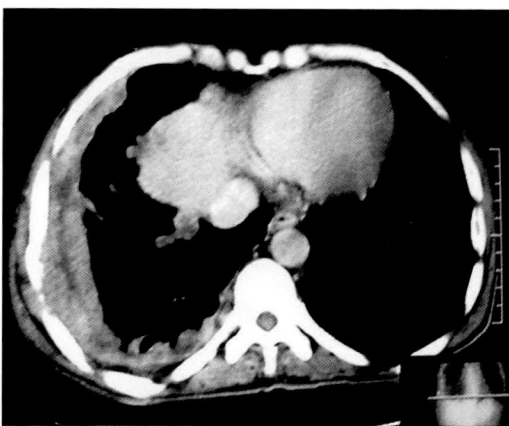

FIG. 7E.3: Malignant pleural thickening.

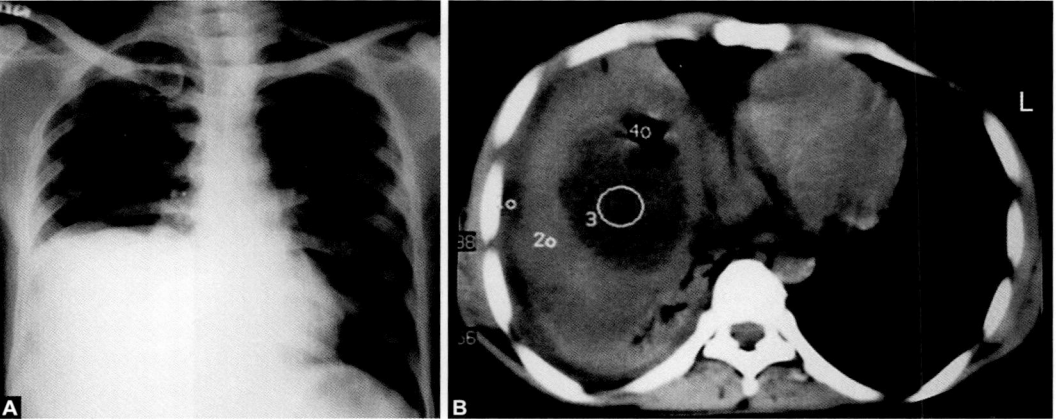

FIGS. 7E.4A AND B: Computed tomography (CT) scan showing accidental detection of liver abscess as a cause of pleural effusion.

CT scan may accidentally detect extrapulmonary pathology as a cause of pleural effusion **(Figs. 7E.4A and B)**. Most empyemas have a lenticular shape and demonstrate "split pleura" sign which refers to thickened and enhanced visceral pleura and parietal pleura separated by fluid **(Fig. 7E.5)**. With empyema, the cavity walls are of uniform thickness, the adjacent lung is compressed, and the angle of contact with the chest wall is usually obtuse. Taking care to look at the liver **(Fig. 7E.5)** soft tissue and vertebrae **(Figs. 7E.6A and B)**, contralateral lung **(Fig. 7E.7)** and ribs **(Figs. 7E.8A and B)**, in a CECT scan of thorax is often rewarding.

In the evaluation of PE in a patient with pleural effusion, if the Doppler ultrasound of the lower extremities is negative, CT pulmonary angiography (CTPA) is recommended.

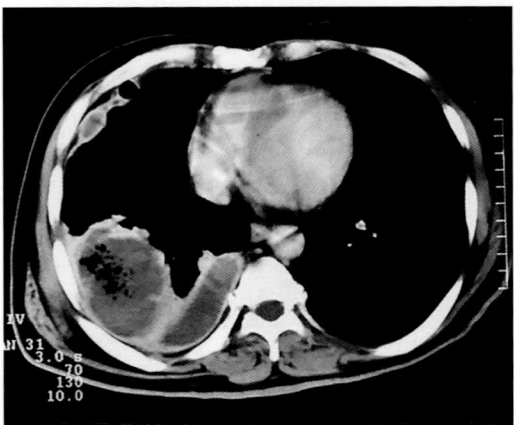

FIG. 7E.5: The "split pleura sign"—thickened enhancing parietal and visceral pleura separated by fluid with loculations.

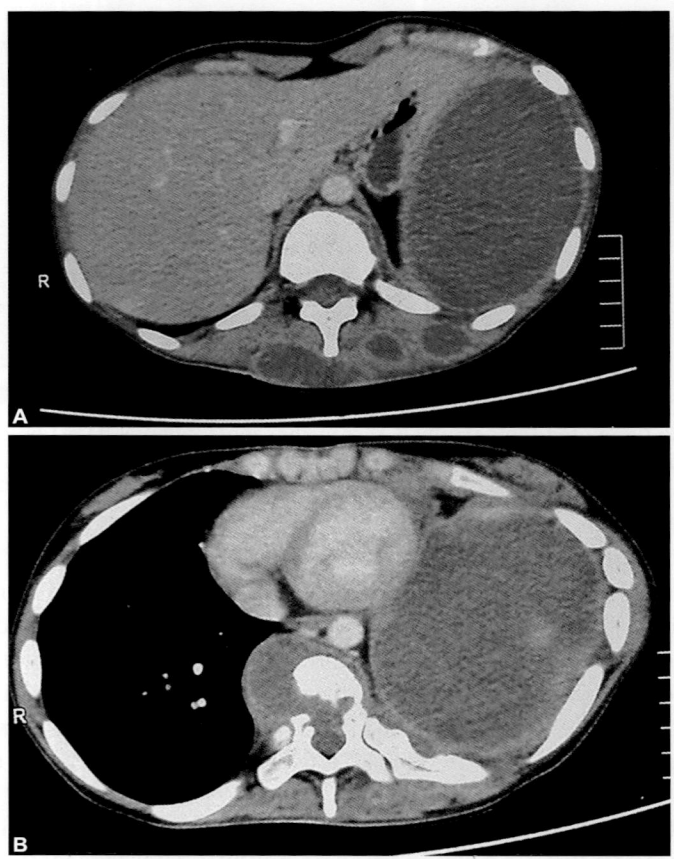

FIGS. 7E.6A AND B: Computed tomography (CT) scan showing lytic vertebral obstruction along with left-sided pleural effusion.

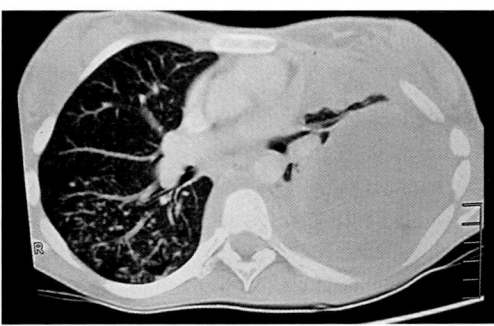

FIG. 7E.7: Left lung showing pleural effusion and "tree-in-bud" appearance in opposite lung.

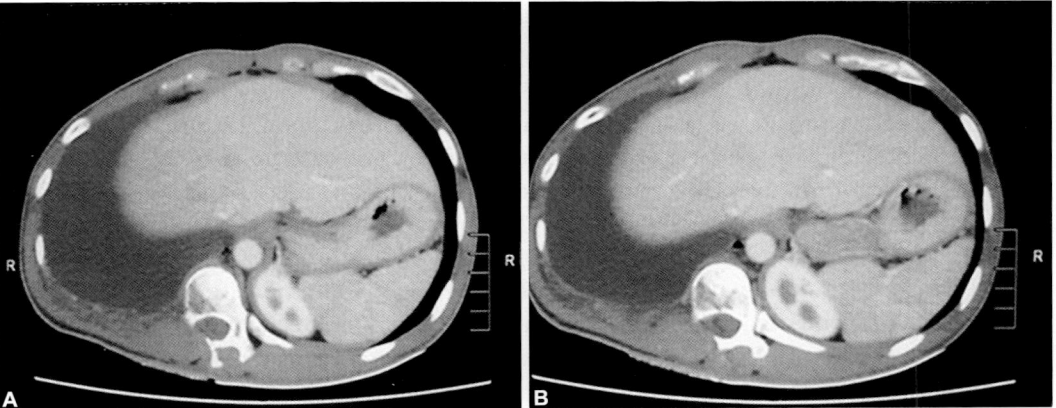

FIG. 7E.8A AND B: Contrast-enhanced computed tomography (CECT) scan showing right-sided chylothorax with rib and vertebral obstruction suggestive of Gorham's syndrome.

■ PLEURAL BIOPSY

In a suspected patient of malignant effusions, pleural biopsy can be done if the cytology at initial diagnostic thoracentesis is negative. In malignant pleural disease, needle biopsy of the pleura will be positive in 40–60% of patients. If CT or ultrasound shows diffuse pleural thickening or nodularity, the biopsy yield is higher.

Needle biopsy is more useful in diagnosis of tuberculosis with initial biopsy being positive for granulomas in 50–80% of patients. When tuberculous pleuritis is suspected, a portion of the pleural biopsy specimen should be cultured for mycobacteria and drug sensitivity testing obtained.

Medical thoracoscopy has a higher yield than blind needle biopsy especially if the pleural involvement is patchy and is discussed in the chapter on invasive procedures. Fiberoptic bronchoscopy can be considered in a patient with undiagnosed pleural effusion if there are associated parenchymal lesions/collapse or if there is history of hemoptysis.

■ UNDIAGNOSED PLEURAL EFFUSION

When faced with a patient with an undiagnosed pleural effusion, we should review the patient for clues for a diagnosis of CHF such as dyspnea on effort, history of paroxysmal nocturnal dyspnea, leg edema, raised jugular venous pressure (JVP), S3 gallop, murmurs, and investigate with electrocardiogram (ECG), CXR (enlarged cardiac silhouette), echocardiography, and NT-proBNP. We have to keep in mind possibilities of constrictive pericarditis, nephrotic syndrome (evaluate for proteinuria, hypoproteinemia), myxedema (concomitant pericardial effusion), and cirrhosis when evaluating patients with transudative effusion. Hepatic hydrothorax may not be associated with ascites in some cases where the peritoneal fluid immediately decompresses into the pleural space, making these patients difficult to diagnose. A history of chronic liver disease, alcoholism, chronic pancreatic disease, cholangitis, and abdominal surgeries should be taken and ultrasound of abdomen done keeping in mind causes such as chronic pancreatic pleural effusion, liver abscess, and intra-abdominal abscess. Breast and gynecologic examination (ovarian malignancy and Meigs's syndrome) and ultrasound imaging constitute an important step in the workup. A history of asbestos exposure, previous history of malignancy and its treatment, history of esophageal instrumentation, and drug history (nitrofurantoin, dantrolene, and more recently dasatinib) are considered informative. History of rash, joint pains, palatal ulcer in a young female, or deformed joints should raise suspicion of CTD. An accessible supraclavicular lymph node lends itself to cytologic and biopsy examination. Patients with chronic kidney disease develop pleural effusion commonly due to fluid overload or CHF. Sometimes those on peritoneal dialysis develop acute hydrothorax due to transdiaphragmatic leak. Uremic pleuritis may give rise to an exudative pleural effusion, requiring a pleural biopsy to differentiate it from tuberculous pleuritis, a common problem in a developing country.

In patients with persistent exudative pleural effusion, if no diagnosis is forthcoming (after routine laboratory tests including cytology and a pleural biopsy) and if the clinical picture is not suggestive of malignancy, the best course of management is by observation. In those with symptoms suggestive of malignancy, thoracoscopy is probably the procedure of choice.

SUGGESTED READINGS

1. Petersen WG, Zimmerman R. Limited utility of chest radiograph after thoracentesis. Chest. 2000;117:1038-42.
2. Light RW, Macgregor MI, Luchsinger PC, Ball W C Jr. Pleural effusions: the diagnostic separation of transudates and exudates. Ann Intern Med. 1972;77(4):507-13.
3. Shan SA. Pleural effusions of extravascular origin. Clin Chest Med. 2006;27:285-308.
4. Broaddus VC, Light RW. Pleural Effusion. In: Mason RJ, Ernst JD, King TE, Lazarus SC, Murray JF, Nadel JA, Slutsky AS (Eds). Murray & Nadel's Textbook of Respiratory Medicine, 6th edition. Philadelphia: Elsevier Saunders; 2016. pp. 1396-424.
5. Romero-Candeira S. Influence of diuretics on the concentration of proteins and other components of pleural transudates in patients with heart failure. Am J Med. 2001;110:681-6.
6. Porcel J, Martinez-Alonso M, Cai G. Biomarkers of heart failure in pleural fluid. Chest. 2009;136:671-7.
7. Light RW, Erozan YS, Ball WC. Cells in pleural fluid: their value in differential diagnosis. Arch Intern Med. 1973;132:854-60.
8. Staats BA, Ellefson RW, Budhan LL. The lipoprotein profile of chylous and non-chylous pleural effusions. Mayo Clin Proc. 1980;55:700-04.
9. Maltais F, Laberge F, Cormier Y. Blood hypereosinophilia in the course of post-traumatic pleural effusion. Chest. 1990;98:348-51.

10. Light RW. Pleural diseases, 6th edition. Philadelphia, PA: Lippincott, Williams & Wilkins; 2013.
11. Light RW, Girard WM, Jenkinson SG, George RB. Parapneumonic effusions. Am J Med. 1980;69:507-12.
12. Potts DE, Willcox MA, Good JT Jr, Taryle DA, Sahn S A . The acidosis of low-glucose pleural effusions. Am Rev Respir Dis. 1978;117:665-71.
13. Rahaman NM, Chapman BM, Davis RJO. The approach to a patient with a parapneumonic effusion. Clin Chest Med. 2006;27:253-66.
14. Ferrer JS, Muñoz XG, Orriols RM, Light RW, Morell FB. Evolution of idiopathic pleural effusion: a prospective, long-term follow-up study. Chest. 1996;109(6):1508-13.
15. Porcel JM, Esquerda A, Bielsa S. Diagnostic performance of adenosine deaminase activity in pleural fluid: a single-center experience with over 2100 consecutive patients. Eur J Intern Med. 2010;21:419-23.
16. Järvi OH, Kunnas RJ, Laitio MT, Tyrkkö JE. The accuracy and significance of cytologic cancer diagnosis of pleural effusions. (A follow up study of 338 patients). Acta Cytol. 1972;16:152-8.
17. Dekker A, Bupp PA. Cytology of serous effusions: An investigation into the usefulness of cell blocks versus smears. Am J Clin Pathol. 1978;70:855-60.
18. Ordonez NG. What are the current best immunohistochemical markers for the diagnosis of epithelioid mesothelioma. A review and update. Hum Pathol. 2007;3:1-16.
19. Fetsch PA, Abati A. Immunocytochemistry in effusion cytology: a contemporary review. Cancer. 2001;93: 293-308.
20. Hooper CE, Morley AJ, Virgo P, Harvey JE, Kahan B, Maskell NA. A prospective trial evaluating the role of mesothelin in undiagnosed pleural effusions. Eur Respir J. 2013;41:18-24.
21. Fiegl M, Kaufmann H, Zojer N, Schuster R, Wiener H, Müllauer L, et al. Malignant cell detection by fluorescence in situ hybridization (FISH) in effusions from patients with carcinoma. Hum Pathol. 2000;31:448-55.
22. Porcel JM, Ordi-Ros J, Esquerda A, Vives M, Madronero AB, Bielsa S, et al. Antinuclear antibody testing in pleural fluid for the diagnosis of lupus pleuritis. Lupus. 2007;16:25-7.
23. Halla JT, Schrohenloher RE, Volanakis JE. Immune complexes and other laboratory features of pleural effusions. Ann Intern Med. 1980;92:748-52.
24. Forbes BA. Critical assessment of gene amplification approaches on the diagnosis of tuberculosis. Immunol Invest. 1997;26:105-16.
25. World Health Organization. Using the Xpert MTB/RIF assay to detect pulmonary and extrapulmonary tuberculosis and rifampicin resistance in adults and children: Expert Group meeting report. (2013) Geneva. [online] Available from http://www.who.int/tb/laboratory/ policy_statements/en/ [Accessed January 2018].
26. Mayo PH, Doelken P. Pleural Ultrasonography. Clin Chest Med. 2006;27:215-27.
27. Bressler EL, Francis IR, Glazer GM, et al. Bolus contrast medium enhancement for distinguishing pleural from parenchymal lung disease: CT features. J Comput Assist Tomogr. 1987;11:436-40.
28. Leung AN, Muller NL, Miller RR. CT in differential diagnosis of diffuse pleural disease. Am J Roentgenol. 1990;154:487-92.
29. Stark DD, Federle MP, Goodman PC, Podrasky AE, Webb WR. Differentiating lung abscess and empyema: radiography and computed tomography. Am J Roentgenol. 1983;141:163-7.
30. Prakash UBS, Relman HM. Comparison of needle biopsy with cytologic analysis for the evaluation of pleural effusion: analysis of 414 cases. Mayo Clin Proc. 1985;60:158-64.
31. Bhattacharya S, Bairagya TD, Das A, Mandal A, Das SK. Closed pleural biopsy is still useful in the evaluation of malignant pleural effusion. J Lab Physicians. 2012;4:35-8.
32. Scerbo J, Keltz H, Stone DJ. A prospective study of closed pleural biopsies. JAMA. 1971;218:377-80.
33. Chang SC, Perng RP. The role of fiberoptic bronchoscopy in evaluating the causes of pleural effusions. Arch Intern Med. 1989;149:855-7.
34. Ray S, Mukherjee S, Ganguly J, et al. A cross-sectional prospective study of pleural effusion among cases of chronic kidney disease. Indian J Chest Dis Allied Sci. 2013;55:205-10.
35. Poe RH, Israel RH, Utell MJ, Hall WJ, Greenblatt DW, Kallay MC. Sensitivity, specificity, and predictive values of closed pleural biopsy. Arch Intern Med. 1984;144:325-8.

F. BASIC APPROACH TO COMPUTED TOMOGRAPHY OF THORAX

Bhoomi Angirish

■ INTRODUCTION

Thoracic diseases can be divided into diseases of the lungs, airways, pleura, mediastinum, and chest wall. Computed tomography (CT) of thorax is indicated in various conditions such as infection, masses, and airways disease. It is primarily done for anatomical localization and characterization of the disease. CT images also acts as a guideline map to plan for further investigation of the intrathoracic lesion.

Contrast-enhanced CT (CECT) is indicated in lesions arising from pulmonary parenchyma, mediastinum, pleura, or extrathoracic areas to look for their involvement and extension.

High-resolution CT (HRCT) is advised for the pulmonary parenchymal abnormalities such as interstitial lung disease. It is also indicated to look for airway disorders.

■ TECHNIQUE

The recommended scanning protocol for HRCT of thorax is as follows: Volumetric acquisition is done with submillimetric collimation (1.5–3 mm), shortest rotation time, and highest pitch. Tube potential is typically 120 kVp, and tube current is 240 mAs. High spatial frequency reconstruction algorithm is used.

The patient lies in supine position. Prone position is required for certain conditions such as interstitial lung disease and to evaluate fungal ball. On routine supine images, dependent densities/atelectasis can mimic pathology. In such cases, imaging in prone position will be useful because dependent densities will disappear on prone images, whereas true abnormality will persist in both positions **(Figs. 7F.1A and B)**.

Scan is acquired in full inspiration. Expiratory scan is also done in certain conditions such as interstitial lung disease and airways disorders **(Figs. 7F.2A and B)**.

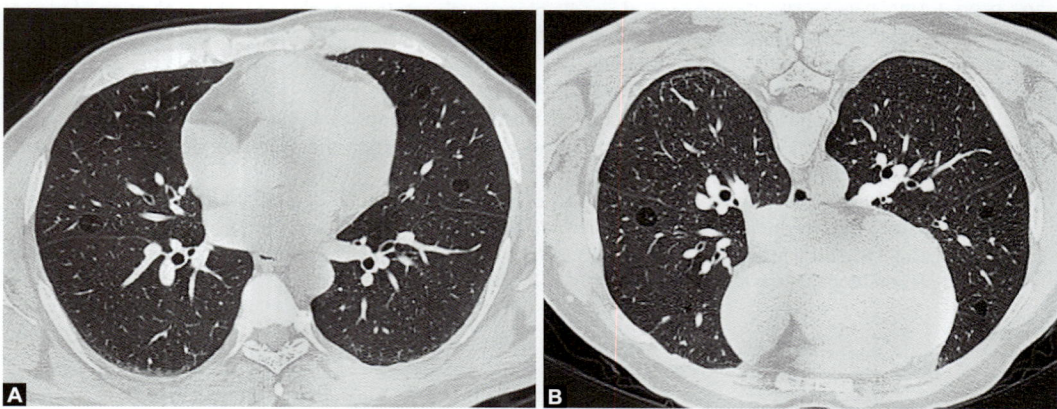

FIGS. 7F.1A AND B: Ground glass opacities are seen in dependent subpleural location in right lower lobe (A) which disappear on prone images (B).

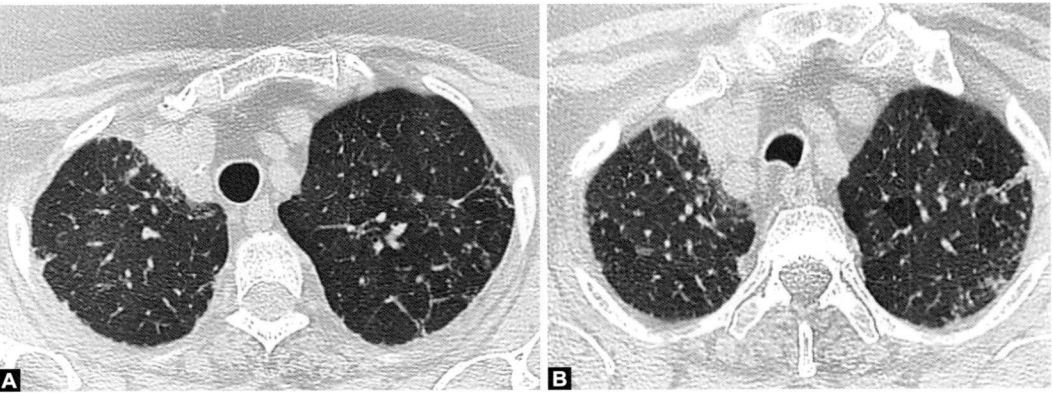

FIGS. 7F.2A AND B: Inspiratory image shows rounded appearance of posterior wall of trachea (A), expiratory image shows concave appearance of posterior wall of trachea (B). On expiratory scan, the areas of air trapping are better appreciated in this case of small airways disease.

■ IMAGE RECONSTRUCTION TECHNIQUES

After acquisition of images, the volumetric data can be processed to obtain multiplanar reformation (MPR), maximum intensity projection (MIP), and minimum intensity projection (MinIP).

- *MPR*: Volumetric image acquisition allows for MPR reconstruction of axial images into other planes such as coronal, sagittal, or oblique.
- *MIP*: MIP images are generated by projecting the maximum attenuation value voxel along each ray from the volume data onto a 2D image. These are useful in the assessment of lung nodules **(Fig. 7F.3)**.
- *MinIP*: MinIP images are generated by displaying the lowest attenuation value voxel along each ray from the volume data onto a 2D image. These are useful in the assessment of airways and detecting subtle mosaic attenuation and cystic lung diseases **(Fig. 7F.4)**.

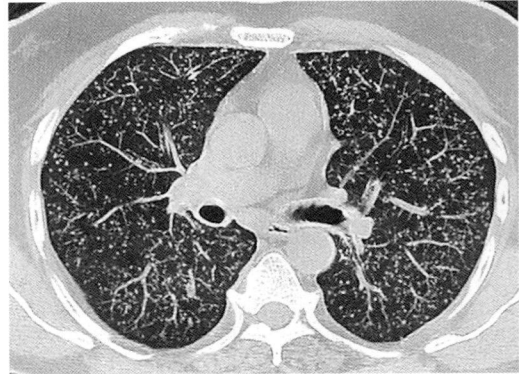

FIG. 7F.3: Maximum intensity projection (MIP) reconstruction of axial images shows better identification of randomly distributed miliary nodules.

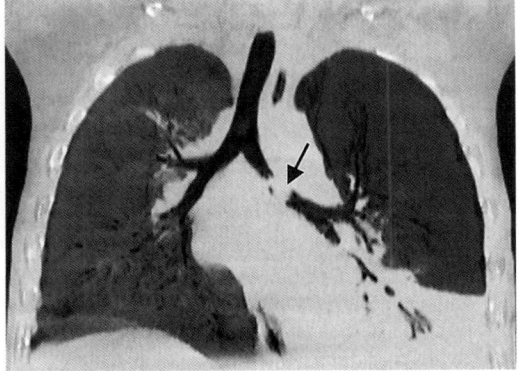

FIG. 7F.4: Minimum intensity projection (MinIP) reconstruction of airways is done. Foreign body is seen in the left main bronchus (arrow).

HIGH-RESOLUTION CT ANATOMY

Evaluation of lung parenchyma is central to any chest CT evaluation. Secondary pulmonary lobule is the fundamental anatomical unit of lung. Each secondary pulmonary lobule is supplied by a central bronchiole and a pulmonary artery branch along the peribronchovascular interstitium. The periphery of each secondary pulmonary lobule is bounded by interlobular septa that contain the pulmonary vein and lymphatics **(Fig. 7F.5)**.

PATTERNS ON HIGH-RESOLUTION CT

There are four basic patterns seen in HRCT of thorax—nodular, reticular, increased lung attenuation, and decreased lung attenuation.

Nodular Pattern

A nodule is a circumscribed, typically round opacity, ≤30 mm in average diameter. A rounded lesion < 6 mm in diameter should be called micronodule.

Distribution: Perilymphatic, centrilobular, and random **(Table 7F.1)**.
- *Perilymphatic nodules*: They are seen in relation to pleural surfaces, interlobular septa, and peribronchovascular interstitium. Nodules are visible in subpleural location and in relation to fissures **(Fig. 7F.6A to C)**. It is seen in sarcoidosis, silicosis, lymphangitic carcinomatosis, and lymphocytic interstitial pneumonia (LIP).

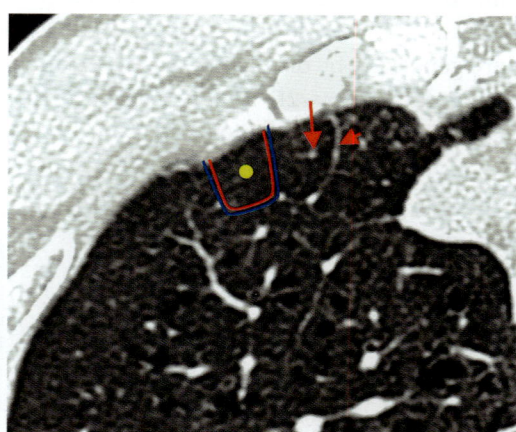

FIG. 7F.5: Secondary pulmonary lobule: Central bronchiole and pulmonary artery (yellow dot) surrounded by interlobular septa that contain the pulmonary vein and lymphatics (blue). The centrilobular artery is visible as a dot (red arrow) while the pulmonary vein branch (arrowhead) is visible in relation to the periphery of the lobule.

CHAPTER 7: Basic Investigations: Indications and Interpretations

- *Centrilobular nodules*: The nodules are limited to centrilobular region and spare the pleural surfaces **(Fig. 7F.7)**. The most peripheral nodules are centered 5–10 mm from fissures and pleural surfaces. These are seen in bronchopneumonia, hypersensitivity pneumonitis, respiratory bronchiolitis interstitial lung disease (RB-ILD), follicular bronchiolitis, and LIP.
- *Tree-in-bud branching pattern* of nodules is seen in endobronchial infection **(Fig. 7F.8)**. It is commonly seen in tuberculosis, postaspiration, and bronchiectasis with infection [e.g., allergic bronchopulmonary aspergillosis (ABPA) and cystic fibrosis).
- *Random nodules*: They can be seen along fissures, peribronchovascular structures, subpleural region, center of lobule, or interlobular septa **(Fig. 7F.9)**. These do not

Table 7F.1: Pattern of distribution of nodules.	
Perilymphatic nodules	• Sarcoidosis • Lymphangitic carcinomatosis • Silicosis • Coal workers' pneumoconiosis • Lymphocytic interstitial pneumonia • Lymphoma/leukemia • Siderosis
Centrilobular nodules	*Without tree-in-bud pattern*: • Bronchopneumonia • Hypersensitivity pneumonitis • Respiratory bronchiolitis • Follicular bronchiolitis • Lymphoid interstitial pneumonia • Langerhans cell histiocytosis • Pulmonary edema • Pulmonary hemorrhage • Pulmonary veno-occlusive disease
	With tree-in-bud pattern: • Endobronchial spread of infection • Tuberculosis • Postaspiration • Cystic fibrosis
Random nodules	*Miliary nodules*: • Miliary tuberculosis • Hematogenous metastasis (e.g., thyroid carcinoma and renal carcinoma) • Varicella pneumonia
	Large random nodules: • Metastasis • Septic emboli • Wegener granulomatosis • Fungal infection • IgG4 disease

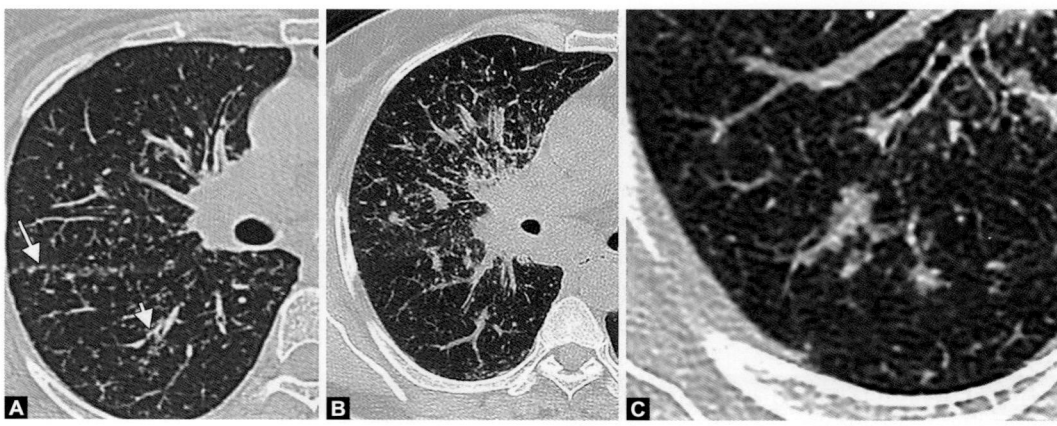

FIGS. 7F.6A TO C: Perilymphatic distribution of nodules: Nodules are seen in peribronchovascular (arrowhead) and perifissural distribution (arrow) in these cases of sarcoidosis.

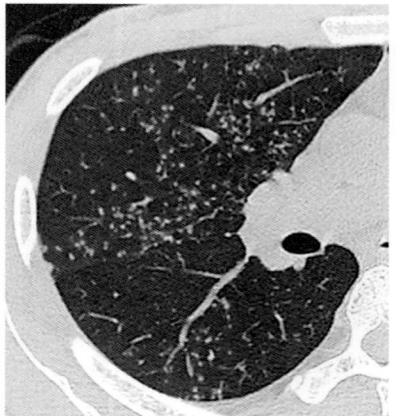

FIG. 7F.7: Centrilobular distribution of nodules in a patient with bronchopneumonia.

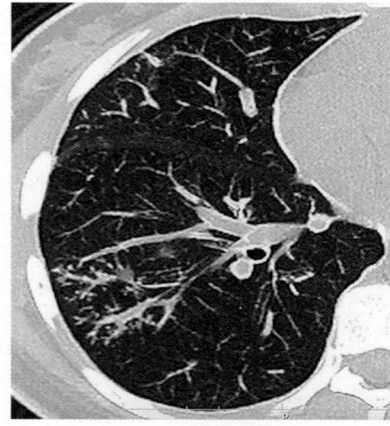

FIG. 7F.8: Tree-in-bud branching pattern of nodules as seen in tuberculosis.

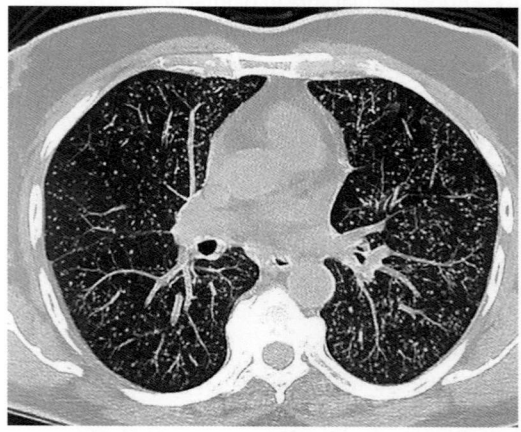

FIG. 7F.9: Random distribution of nodules as seen in miliary tuberculosis.

have a consistent relationship with any of the structures of the secondary pulmonary lobule. These are seen in miliary tuberculosis, hematogenous metastasis, and varicella pneumonia.

Attenuation: Solid and ground glass **(Figs. 7F.10A and B)**
Solid nodules are seen in tuberculosis, endobronchial infection, silicosis, sarcoidosis while ground glass nodules are seen in hypersensitivity pneumonitis, respiratory bronchiolitis, and follicular bronchiolitis.

Size: Miliary and other large nodules
Miliary nodules are discrete 2–3 mm sized nodules (millet sized). These are seen in miliary tuberculosis, miliary metastasis, miliary fungal infections. Other large nodules can be seen in metastasis, septic embolic, granulomatosis with polyangiitis.

Reticular Pattern

Reticulations are a form of pulmonary opacification seen because the disease process involves the pulmonary interstitium. Reticular abnormalities include the following:
- *Interlobular and intralobular septal thickening*: It can be due to fluid, cell proliferation, or fibrosis **(Table 7F.2)**. There is smooth or nodular septal thickening **(Figs. 7F.11A and B)**. Smooth septal thickening is seen in pulmonary edema, pulmonary hemorrhage, pulmonary veno-occlusive disease, whereas nodular septal thickening is seen in lymphangitic carcinomatosis, sarcoidosis, and silicosis **(Table 7F.3)**.
- Subpleural lines
- Parenchymal bands
- *Architectural distortion*:
  ○ Traction bronchiectasis
  ○ Honeycombing appears as enlarged airspaces, often subpleural, that are irregular in size, share thick walls, and are stacked upon one another. These can be single layer or multilayered. The cysts are typically 3–10 mm in diameter but can be as large as 2.5 cm.

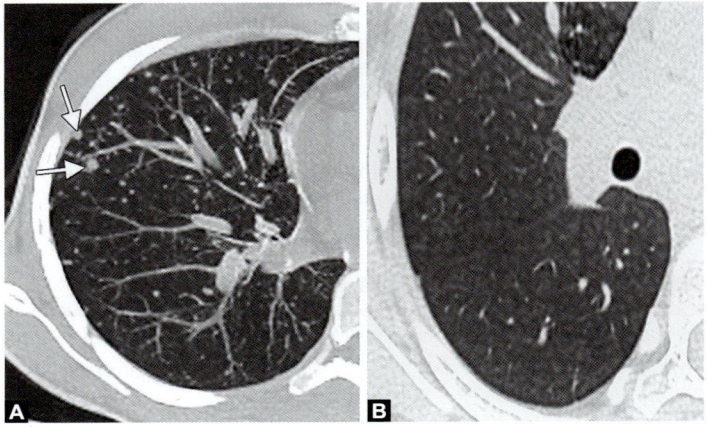

FIGS. 7F.10A AND B: Solid well defined nodules (both white arrows) seen in miliary metastasis (A) whereas ground glass nodules seen in acute hypersensitivity pneumonitis (B).

Table 7F.2: Summary of high-resolution computed tomography (HRCT) pattern of reticular opacities.

Interstitial thickening due to fibrosis	
Usual interstitial pneumonia	Peripheral (subpleural) and basal predominant reticular opacities, honeycombing with or without traction bronchiectasis
Nonspecific interstitial pneumonia	Subpleural sparing, ground glass opacities +/− traction bronchiectasis
Chronic fibrotic hypersensitivity pneumonitis	Reticular opacities, honeycombing, traction bronchiectasis in axial and peripheral distribution, ground glass opacities, centrilobular nodules, and lobular air trapping (triple density sign)
Fibrotic sarcoidosis	Reticular opacities in peribronchovascular distribution, peribronchovascular/perilymphatic nodules, upper lobe, and central distribution
Interstitial thickening due to other causes (fluid/infiltration)	
Pulmonary edema	Smooth interlobular septal thickening, ground glass opacities, and central distribution +/pleural effusion
Pulmonary hemorrhage	Smooth septal thickening with ground glass opacities
Lymphangitic carcinomatosis	Nodular septal thickening + mass lesion
Alveolar proteinosis	Smooth septal thickening with ground glass opacities

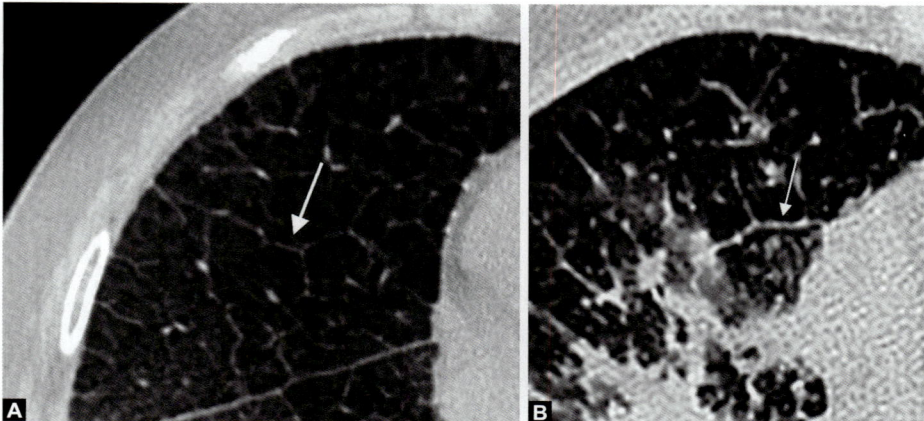

FIGS. 7F.11A AND B: Smooth interlobular septal thickening (white arrow) seen in pulmonary edema (A), nodular interlobular septal thickening (white arrow) seen in sarcoidosis (B).

Table 7F.3: Reticular pattern—interlobular septal thickening.

Smooth interlobular septal thickening:	Nodular interlobular septal thickening:
• Pulmonary edema • Pulmonary hemorrhage • Lymphoproliferative diseases • Pulmonary veno-occlusive disease	• Lymphangitic carcinomatosis • Sarcoidosis • Silicosis • Lymphoma

CHAPTER 7: Basic Investigations: Indications and Interpretations

Although honeycombing can be seen in any disease involving significant fibrosis, a basilar predominant honeycombing is a hallmark of a usual interstitial pneumonia (UIP) pattern **(Table 7F.4) (Figs. 7F.12A to C)**.

Increased Lung Attenuation

Increased lung attenuation **(Table 7F.5)** can be due to:
- *Ground-glass opacity*: Hazy increase in lung attenuation that does not obscure the underlying pulmonary vessels **(Figs. 7F.13A and B)**. Ground glass opacities can be seen in acute conditions such as viral pneumonia, pulmonary edema, pulmonary hemorrhage, drug toxicity, and in chronic conditions such as hypersensitivity pneumonitis, nonspecific interstitial pneumonia, and invasive mucinous adenocarcinoma.
- *Consolidation*: Increased lung attenuation because of filling of the alveoli obscuring the underlying vessels. Air bronchograms are seen, which is a characteristic feature **(Fig. 7F.14)**. Consolidation can be seen in acute conditions such as pneumonia (viral/bacterial/fungal), pulmonary edema, acute lung injury/acute respiratory distress syndrome, aspiration and in chronic conditions such as cryptogenic organizing pneumonia, lipoid pneumonia, invasive mucinous adenocarcinoma, and lymphoma.

Table 7F.4: UIP/IPF evaluation—ATS/ERS guidelines 2018.	
Usual interstitial pneumonia	Peripheral (subpleural) and basal predominant reticular opacities, honeycombing with or without traction bronchiectasis
Probable usual interstitial pneumonia	Peripheral (subpleural) and basal predominant reticular opacities with traction bronchiectasis
Indeterminate for UIP	Subpleural and basal predominant, subtle reticulation

Alternate diagnosis	Findings suggestive of another diagnosis:
	• *CT features*:
	  ○ Cysts
	  ○ Marked mosaic attenuation
	  ○ Predominant GGO
	  ○ Profuse micronodules
	  ○ Centrilobular nodules
	  ○ Nodules
	  ○ Consolidation
	• *Predominant distribution*:
	  ○ Peribronchovascular
	  ○ Perilymphatic
	  ○ Upper or mid lung
	• *Other*:
	  ○ Pleural plaques (consider asbestosis)
	  ○ Dilated esophagus [consider connective tissue disorder (CTD)]
	  ○ Distal clavicular erosions (consider rheumatoid arthritis)
	  ○ Extensive lymph node enlargement (consider other etiologies)
	  ○ Pleural effusions and pleural thickening (consider CTD/drugs)

(IPF: idiopathic pulmonary fibrosis; UIP: usual interstitial pneumonia)

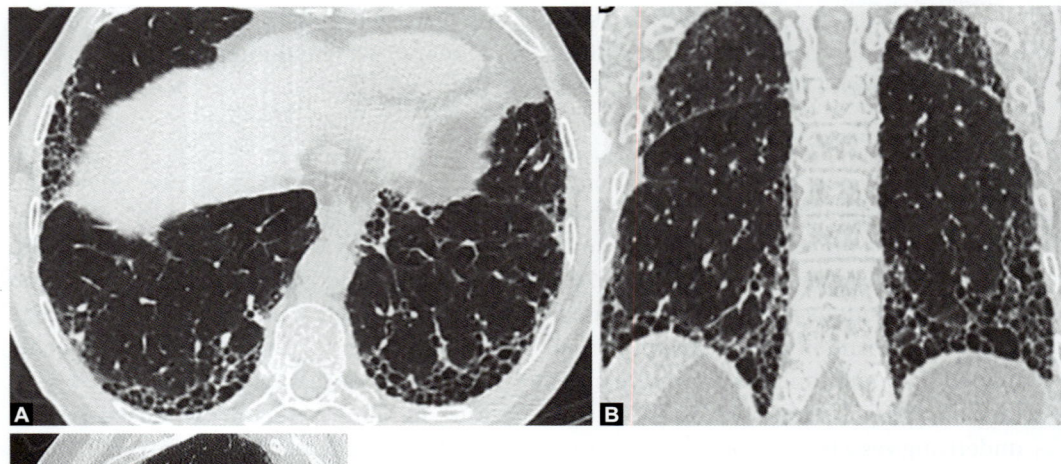
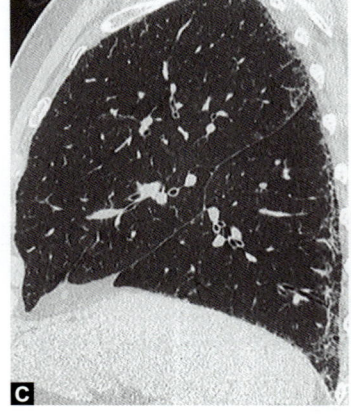

FIGS. 7F.12A TO C: Honeycombing (A and B) is seen as multiple well-defined airspaces in subpleural location with shared walls and stacked upon one another. This classic basal distribution pattern is seen in UIP. Traction bronchiectasis (C) is seen in subpleural distribution in the presence of interstitial septal thickening.

Table 7F.5: Increased lung attenuation.	
Ground glass opacities	• Viral pneumonias • Pulmonary edema • Pulmonary hemorrhage • Acute respiratory distress syndrome • Drug toxicity • Acute hypersensitivity pneumonitis • Nonspecific interstitial pneumonia • Invasive mucinous adenocarcinoma (BAC)
Consolidation	• *Pneumonias*: Viral/bacterial/fungal • Pulmonary edema • Acute lung injury/acute respiratory distress syndrome • Aspiration • Cryptogenic organizing pneumonia • Lipoid pneumonia • Invasive mucinous adenocarcinoma (BAC) • Lymphoma • Pulmonary infarcts
Crazy paving pattern	• Acute respiratory distress syndrome • Pulmonary alveolar proteinosis • Bacterial pneumonia

CHAPTER 7: Basic Investigations: Indications and Interpretations

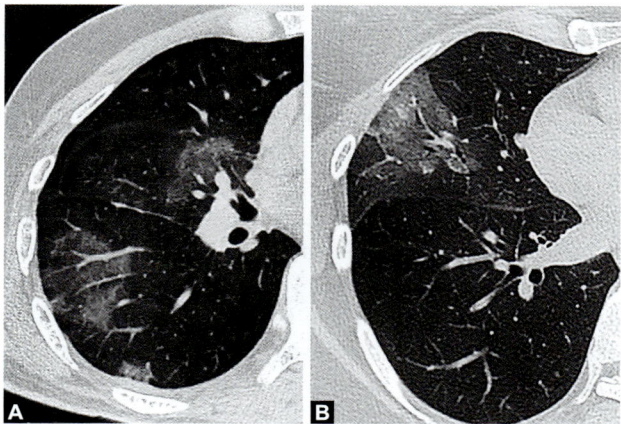

FIGS. 7F.13A AND B: Ground glass opacities are seen as hazy increase in lung attenuation that does not obscure the underlying pulmonary vessels. In contrast, the underlying vessels are obscured in consolidation.

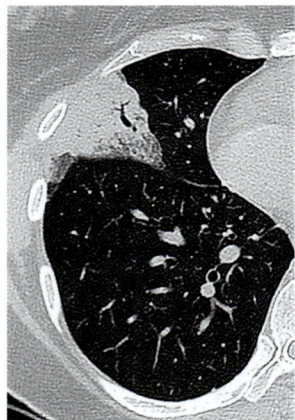

FIG. 7F.14: Consolidation is seen as increased lung attenuation due to filling of alveoli. There is obscuration of underlying vessels; however, air bronchograms are seen.

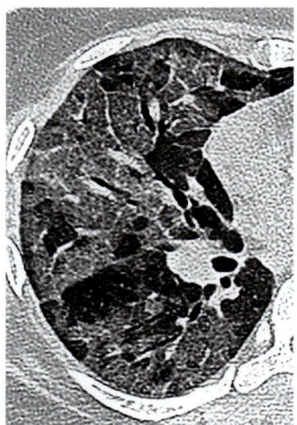

FIG. 7F.15: Ground glass opacities with interlobular septal thickening (crazy-paving pattern) in this patient with pulmonary alveolar proteinosis.

- *Crazy paving*: Appearance of ground-glass density with superimposed interlobular septal thickening **(Fig. 7F.15)**. Crazy-paving pattern is seen in pulmonary alveolar proteinosis, acute respiratory distress syndrome.

Decreased Lung Attenuation

The density of normal lung parenchyma depends on the amount of air in airspaces, volume of blood flow in small vessels, and density of lung tissue itself. Therefore, lung attenuation can be decreased in the following conditions:
- Decrease in parenchymal perfusion (mosaic perfusion)
- Abnormal increase in the amount of air in lung parenchyma (air trapping/cysts)
- Destruction of lung tissue (emphysema)

Mosaic attenuation is a general nonspecific term used to describe different lung attenuations in different regions of the lung, which may be a result of ground-glass opacity, small airway disease, or vascular cause. Mosaic perfusion is a more specific term which means different lung attenuation caused by airway or vascular cause and not because of ground-glass density. In mosaic perfusion, the pulmonary vessels appear smaller in caliber in areas of decreased density **(Fig. 7F.16)**. In small airways disease, air trapping will be present on expiratory scans, distinguishing it from mosaic perfusion secondary to vascular cause. The vascular causes of mosaic perfusion are pulmonary hypertension and chronic pulmonary embolism **(Table 7F.6)**.

Air trapping could be due to obliterative bronchiolitis, postinfectious (Swyer–James syndrome), toxic fumes exposure, bronchiectasis, cystic fibrosis. Expiratory scans in addition to routine inspiratory scans are must to look for air trapping. Lobular air trapping can be seen in chronic hypersensitivity pneumonitis **(Figs. 7F.17A and B)**.

Cysts are parenchymal lucencies or low-attenuation areas with a well-defined interface with surrounding normal lung parenchyma. They have variable wall thickness but are usually thin-walled (<2 mm). Cysts are often confused with other cyst-like lucencies such as cavity, pneumatocele, bulla, emphysema, and honeycombing **(Figs. 7F.18A to C)**. Multiple cysts without other parenchymal abnormalities are seen in cystic lung disease **(Box 7F.1)** such as Langerhans cell histiocytosis (LCH), lymphangioleiomyomatosis (LAM), Birt–Hogg–Dube (BHD) syndrome, and LIP.

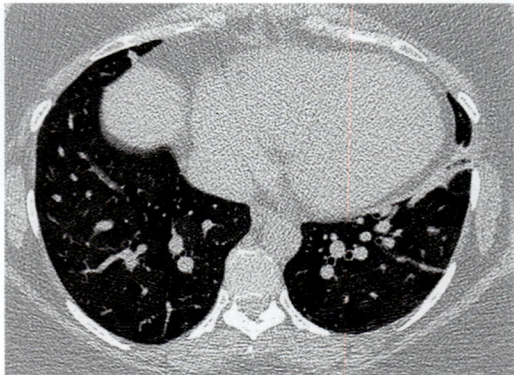

FIG. 7F.16: Mosaic perfusion: There is narrow caliber of pulmonary artery in the areas of reduced density compared to normal lung parenchyma. Here the black lung is abnormal due to reduced perfusion whereas the white lung is the normal lung parenchyma.

Table 7F.6: Mosaic perfusion.	
Airway causes:	*Vascular causes*:
• Obliterative bronchiolitis • *Postinfectious*: Viral/*mycoplasma* (Swyer–James syndrome) • Bronchiectasis • Cystic fibrosis • Collagen vascular diseases	• Chronic pulmonary thromboembolism • Primary pulmonary hypertension

CHAPTER 7: Basic Investigations: Indications and Interpretations

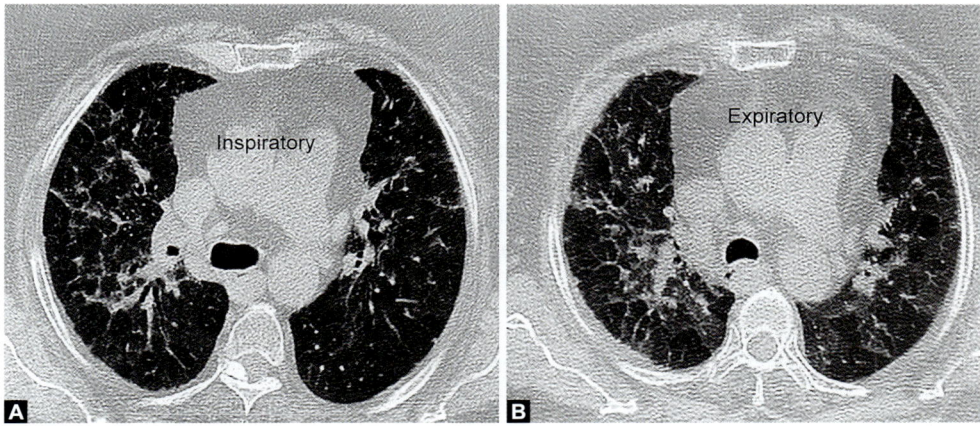

FIGS. 7F.17A AND B: Inspiratory and expiratory scans in this patient with chronic fibrotic hypersensitivity pneumonitis show axial distribution of interstitial septal thickening with ground glass opacities and lobular air trapping.

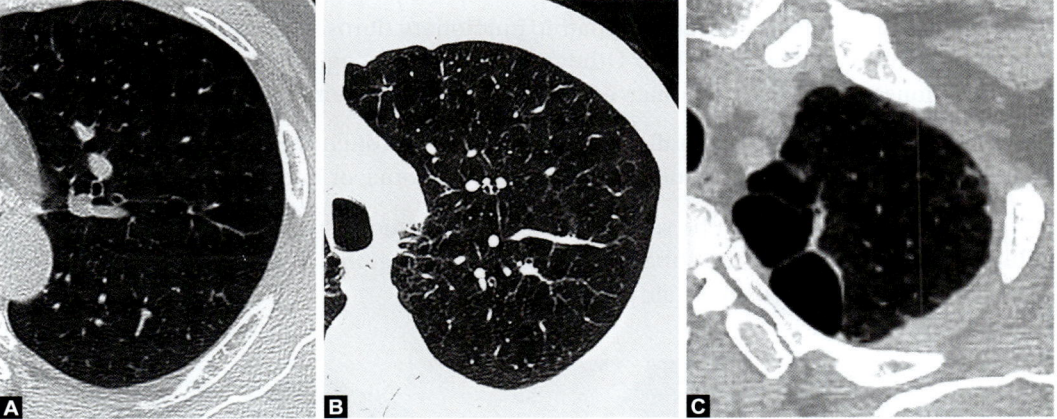

FIGS. 7F.18 A TO C: Parenchymal cyst with thin imperceptible walls (A), centrilobular emphysema, (B) paraseptal emphysema (C).

BOX 7F.1	Cystic lung disease.

- Langerhans cell histiocytosis (LCH)
- Lymphangioleiomyomatosis (LAM)
- Lymphocytic interstitial pneumonia (LIP)
- Birt–Hogg–Dubé down syndrome
- Tuberculosis
- Amyloidosis
- Cystic metastasis—from angiosarcoma and squamous cell carcinoma

Centrilobular emphysema is seen as focal areas of decreased attenuation, usually without visible walls and has a predilection for the upper lobes. It is usually combined with a central dot, which is a central vessel in the secondary pulmonary lobule. It is commonly associated with smoking. Emphysema is classified into three major subtypes: Centrilobular or centriacinar emphysema, panlobular or panacinar emphysema, and paraseptal or distal acinar emphysema. Panlobular emphysema has lower lobe predominance. It is seen in alpha-1 antitrypsin deficiency but can also be seen in smokers in advanced emphysema. Paraseptal emphysema is seen along fissures and pleura. It is associated with bullae formation which can rupture leading to pneumothorax.

■ SPATIAL DISTRIBUTION OF DISEASE

Both the craniocaudal and the central/peripheral extent of disease are important to determine formulating a differential diagnosis of diffuse lung disease **(Figs. 7F.19A and B)**.

Upper lobe distribution: It is seen commonly in inhalational disease. Silicosis, sarcoidosis, coal workers pneumoconiosis, centrilobular emphysema, LCH, and tuberculosis are commonly seen in upper lobes.

Lower lobe distribution: Classically idiopathic pulmonary fibrosis (IPF) showing UIP pattern has a predilection for lower lobes. Other common pathologies seen in lower lobes are hematogenous metastasis, pulmonary edema, and panlobular emphysema.

Central distribution: It is seen in diseases related to the bronchovascular bundles; example includes pulmonary edema, sarcoidosis, silicosis, lymphoma, or Kaposi's sarcoma.

Peripheral distribution: It can be seen in acute diseases such as pulmonary infection, septic emboli, and aspiration. In the subacute or chronic setting, this distribution can be seen in organizing pneumonia, eosinophilic pneumonia, and IPF.

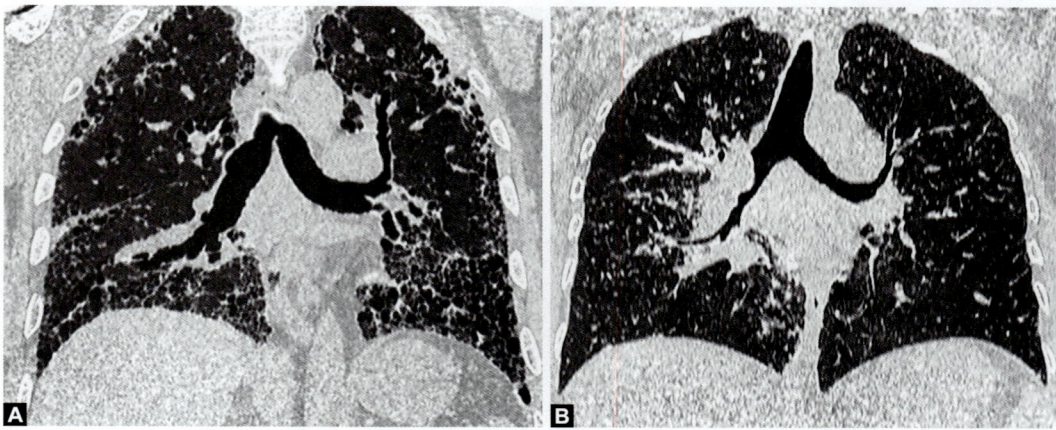

FIGS. 7F.19A AND B: Lower lobe and peripheral distribution seen in usual interstitial pneumonia (A), central distribution seen in sarcoidosis (B).

AIRWAYS DISEASE

The central airways consist of trachea and main bronchi.

Numerous pathologies are seen in central airways such as tuberculosis, relapsing polychondritis, granulomatosis with polyangiitis, foreign body, postintubation stenosis, neoplasms (such as carcinoid, squamous cell carcinoma, and metastasis), and tracheobronchomegaly **(Figs. 7F.20A and B)**.

Bronchiectasis is the irreversible localized or diffuse bronchial dilatation, usually resulting from chronic infection, proximal airway obstruction, or congenital bronchial abnormality. Bronchiolectasis is defined as dilatation of bronchioles. It is caused by inflammatory airways disease, more frequently due to fibrosis.

The direct signs of bronchiectasis are: Inner airway—artery diameter ≥ 1, outer airway—artery diameter ≥ 1, lack of tapering of airways > 2 cm distal to the point of bifurcation, and visibility of peripheral airways within 1 cm of costal pleura or fissures. The association of a dilated bronchus with a much smaller adjacent pulmonary artery branch has been termed the signet ring sign. Other indirect associations are bronchial wall thickening, mucoid impaction, inflammatory/infectious bronchiolitis and air trapping—constrictive bronchiolitis. Bronchiectasis can be cylindrical, varicose, or cystic **(Figs. 7F.21A to C)**.

Traction bronchiectasis is the dilatation of the bronchial lumen associated with thickened, irregular bronchial walls, which is caused by fibrosis and is seen in interstitial lung disease.

Cystic fibrosis presents as bronchiectasis with predilection for central/perihilar distribution in upper lobes and superior segment of lower lobes.

Williams–Campbell syndrome is characterized by congenital cystic bronchiectasis. It is caused by cartilage deficiency in the subsegmental bronchi of fourth to sixth order. There is diffuse bronchiectasis with sparing of the lower order bronchi and trachea.

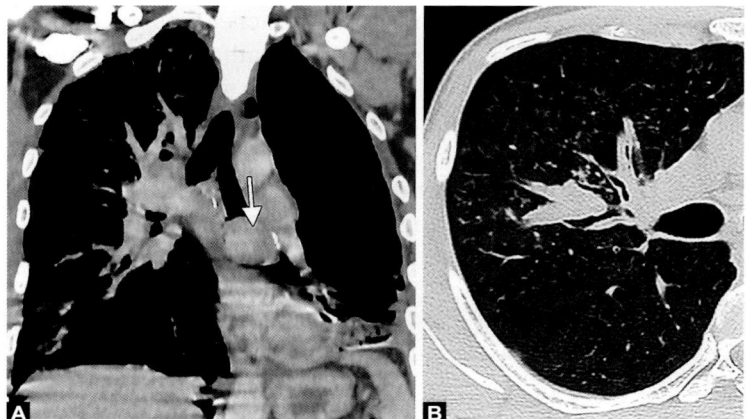

FIGS. 7F.20A AND B: Well-defined enhancing endobronchial mass (arrow) seen in left main bronchus which on biopsy was carcinoid (A), bronchiectasis with mucoid impaction giving finger in glove appearance in allergic bronchopulmonary aspergillosis (B).

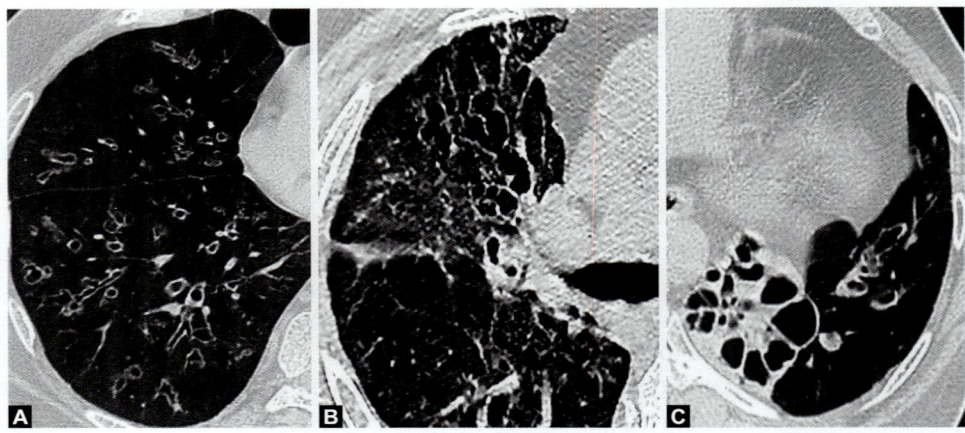

FIGS. 7F.21A TO C: Bronchiectasis: Cylindrical or tubular bronchiectasis seen as tram-track appearance (A), varicose bronchiectasis (B), cystic bronchiectasis (C).

■ MEDIASTINUM

The mediastinum is divided into anterior, middle, and posterior compartments **(Table 7F.7)** by imaginary lines on lateral chest radiograph. The ITMIG classification is used on cross-sectional images for dividing the mediastinum into prevascular, visceral, and paravertebral compartments.

The anterior mediastinum contains thymus, lymph nodes, ascending aorta, pulmonary artery, phrenic nerves, and thyroid. Lesions of anterior mediastinum commonly arise from thymus or lymph node. The common pathologies seen in anterior mediastinum are thymoma, lymphoma, and germ cell tumors **(Figs. 7F.22A and B)**.

The middle mediastinum contains lymph nodes, trachea, esophagus, vena cava, azygos vein, posterior heart, and aortic arch. Most common pathology of middle mediastinum is lymphadenopathy **(Fig. 7F.23)**. Other middle mediastinum masses are esophageal duplication cyst, bronchogenic cyst, esophageal malignancy, vascular lesions, etc.

The posterior mediastinum contains nerve roots, sympathetic ganglia, parasympathetic chain, lymph nodes, thoracic duct, descending thoracic aorta, and vertebrae. Most masses in the posterior mediastinum are neurogenic in origin (neuroblastoma, schwannoma,

Table 7F.7: Mediastinal masses.		
Anterior mediastinum	**Middle mediastinum**	**Posterior mediastinum**
• Thymoma • Thymic cyst • Lymphoma • Germ cell tumor • Thyroid lesions • Thymolipoma	• Lymph nodes • Duplication cyst • Arch anomaly	• Neuroblastoma • Schwannoma • Neurofibroma • Neuroenteric cysts • Meningoceles • Lymphadenopathy • Extramedullary hematopoiesis

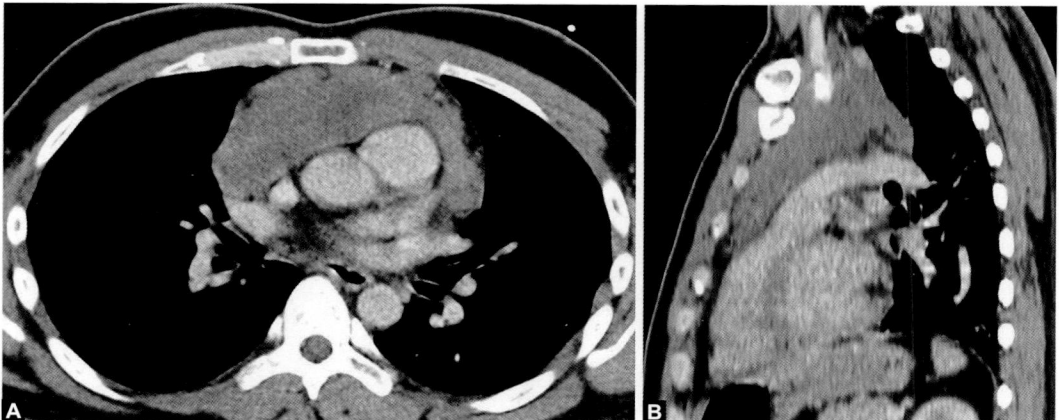

FIGS. 7F.22A AND B: Anterior mediastinal mass seen in prevascular space in this biopsy proven case of lymphoma.

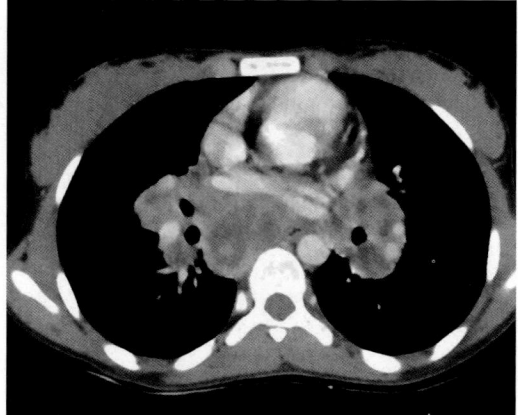

FIG. 7F.23: Middle mediastinal mass seen as enlarged necrotic subcarinal and bilateral hilar lymph nodes in this patient with tuberculosis.

or neurofibroma). Cystic lesions of posterior mediastinum include neuroenteric cysts, schwannomas, or meningoceles. Lymphadenopathy and extramedullary hematopoiesis are other common lesions of posterior mediastinum.

■ PLEURA

Chest CT is an excellent modality for examination of pleura. Pleural effusion may be loculated or free **(Figs. 7F.24A and B)**. Encysted pleural effusion may become loculated in interlobar fissure as seen in heart failure. Contrast CT helps in localization of empyema and differentiation of lung abscess from loculated empyema.

Pleural thickening is seen in variety of benign and malignant conditions. Most common cause of pleural thickening is as sequelae of prior infection such as tuberculosis or sequelae

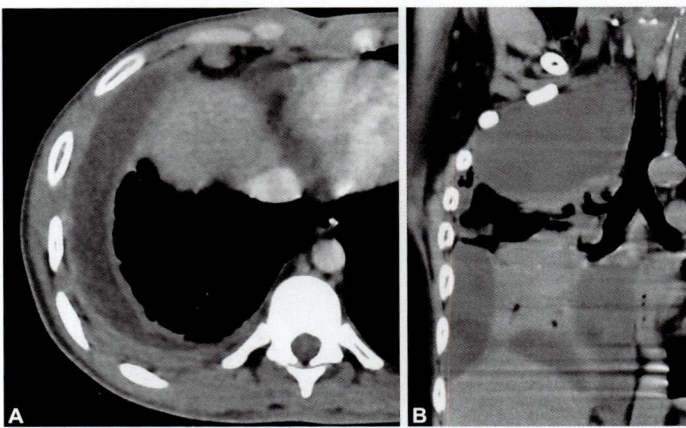

FIGS. 7F.24A AND B: Pleural effusion seen in right hemithorax with enhancing parietal pleural thickening (A), multiloculated pleural effusion seen along right upper and lower hemithorax (B).

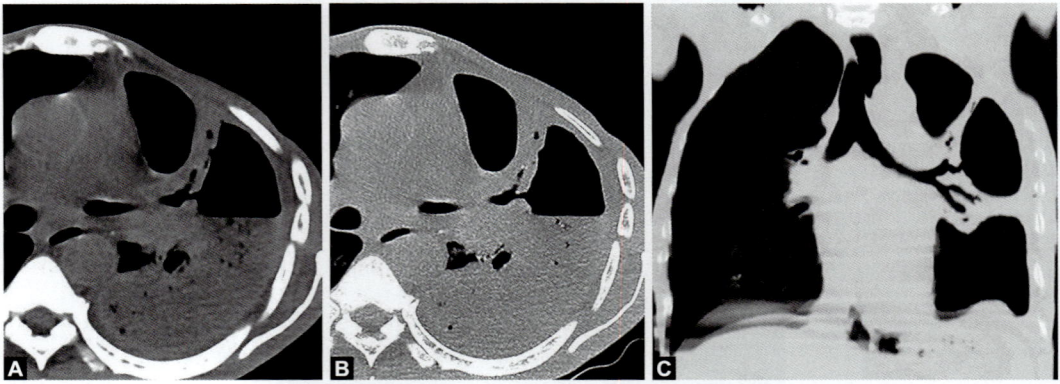

FIGS. 7F.25A TO C: This patient with past history of tuberculosis had recurrent left pleural effusion with air fluid levels within. CT scan was performed which showed bronchopleural fistula.

of pleural effusion. Nodular enhancing pleural thickening usually points to an underlying malignant cause such as pleural metastasis, mesothelioma, and pancoast tumor.

Unilateral pleural calcification is usually a result of previous empyema, hemothorax, and pleural effusion. Multiple bilateral pleural calcification/pleural plaques are seen in asbestos exposure.

Bronchopleural fistula can also be well identified with the help of CT scan and should be suspected in cases with chronic/recurrent pleural effusion **(Figs. 7F.25A to C)**.

■ CHEST WALL

A variety of primary bone and soft tissue diseases and manifestations of systemic disease can be characterized at CT reviewed with bone window setting. The common pathologies of ribs are fractures, fibrous dysplasia, chondrosarcoma, and Ewing's sarcoma **(Figs. 7F.26A and B)**.

CHAPTER 7: Basic Investigations: Indications and Interpretations

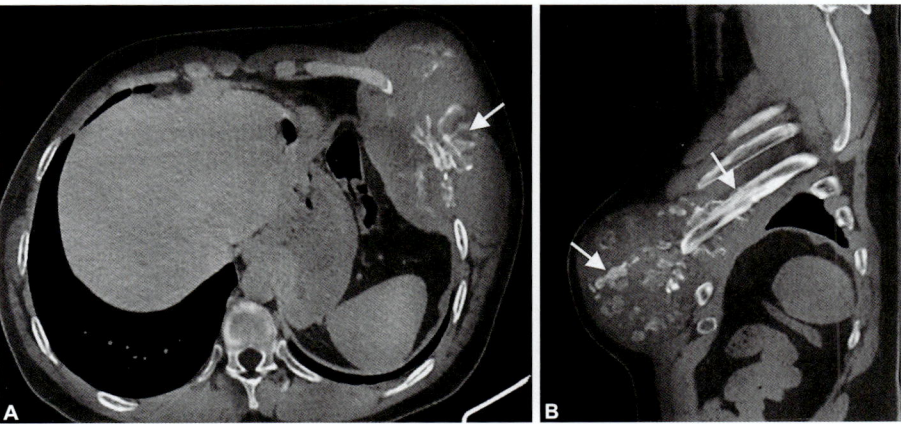

FIGS. 7F.26A AND B: Chrondrosarcoma of rib seen as osteolytic lesion of rib (white arrow pointing to rib) associated with soft tissue component showing multiple internal areas of calcification (arrows in A and B).

CT scan of thorax is also helpful in cases of cold abscess to look for deeper extension and communication of the chest wall abscess. Other soft tissue lesions of chest wall such as lipoma rhabdomyosarcoma can also be well characterized with CT of thorax.

■ CONCLUSION

CT scan of thorax has a very important role in the diagnosis of various conditions related to lungs, airways, mediastinum and chest wall. A good understanding of the basic patterns of HRCT of the lungs is very essential for accurate diagnosis.

SUGGESTED READINGS

1. Irodi A, Jagia P, Rajeshkannan R, Mohan C, Someshwar V, Sharma P. Comprehensive Textbook of Clinical Radiology: Chest and Cardiovascular System. Volume 3 - eBook. Elsevier Health Sciences; 2023.
2. Jankharia B. Computed Tomography of Interstitial Lung Diseases. 1st edition. In: Tree Life Media. 2019.
3. Richard W. High-resolution CT of the lung. 5th edition. Wolters Kluwer. 2015.

G. MOLECULAR DIAGNOSIS OF TUBERCULOSIS

Sumit Roy Tapadar

■ INTRODUCTION

Conventional tests for detection of mycobacterial drug resistance are slow, complicated, expensive, and difficult to perform in field conditions. The long-standing need for new, rapid, accurate, and convenient tests for tuberculosis (TB) diagnosis and drug resistance is addressed by different molecular tests. This article intends to focus on the basic features of such molecular tests with emphasis on their clinical applications.

■ NUCLEIC ACID AMPLIFICATION TEST

It is also known as direct amplification test. Here, the nucleic acid regions specific for *Mycobacterium tuberculosi*s complex (MTBC) are amplified. These tests may be applied directly on clinical samples such as sputum or gastric aspirate (in children).

For nucleic acid amplification test (NAAT), two types of arrangements are there: (1) Commercial kits such as Ampicor, GeneXpert and *M. tuberculosis* direct test, which are widely used; and (2) institutional in-house assay, which is basically laboratory-developed polymerase chain reaction (PCR) assay. They used to vary widely in laboratory methods and are used in research activities or resource-limited countries.

In India under Revised National TB Control Program (RNTCP), cartridge-based GeneXpert is widely used. It has been developed by the Foundation for Innovative New Diagnostics (FIND) in partnership with Cepheid Corporation and University of Medicine and Dentistry of New Jersey.

■ CBNAAT (Xpert MTB/RIF)

Standard Assay Procedure of CBNAAT (GeneXpert)

It is a single use plastic cartridge with multiple chambers reloaded with a mixture of lyophilized agent bids in liquid buffers for processing of the sample **(Fig. 7G.1)**. Within this cartridge, deoxyribonucleic acid (DNA) extraction and hemi-nested RT-PCR (reverse transcriptase-PCR) take place. The cartridge incorporates a syringe drive, a rotary drive, and a filter on which MTB bacilli are deposited after getting liberated from clinical material. The test platform is equipped with a sonic horn which gets inserted within the cartridge base and cause ultrasonic lysis of the bacilli for releasing the genetic material. The assay then amplifies a 192 bp (base pair) segment of the *rpoB* gene using a hemi-nested RT-PCR reaction 8,9. MTB is detected by the five overlapping molecular probes (probes A–E) that collectively are complementary to the entire 81 bp *rpoB* core region 8,9. MTB is identified when at least two of the five probes give positive signals with a cycle threshold (CT) of d"38 cycles that differ no more than a prespecified number of cycles. The basis for detection of rifampicin resistance is the difference

CHAPTER 7: Basic Investigations: Indications and Interpretations

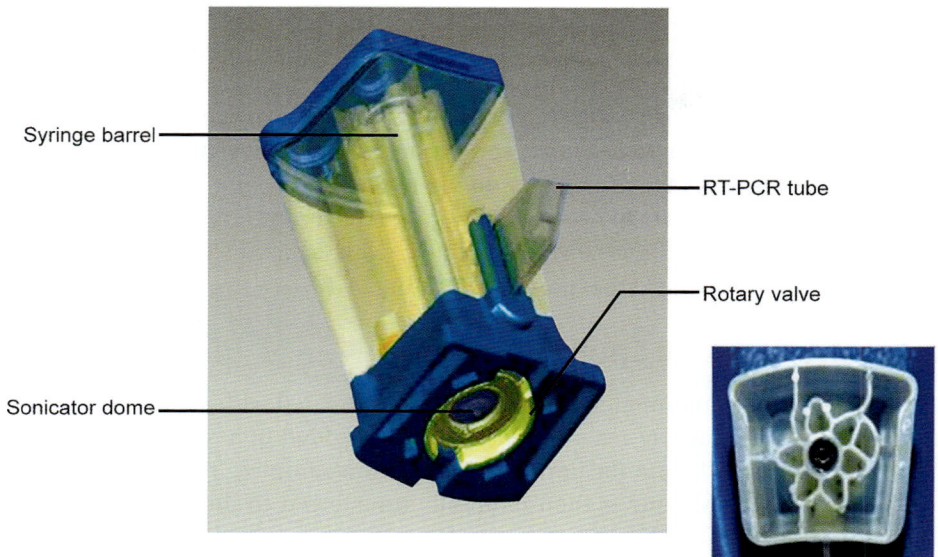

FIG. 7G.1: Cartridge design and operating principle.
(RT-PCR: reverse transcriptase-polymerase chain reaction)

between the first (early CT) and the last (late CT) MTB specific beacon [amplification cycle threshold (ACT)]. The test is configured in such a way that resistance was reported if ACT is >3.5 cycles and sensitive if d" 3.5 cycles.

Indications of CBNAAT

As per World Health Organization (WHO) recommendations, this test may be used for:
- Initial diagnostic test for suspected multidrug-resistant tuberculosis (MDR-TB) and human immunodeficiency virus (HIV) associated TB
- Previously treated suspected sputum negative cases
- Almost all/any extrapulmonary TB (EPTB) cases
- To diagnose pediatric TB (by testing gastric aspirates and sputum)

Method of Sample Collection for CBNAAT

"Falcon-tube" (supplied by RNTCP) is commonly used for the following purposes:
- *Sample for pulmonary TB*: Respiratory samples such as sputum or bronchoalveolar lavage (BAL) fluid are commonly used as sample. Sputum should be mucoid (to avoid saliva), quantity 2–10 mL, without contamination of food, *pan, supari*, tobacco, etc. Older and sick people may be asked for "induced sputum" by nebulization with 3% sodium chloride.
- *Pediatric pulmonary TB*: Single morning sample of empty stomach gastric aspirate is preferable. It must be immediately transported to laboratory, because acidity of gastric juice may affect it. Sample collected in a "fed" state is rejected. Older children who can expectorate should be encouraged for sputum sample.

- *Sample for EPTB*: Samples from representative sites of tubercular activity such as cerebrospinal fluid (CSF), body fluid, and pus are to be sent to laboratory. Pus, biopsy material, and blood-containing samples are thick and may have inhibitory proteins. So they take long time for processing and sometimes may be rejected by the system. Unacceptable samples include blood, serum, urine, needle washings, and fine-needle aspiration cytology (FNAC) if there is no visible aspirate. In a nutshell, a sample of EPTB diagnosis should be: (1) As much as possible in amount, (2) minimum blood contamination, (3) no additives, (4) to send in a screw-capped sterile container such as "Falcon tube", and (5) quick transport to laboratory.

Initiating the Test with Sputum Sample

Sputum samples or decontaminated sputum pellets are treated with sodium hydroxide and isopropanol-containing sample reagent (SR). This SR is added in a recommended 3:1 ratio for sputum pellets and 2:1 ratio for unprocessed sputum samples. Then it is incubated for 15 minutes. The treated sample is then manually transferred to the cartridge. Lastly, the cartridge is loaded in the GeneXpert instrument **(Fig. 7G.2)**.

A Brief Account of CBNAAT Reporting Format of RNTCP

The reporting format presently has the following components:
- Identity and particulars of the patient
- Description of type of sample (e.g., sputum, gastric aspirate, body fluid, etc.)
- *Purpose of testing*: Diagnosis [presumptive TB, repeat examination, presumptive nontuberculous mycobacteria (NTM)], follow-up (end of continuation phase and posttreatment) and others
- Laboratory number, CDL NIKSHAY ID
- Test validity—valid/invalid
- *M. tuberculosis*—detected/not detected/not available (error)

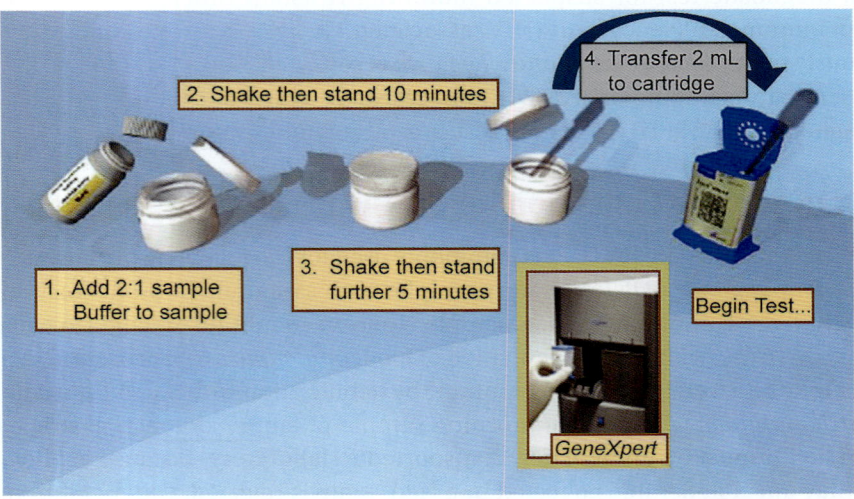

FIG. 7G.2: Simple sample processing—direct sputum.

- Rifampicin resistance—detected (low, medium, and high)/not detected/not available/indeterminate
- Test—no result/invalid/error (with error code)

■ CBNAAT REPORT INTERPRETATION—SOME EXAMPLES

Some common problematic situations that are faced by practicing physicians with CBNAAT report and the trouble shooting:

Situation 1

A patient having sputum smear positive for acid-fast bacilli (AFB) but CBNAAT reports negative: In such a situation, there is no need to repeat CBNAAT. A fresh sputum sample should be sent to the laboratory with a request to examine the smear for AFB. Interestingly, there exists a sample to sample variation in AFB positivity of sputum samples. If this sample comes as AFB smear positive then line probe assay (LPA) is to be done with it. Conversely, if it is AFB smear negative this time then liquid culture is the best option. One must be aware of the fact that smear positivity may be found in NTM. 5–7% of mycobacterial isolates are NTM. LPA can only suggest but cannot confirm NTM. It is confirmed by culture only.

Situation 2

A patient is having (suspected) tubercular lesions in more than one site. How many samples are to be sent for CBNAAT? As per RNTCP protocol, usually a sample from only one site of a patient is tested at a time. So the concerned physician has to decide which site is most likely to harbor active disease as well as accessible for sufficient and good quality sample. However, if the first sample comes as CBNNAT negative, then another sample from other site may be sent.

Situation 3

The CBNAAT report is showing rifampicin sensitive organism but sputum conversion is not achieved by first-line anti-tubercular drugs: A culture and drug sensitivity testing (CDST) is advisable here. "Phenotypic" DST report is more accurate in case of MTB. In this regard, it is worth remembering that no genotypic test is 100% accurate. Average sensitivity and specificity of CBNAAT is around 95%.

Situation 4

The CBNAAT report comes as "MTB detected", rifampicin resistance is "indeterminate": In such situation, a repeat CBNAAT test is to be done with a second sample. If it still comes as "indeterminate", then the only option is to collect a new specimen and to send for CDST.

Situation 5

The treating physician sends for CBNAAT test with a high hope but report comes as "invalid test" or "error" or "no result": In such situation, a repeat CBNAAT with a second sample is to be done.

Table 7G.1: Turnaround time (TAT) and strength of sample with common mycobacterial tests.				
	Sputum smear examination (Z-N/A-R staining)	Mycobacterial culture (solid/ liquid)	NAAT (conventional/RT)	CBNAAT
TAT	2 hours	2 days to 8 weeks	2 days	4 hours
Strength of sample	1,000 bacilli/mL	100 bacilli/mL	10 bacilli/mL	10 bacilli/mL

(NAAT: nucleic acid amplification test; CBNAAT: cartridge-based NAAT; RT: reverse transcriptase)

Situation 6

The CBNAAT report comes as "MTB not detected" in an extrapulmonary TB sample (e.g., body fluids, lymph node aspirate, etc.): Here, it is advisable to send sample for liquid culture for cross-checking the result of CBNAAT before announcing it as "nontubercular" etiology. Obviously, further relevant investigations and specialist's clinical judgment are also necessary.

Situation 7

There is strong clinical suspicion of TB, but CBNAAT result show "MTB not detected": In such a confusing situation, we should do a repeat sputum smear examination with a new specimen. If smear comes positive for AFB, then it should be send for LPA, while if it is negative then mycobacterial culture should be the next step.

Before concluding our discussion on CBNAAT, let us take an account of "turnaround time" (TAT) and strength of sample in a comparative manner with common mycobacterial tests **(Table 7G.1)**.

This comparison shows conspicuous supremacy of CBNAAT over other commonly employed tests. Moreover, it provides additional information of rifampicin resistance. From operational view point, its privilege is a fully automated system, needing minimal biosafety arrangements, training, and nonconventional laboratory arrangements.

■ LINE PROBE ASSAY

Molecular LPA focuses on rapid detection of rifampicin resistance (alone or in combination with isoniazid). It involves following steps as described here.

Initially DNA is extracted from *M. tuberculosis* culture isolate or directly from clinical specimens. Then PCR amplification of the resistance determining genetic region is done by biotinylated primers. Now labeled PCR products are hybridized with specific oligonucleotide probes which are immobilized in a strip. Labeled captured hybrids are now detected by colorimetric methods. Thus, the presence of *M. tuberculosis* is detectable as well as presence of resistance by mutation probes. If mutation is present in only one target region, then the amplicon will not hybridize with the relevant probe. Mutations are detected by lack of binding to wild type of probes and binding to specific probes for the most commonly occurring mutations. Posthybridization reaction leads to development of colored bands on strip at the site of probe binding and observed by eye.

Presently, two commercial LPA products are available, both of which are manufactured under ISO 13485:2003 certification and approved by regulatory authority in Europe. In-house LPAs, which are developed in a few academic settings only, have not adequately validated or evaluated. So their use in patient care is not recommended.

Systematic reviews and meta-analysis show LPA assay performance result as against conventional DST is highly sensitive (≥97%) and specific (≥99%), for detection of rifampicin resistance alone or in combination with isoniazid (sensitivity ≥90% and specificity ≥99%).

Application of Line Probe Assay

Line probe assay test is applicable on:
- Sputum positive sputum sample
- *M. tuberculosis* isolates in culture

Biosafety

Line probe assay requires digestion, decontamination, and concentration of clinical material prior to DNA extraction. These processes involve aerosol production and cross-contamination of specimens. WHO recommends this specimen processing is to be done in a biological safety cabinet (BSC) under at least biosafety level-2 (BSL-2) conditions. While performing the assay on positive cultures requires BSL-3 facilities.

Adoption of CBNAAT and LPA does not eliminate the need for conventional culture and DST as they remain necessary for diagnosis of TB in smear negative patients and diagnosis of extensively drug-resistant TB (XDR-TB).

SUGGESTED READINGS

1. Long MH, Johansson E, Lonnroth K, Eriksson B, Winkvist A, Diwan VK. Longer delays in tuberculosis diagnosis among women in Vietnam. Int J Tuberc Lung Dis. 1999;3(5):388-93.
2. Gupta KB, Garg S. Sputum induction—a useful tool in diagnosis of respiratory diseases. Lung India. 2006; 23:82-6
3. Tadolini M, Centis R, D'Ambrosio L, et al. Clinical diagnosis of TB and role of GeneXpert. Breathe. 2012;9:104.

CHAPTER 8

National Tuberculosis Elimination Program

Supriya Sarkar, Surya Kant, Arunava Dutta Choudhury

■ INTRODUCTION

Our fight against tuberculosis (TB) started with rituals followed by sanatorium treatment with rest, fresh air, and good diet then with surgery and anti-TB medicines. Revolutionary findings of Madras Chemotherapeutic Centre in 1956 led us to domiciliary treatment of TB. In 1962, *National TB Control Program (NTP)* was launched to control the curse in India. An organizational set-up was established with Central TB Division (CTD), district TB units, and chest clinics. In 1983, short course chemotherapy (SCC) with rifampicin (R) was introduced in NTP. But NTP failed miserably with only 30% case detection and 30% success rate. In 1993, World Health Organization (WHO) declared TB as *global public health emergency*.

■ REVISED NATIONAL TB CONTROL PROGRAM

In 1993, Revised National TB Control Program (RNTCP) was launched as pilot project and subsequently entire country was covered by 1997. RNTCP encompassed "Directly Observed Treatment Short-course (DOTS)", "Fixed Drug Combination (FDC)", "Stop TB Strategy", and "NIKSHAY portal". In 2012, TB was proclaimed as notifiable disease. Subsequently, molecular diagnostic tests were introduced that include cartridge-based nucleic acid amplification test (CBNAAT) and Truenat (a chip-based test) as point-of-care test (POCT) and line probe assay (LPA) [first line (FL-LPA) and second line (SL-LPA)] at intermittent reference laboratories (IRL). Subsequently, several changes were undertaken such as abolition of Category III (2010) and Category II regimens (2018); introduction of daily regimen (2016); addition of ethambutol (E) in continuation phase (CP); and long-term follow-up.

Anti-TB chemotherapy has achieved high cure and has reduced mortality but has failed to reduce the epidemiologically significant pool (patients survived with sputum positivity), responsible for spread of disease. Moreover, the problem has been complicated by human immunodeficiency virus (HIV) infection, diabetes mellitus (DM), drug-resistant TB (DR-TB), and COVID-19 pandemic.

NATIONAL TUBERCULOSIS ELIMINATION PROGRAM

World Health Organization advocated END TB strategy with a vision to end TB, zero death, and rescuing families from catastrophic costs by 2030. NTEP was introduced and incorporated in National Health Mission with an aim of "TB-Free India"/"*TB-Mukt Bharat*" by 2025, 5 years earlier than global target. NTEP set certain target to be achieved by 2025.

The Objective of National Tuberculosis Elimination Program

- To reduce estimated TB incidence rate to 44 (36–158) per 100,000
- To reduce estimated TB prevalence rate to 65 (56–93) per 100,000
- To reduce estimated mortality due to TB to 3 (3–4) per 100,000
- To achieve zero catastrophic cost for affected families due to TB

To attain those *objectives* following milestones were set those to be achieved by 2025:
- We must achieve treatment success rate to 92% among drug-sensitive TB (DS-TB) and at least 75% among drug-resistant TB (DR-TB).
- We must implement active case finding (ACF) among the targeted population.
- We must notify all TB patients before starting treatment and at least 90% of them must receive financial support through direct benefit transfer.
- We must start TB preventive treatment (TPT) in at least 95% of eligible population (all house hold contacts and high-risk population).

Pillars of National Tuberculosis Elimination Program

National Tuberculosis Elimination Program is based on four strategic pillars:
1. To *"Prevent"* by ensuring airborne infection control, prevention of emergence of TB in susceptible populations by TPT, and implementation of strategies to prevent DR-TB.
2. To *"Detect"* by early identification of presumptive TB and early detection of DS-TB and DR-TB by highly sensitive diagnostic tools.
3. To *"Treat"* by initiating and sustaining free and appropriate anti-TB treatment in all cases, implementation of programmatic management of DR-TB (PMDT), and management of comorbidities.
4. To *"Build"* by appropriate infrastructure and ecosystem by ensuring adequate funding, human resources, community engagement, and research activities.

NATIONAL TB PREVALENCE SURVEY 2019–2021

Long after National Sample Survey (1955–1957), National TB Prevalence Survey was conducted in 2019–2021. The findings were eye opener and helped the program in modifying and planning NTEP in India.
- About 64% of patients with respiratory symptoms did not seek healthcare services and that leads to the change from passive case finding to ACF.
- The yield of CBNAAT was found to be twice than that of smear microscopy (2.0–1.1%) and that leads to CBNAAT first policy (CBNAAT is a diagnostic tool and cannot be used for follow-up).

- Chest X-ray (CXR) had 42.6% additional yield, leading to reintroduction of CXR as a diagnostic as well as follow-up tool.
- About 23.4% patients had past history of TB, leading to incorporation of long-term follow-up of TB patients.
- Notification ratio was 2.84 (indicating for each notified case there were two missed cases) and that led to mandatory notification of TB cases.
- Prevalence of latent TB infection was 31.4%. There was a 10% lifetime chance of conversion to active disease, and 60% of conversion occurs by the first year. The TPT was introduced.
- Patients preferred public and private facilities equally (49% vs. 49%) despite of cost incurred Rs. 7,500/patient in public sector bared by government versus Rs. 20,000/patient in private sector. TB elimination program gave extra emphasis on private sectors.
- Important comorbidities of TB were social problems such as malnutrition, smoking, alcohol intake, diabetes, and silicosis, and all were incorporated in National Health Mission.

■ DIAGNOSIS OF TB IN NATIONAL TUBERCULOSIS ELIMINATION PROGRAM

New classification of TB: TB cases are reclassified into:
- "Microbiologically confirmed TB" where the diagnosis is confirmed by smear, culture, or molecular tests.
- "Clinically diagnosed TB" where TB is diagnosed by clinical, radiological, biochemical, histopathological, or a combined method.

Cartridge-based nucleic acid amplification test/Truenat is recommended in all presumptive TB cases and in high-risk subjects. Presumptive TB for adult includes: (1) Cough for more than 2 weeks, (2) unexplained fever for more than 2 weeks, (3) significant weight loss, (4) hemoptysis, and (5) abnormal CXR. In children, failure to gain weight and contact with known case of TB are additionally included. For extrapulmonary TB (EPTB) site specific manifestations with or without constitutional symptoms are included. High-risk subjects include close contacts with HIV-infected persons, patients with diabetes, renal disease, malignancies and other immunosuppressive conditions, and patients on immunosuppressive medications.

Next step is to collect appropriate clinical materials. Clinical materials include sputum, bronchoalveolar lavage (BAL) and transbronchial lung biopsy (TBLB) for pulmonary TB and miliary TB. For EPTB, clinical materials include aspirated fluid from pleural effusion, pericardial effusion, cerebrospinal fluid and ascites; and fine-needle aspiration (FNA) and biopsy samples from solid lesions (lymph nodes, tumors, etc). Clinical materials should be sent to laboratories in Falcon tube. Biopsy samples should be sent in normal saline (just deep).

Cartridge-based nucleic acid amplification test can confirm TB as well as detect R sensitivity. Accordingly, TB cases are classified as R sensitive (RS-TB) and R resistant TB (RR-TB). FL-LPA can divide RS-TB into DS-TB and isoniazid (H) mono-resistant TB. RR-TBs are subjected to FL-LPA, SL-LPA, and liquid culture with drug sensitivity test (LC-DST) to diagnose multi-drug-resistant TB (MDR-TB) and extensively drug-resistant TB (XDR-TB)

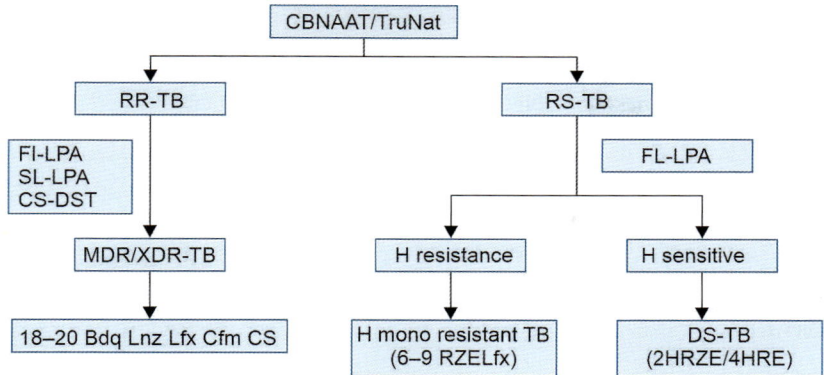

FLOWCHART 8.1: The diagnosis and treatment regimens of TB.
(CBNAAT: cartridge-based nucleic acid amplification test; DS-TB: drug-sensitive TB; FL-LPA: first-line LPA; LPA: line probe assay; MDR: multi-drug-resistant; RR-TB: R-resistant TB; RS-TB: R-sensitive TB; SL-LPA: second line LPA; XDR: extensively drug-resistant)

(**Flowchart 8.1**). MDR-TB is defined as resistance to H and R with or without other drugs. Whereas, XDR-TB is defined MDR/RR-TB with resistant to any fluoroquinolone and at least one additional Group A drug [bedaquiline (Bdq) or linezolid].

MANAGEMENT OF TB IN NATIONAL TUBERCULOSIS ELIMINATION PROGRAMME

Drug-sensitive TB is treated with 2 months of HREZ (where E means ethambutol and Z means pyrazinamide) followed by 4 months of HRE. E is a companion drug, and its main function is to prevent the development of R resistance in endemic H-resistant countries such as India. No extension of intensive phase (IP) is permissible, whereas 3–6 months of extension of continuation phase (CP) is allowed in selected cases, particularly in slow responders, disseminated TB, skeletal, and central nervous system TB (CNS-TB). Each FDC tablet (adult) contains 75 mg H, 150 mg R, 400 mg Z and 275 mg E for IP and FDC containing same doses of HRE for CP. Children FDC tablet contains 50 mg H, 75 mg R, 150 mg Z, and 100 mg E for IP and FDC containing same doses of HRE for CP. E is usually supplied separately. The number of FDC in adult is depicted in **Table 8.1** and that in children is depicted in **Table 8.2**.

Table 8.1: The number of Fixed Drug Combination (FDC) table in adult as per weight band.		
Weight band	**Intensive phase**	**Continuation phase**
25–34 kg	2 tablets	2 tablets
35–49 kg	3 tablets	3 tablets
50–64 kg	4 tablets	4 tablets
65–75 kg	5 tablets	5 tablets
>75 kg	6 tablets	6 tablets

Table 8.2: The number of tablets in children.		
Weight band	Intensive phase	Continuation phase
4–7 kg	1 tablet	1 tablet
8–11 kg	2 tablets	2 tablets
12–15 kg	3 tablets	3 tablets
16–24 kg	4 tablets	4 tablets
25–29 kg	3 + 1A* tablets	3 + 1A* tablets
30–39 kg	2 + 2A* tablets	2 + 2A* tablets

*A means adult Fixed Drug Combination (FDC) tablet.

FOLLOW-UP OF TB PATIENTS

Assessment of Response to Treatment

- *Clinical follow-up at least monthly*: For improvement of chest symptoms, weight gain, control of comorbid condition such as HIV and DM and adverse reaction to ATD
- Laboratory investigation including sputum smear examination at the end of IP and end of treatment or when medical officer considers during continuation phase and other laboratory investigations, for example, liver function tests
- CXR and other radiological investigations as and when necessary [magnetic resonance imaging (MRI) spine at the end of treatment or earlier in partial responders]

Long-term Follow-up

As 23.4% of TB patients have past history of TB, a long-term follow-up for 2 years is recommended in NTEP. After completion of treatment, each patient should be followed up at the end of 6, 12, 18, and 24 months, and appropriate investigations should be offered.

MANAGEMENT OF DRUG-RESISTANT TB

H mono-resistant TB is treated with 6–9 months of RZE and levofloxacin. RR-TB/MDR-TB are treated with "all oral longer MDR regimen" containing all group A and group B drugs **(Table 8.3)**. The regimen contains 18–20 months of Bdq (for 6 months), linezolid, levofloxacin, clofazimine, and cycloserine. Group C drugs are used when any drug has to be replaced due to intolerance, side effects, or contraindications. Selected cases may be treated with "all oral Bdq containing shorter regimen" for patient > 5 years and body weight > 15 kg. Patient should not have extensive pulmonary TB, severe EP-TB, pregnancy and lactation, bacilli resistant to FQ or other drugs and *KatG* gene or *InhA* gene mutation (not both). All oral shorter regimen is a 9–11 months regimen containing 4–6 months of Bdq (6 m), Lfx, Cfz, Z, E, H^h, Eto; followed by 5 months of Lfx, Cfz, Z, and E. Regimens used in the management of TB are depicted in **Table 8.4**. High dose H (H^h) means 600 mg for weight band 30–45 kg and 900 mg for patients with 46 kg and above body weight.

CHAPTER 8: National Tuberculosis Elimination Program

Table 8.3: Classification of drugs used in drug-resistant TB (DR-TB) with their doses.

Group	Drugs	Doses in adult (45–70 kg body weight)
A (Include all three drugs)	Levofloxacin (LFx) or	1000 mg
	Moxifloxacin (Mfx)	400 mg
	Bedaquiline (Bdq)	400 mg/day for 2 weeks then 400 mg weekly up to 24 weeks
	Linezolid (Lzd)	600 mg/day and 300 mg/day after 6 months
B (Add one or two drugs)	Clofazimine (Cfz)	50 mg/day
	Cycloserine (Cs) or Terizidone (Trd)	750 mg/day
C (Used as a substitute of group A and B drugs)	Ethambutol (E)	1,200 mg/day
	Delanamid (Dlm)	50 mg/day for 24 weeks up to 11 years / 100 mg/day for 24 weeks above 11 years
	Pyrazinamide (Z)	1,750 mg/day
	Ethionamide (Eto) or Prothionamide (Pto)	750 mg/day
	Para-aminosalicylic acid (PAS)	16 g/day
	Amikacin (Ak) or Streptomycin (S)	750 mg/day
	Imipenem (Ipm) + cilastatin (Cln) or	1,000 /1,000 mg twice daily
	Meropenem (Mpm)	1,000 mg thrice daily
	Amoxycillin + clavulanic acid	875/125 mg 2 doses in morning and 1 dose in evening

Table 8.4: Regimens used in National Tuberculosis Elimination Program (NTEP).

Patient group	Intensive phase	Continuation phase
Drug sensitive TB	2 HRZE	4 HRE
H mono resistant TB	6–9 RZE, Lfx	
All oral longer regime for drug-resistant TB	18–20 Bdq (6 m), Lzd, Lfx, Cfz, and Cs	
All oral shorter regime for drug-resistant TB	4–6 Bdq (6 m), Lfx, Cfz, Z, E, H^h, and Eto	5 Lfx, Cfz, Z, and E

Note: High dose H (H^h) is 600–900 mg of H.

It should be done under programmed condition, the programmatic management of DR-TB (PMDT). The drugs used are toxic (needs pretreatment evaluation and regular follow-up), costly (some of them are not available in open market), and the response to treatment is not always satisfactory. Pretreatment and during treatment counseling of patients and family members are an essential step in PMDT program. Pretreatment evaluation includes ocular, psychiatric, and otolaryngological check-up; pregnancy test; ECG (to detect cardiac dysrhythmias and QTc measurement); complete blood count, liver function, renal function, serum electrolyte levels (K, Ca, and Mg), thyroid function tests, blood sugar testing; serum uric acid, amylase, and lipase level; routine urine test; and HIV testing and counseling. QTc > 500 Ms is an absolute and >450 Ms is a relative contraindication for using Bdq. The adverse reactions and their management are depicted in **Table 8.5**.

Table 8.5: Side effects and their management.

Manifestations	Offending drugs	Management
Rash, allergic reactions, and anaphylactic reactions	All anti-TB drugs	• Minor reactions may be managed by antihistamines, sometimes corticosteroids • Major reactions need cessation of therapy, identification of offending drug by one in sequential introduction of drugs as H, R, Z, E, Eto, Cs, PAS, FQ, and injectables
Gastrointestinal symptoms such as nausea, vomiting, pain abdomen, flatulence, and diarrhea	All drugs mainly Z, H, E, Eto, PAS, Cfz, and FQs	• Advice to take drugs with snakes • Use H2-receptor inhibitors (avoid proton pump inhibitors), domperidone, metoclopramide/ ondansetron, and loperamide (in severe diarrhea)
Liver function abnormalities/jaundice	Z, H, R, Eto, PAS, FQ, and Bdq	• Symptomatic management for liver enzyme elevation up to 3–5 times • Stop drugs if enzymes rise > 5 times or jaundice Reintroduce drugs after liver functions come down to normal (avoiding Z) • Use regimes with no or single hepatotoxic drug in severe and life-threatening TB
Giddiness and vertigo	Aminoglycosides, Eto, and FQ	Stopping offending drug or reducing dose
Hematological *abnormalities*	Lzd	Stop Lzd or reduce dose to 300 mg/day
Hypothyroidism	Eto, Pto, and PAS	Use thyroid hormone during therapy
Arthralgia	Z, E, FQ, and Bdq	Use analgesics, measure uric acid, and allopurinol is required in severe arthralgia
Peripheral neuritis	Cs, Lzd, H, S, and FQ	Always add pyridoxin 100 mg in DR-TB, alcoholic, and diabetics
Headache, depression, and psychotic symptoms	Cs, Bdq, H, FQ, and Eto	Lower dose of Cs, use amitriptyline, and fluoxetine
Suicidal ideas	Cs, H, and Eto	Hospitalization and stop Cs
Seizures	Cs, H, and FQ	• Avoid in case of history of seizure disorders • Hold offending drugs. Initiate anticonvulsants
Tendonitis	FQ	Ibuprofen, withdraw FQ
Nephropathy	Injectables	Withdraw injectables. Thrice weekly dose of E
Vestibular toxicity	Injectables, Cs, FQ, H, Eto, and Lzd	Thrice weekly dose or withdrawal of offending drug
Optic neuritis	E, Lzd, Eto, Cfz, rifabutin, H, and S	Stop E and Lzd—do not restart
QTc prolongation	Bdq, Dlm, FQ, Clarithomycin, and Cfz	QTc > 500 Ms stop the drug. Check serum K, Ca, Mg, and correct them
Gynecomastia, acne, and alopecia	Eto, Pto, and H	Usually temporary, counsel patients

EXTRAPULMONARY TB

Extrapulmonary TB means diseases caused by mycobacterium tuberculosis complex involving any organ other than lungs. EPTB occurs by spread of bacilli from lungs through hematogenous, lymphatic or local spread, and their subsequent activation in conducive atmosphere. Recently, EPTB has been focused in National TB Elimination Programme (NTEP).

Diagnosis: EPTB usually presents with site-specific manifestations. Radiological investigations include X-ray, ultrasonography (USG), contrast-enhanced computed tomography (CECT), MRI, etc., and identify the structural changes in EPTB. The confirmation of diagnosis requires: (1) Collection of clinical materials by aspiration, FNA, or biopsy; (2) sending samples in normal saline (just deep); and (3) subjecting them to smear, CS-DST, and molecular diagnostic tests (CBNAAT and LPA). CXR and sputum for CBNAAT (if sputum is available) should be done in all EPTB cases.

Management: Basically, the management of EPTB is same as that of PTB with 2 months of HRZE, followed by 4 months of HRE. The duration may be prolonged for 9–12 months in skeletal and neurological TB. Surgery may be required in selective cases. DR EP-TB is usually treated with all oral longer drug-resistant regimens. All oral shorted regimens may be tried in pleural TB and lymph node TB.

Assessment of response to treatment: Radiological changes may be permanent making follow-up difficult. Moreover, immune reconstitution inflammatory syndrome (IRIS)/paradoxical reaction (enlargement of lymph nodes or appearance of new lymph nodes and increase of serous fluid with or without systemic symptoms) makes EP-TB assessment complex. IRISs are generally managed with continuation of anti-TB drugs, symptomatic management, and sometimes corticosteroids. Corticosteroids are sometimes used to prevent fibrosis in pericardial effusion and meningitis, to prevent structural changes in renal TB, to treat vital structure compression from glands or tumors, and to reduce perilesional edema in tuberculoma of the brain. Differential diagnosis in nonresponders or partially responders includes wrong diagnosis, IRIS, non-TB mycobacterial infections, DR-TB, etc.

NOTIFICATION OF TB

In 2012, TB has been declared as notifiable disease, and in 2018, nondeclarance of TB was made a punishable offence. It has been found that for each reported case, there are two unreported cases. The emphasis is to bring all TB cases, whether treatment in public or private sector, should be brought under program, and the accountability can be fixed. The NIKSHAY portal, http://nikshay.gov.in, has been developed to report TB cases.

TB PREVENTION TREATMENT

The lifetime chance of conversion into active disease is about 10%, and 60% conversion occurs in the first year. In people living with HIV (PL-HIV) the chance of activation is 10% per year. TPT is intended to prevent the development of active disease. TPT will incorporate all house hold contacts of confirmed DS-TB cases and PL-HIV in first phage. Subsequent phases include all high-risk group persons and then household contacts of DR-TB cases. The selection of persons needs: (1) Detection of TB infection by tuberculin test, gamma-interferon release assay, or newer skin test Cy-TB; and (2) exclusion of active TB by appropriate tests. Two regimes are used: (1) Regimen I with H for 6–9 months (10 mg/kg body weight for children <5 years and 5 mg/kg for >5 years of age) and (2) regimen II with a combination of H and rifapentine (P). HP is available as FDC containing 300 mg H and 300 mg P. In adult (above 30 kg body weight), the dose is three tablets weekly for 3 months.

■ ACTIVE CASE FINDING

Revised National TB Control Program advocated passive case finding, meaning patients those seek medical help should be screened for TB. The aim was to achieve 85% cure rate first and then to detect at least 70% cases. Survey showed that only one-third of chest symptomatic seeks medical help. A revolutionized shift from passive to ACF has been advocated in NTEP. ACP includes rigorous TB contact tracing and investigation for TB among household contacts and high-risk groups.

■ CERTIFICATION OF ELIMINATION OF TB

To motivate, encourage competition, and incentivize states and districts, the program of certification has been started. "Bronze award" for > 20%, "Silver award" for >40% and "Gold award" for >60% reduction of TB burden and "TB free district/state" for reduction more than 80% (or ≤44 lakh decline) from that of 2015 data.

■ TRAINING AND RESEARCH ACTIVITIES

Dissertations and operational research (OR) activities are encouraged by timely acceptance and release of funds. Training must include motivation and warmness that will be percolated to patients. Training should include the importance of defaulter retrieval and regular home visit.

■ STRATEGIES FOR PRIVATE SECTOR

As the same number of patients of TB is treated in private sector and public sector, the program has emphasized to bring them into the system. An extra drive has been initiated for private sectors by addressing their concerns. Interface agencies are utilized for offering free drugs and diagnostic facilities, for example, assigning private laboratories in NTEP.

Nikshay Poshan Yojana (started from 2018): The target is to give all patients ₹500 per month during treatment as direct benefit transfer. Doctors, medical staffs, civil society personals, and general people have been encouraged to adopt TB patients and distribute nutritious food to patients during treatment period.

FUTURE SUGGESTED CHANGES IN NATIONAL TUBERCULOSIS ELIMINATION PROGRAM

Diagnosis: CBNAAT will be replaced by Xpert XDR, simply by a 10-color calibration to the existing CBNAAT machine. Xpert XDR, in addition to all, will detect resistance to H, E, fluoroquinolone (FQ), and injectable drugs. Drug susceptibility testing (DST) will include new drugs such as Bdq and linezolid in future. Cy-TB, a skin prick test such as Mantoux test using antigen specific to TB bacilli, will be used to detect TB infection.

Management: In DSTB, where H and FQ resistance not detected, 4 months regime will be recommended with 2 months HPZM (M means moxifloxacin) followed by 2 months HPM. For RR-TB, 6-month regimens will be recommended for age group ≥14 years. BPaL regimen ("B" for bedaquilin, "Pa" for pretomanid and "L" for linezolid) for FQ resistance cases, and BPaLM regimen for FQ sensitive cases.

CONCLUSION

There is a success story in laboratories and program designing, but the program has failed. A potentially curable disease may be going to be incurable. Despite political and administrative commitment and achieving several milestones, we are far away from our set targets. COVID pandemic has taken away more than 2 years. Problem of missing cases and inertia of public sector must be addressed immediately. We must accelerate our endeavor by declaring war on TB and implement the program at the ground level. Let all players in government sectors, private sectors, NGOs and social activists come together to make the program successful.

SUGGESTED READINGS

1. Katri GR. National Tuberculosis Control Programme. J Indian Med Assoc. 1996;94(10):372-5.
2. Revised National Tuberculosis Control Programme. National Strategic Plan for TB Elimination 2017–2025, March 2017, Central TB Division, Directorate General of Health Services, Ministry of Health with Family Welfare, Nirman Bhawan, New Delhi–110 108.
3. National Tuberculosis Elimination Programme. National Strategic Plan to End Tuberculosis in India. Accelerating the National Response for Expanded Coverage and Sustained Impact at Scale to End TB in India. June 2020. Ministry of Health with Family Welfare, Nirman Bhawan, New Delhi–110 108.
4. National TB Prevalence Survey in India 2019 – 2021. Indian Council of Medical Research (ICMR), New Delhi; ICMR-National Institute for Research in Tuberculosis (NIRT), Chennai, Ministry of Health and Family Welfare, Government of India.
5. Guidelines for Programmatic Management of Drug-Resistant Tuberculosis. March 2021. National Tuberculosis Elimination Program. Central TB Division, Ministry of Health with Family Welfare, Government of India, New Delhi.
6. Training Module on Extrapulmonary Tuberculosis, 2023. Ministry of Health and Family Welfare Government of India. Nirman Bhawan, New Delhi.
7. Guidelines for Programmatic Management of Tuberculosis Preventive Treatment in India. July 2021. National TB Elimination Programme, Central TB Division, Ministry of Health and Family Welfare Government of India, Nirman Bhawan, New Delhi.

Index

Page numbers followed by *b* refer to box, *f* refer to figure, *fc* refer to flowchart, and *t* refer to table.

A

Abdominal paradox 107
Abdominojugular reflux 115, 116*f*
Abscess 111
 intra-abdominal 212
 liver 212
 lung 46, 78
Absorption collapse 38
 common causes of 39
Acid-base
 buffer 25
 disorders, primary 190*t*, 191, 193*t*
 disturbances, mixed 194
Acidemia 191
Acid-fast bacilli 37, 44, 170
Acne 244
Acquired hiatus hernia 14
Acquired immunodeficiency syndrome 33, 172
Acute chest syndrome 53
Acute coronary syndrome 60
Acute cough 32
 management of 32
Acute respiratory distress syndrome 27, 190*t*
Addison's disease 154
Adenosine 34
 deaminase 206
Adie's tonic pupil 139
Air 174
 fluid 230*f*
  level 187*f*
 hunger 105
 trapping 223, 224
Airway 27, 177
 anatomy of 7
 disease 21, 33, 61, 168, 214, 227
 extrathoracic 7
 inflammation 35
  measuring 34
 intrathoracic 28
 obstruction forced expiratory volume, severity of 201*t*
 reconstruction of 215*f*
 subdivision of 16*f*
Albumin 132
Alcohol 93
Alkalemia 191
Allan's test 147
Allergic bronchopulmonary aspergillosis 171, 227*f*
Allergic reactions 244
Allergic rhinitis 32
Alopecia 244
Alveolar cell carcinoma 169
Alveolar ducts 16
Alveolar macrophages 169
Alveolar proteinosis 220
Ambulatory blood pressure monitoring 97, 98*f*
 report 99*f*
Amiodarone 73
Amyloidosis 119, 225
Anaphylactic reactions 244
Anchovy sauce-like sputum 171
Anemia 84
 classification of 85
 clinical presentation of 84
 detection of 84*f*
 examination of 84
 severity of 44
 types of 85*b*
Anemic hypoxia 70
Aneurysm 9
Angina pectoris 49
Angiotensin-converting enzyme inhibitor 32
Angular stomatitis 118
Anion gap metabolic acidosis 196
Ankle-brachial pressure index 97
Ankylosing spondylitis 200
Anorexia 128
Anthem sign 115
Anthropometry 127
Anti-tubercular
 chemotherapy 238
 therapy, complications of 48
Anxiety neurosis 77
Aorta
 coarctation of 103
 giant aneurysms of 117
Aortic aneurysm 14
Aortic arch, aneurysms of 8
Aortic dissection 50, 51*f*, 60
 classifications of 50*t*
 diagnosis of 50
 management of 51
Aortic stenosis 101
Ape hand deformity 150
Aphthous ulcer 119
Apical impulse 160
Apnea
 aentral 107
 deglutition 107
 mixed 108
 monitoring 108
 test 108
Apraxia 83
Arachnodactyly 145
Arch anomaly 228
Architectural distortion 219
Argyll Robertson pupil 139
Arm span 129
Arrhythmia 97, 100
Arsenic hyperpigmentation 145*f*
Arterial blood gas
 analysis 74, 189
 analyze 189
 applications of 189
 normal values of 190*t*
 report 191
Arterial blood sample 189
Arterial hypoxemia 88
Arterial oxygen saturation 70
Arterial vascular systems 42
Artery
 abdominal 29
 bronchial 9
 bronchiole 216*f*

carotid 114*f*
centrilobular 216*f*
palpation of 102, 103
pulmonary 216*f*
thoracic 29
Arthralgia 244
Artifacts 176
Assess oxygenation 191
Asthma 1, 3, 33, 34, 53, 169, 171, 172
 diagnosis of 34
Ataxic gait 120
Atelectasis 180
Athetosis 151
Atrial fibrillation 100
 common causes of 101
Atrial flutter 100
Auscultation 165
Auscultatory gap 96
Autoimmune disorders 43
Autonomic nervous system, tumor of 15
Axillary lymphadenopathy, unilateral 127
Axillary region 124
Azithromycin 36
Azygos vein 116

B

Bacterial endocarditis, subacute 148
Bacterial infection 205
Bacterial meningitis 111
Barometric pressure 22
Beau's line 133
Bilirubin 124
Biochemical tests 44
Biopsy
 lung 4
 needle 208, 211
 pleural 211, 212
Biosafety 237
Biotin 133
Birt–Hogg–Dubé
 Down syndrome 225
 syndrome 224
Blackish sputum 171
Bleeding 118
 profile 44
Blood 180
 counts 44
 eosinophilia, peripheral 205
 gases 21
 pressure 94, 94*t*

diastolic 95
 systolic 52
stained sputum 170
sugar testing 243
supply 9
Blood-cerebrospinal fluid barrier 29
Bochdalek foramen 13
Body fluids 236
Body mass index 130
 calculation 128*t*
Bone 177
 density 174
Bouchard's node 151
Boutonniere deformity 146
Brachial pulse 104*f*
Bradycardia
 causes of 100
 relative 112
Bradypnea 106, 109
Brain suffer 23
Branch pulmonary artery 15
Breath 21
 mechanics of 26
 rate 105*t*
 shortness of 33
 sound 165
Breathing
 apneustic 107
 ataxic 107, 107*f*
 Biot's 64, 107
 Cheyne-Stokes 64, 106, 106*f*, 155
 Kussmaul's 64
 obstructive 106, 106*f*
 paradoxical 107
 rapid deep 106, 107*f*
 rapid shallow 106, 106*f*
 slow 106, 106*f*
Breathlessness 108
Broca's aphasia 81, 83
Bronchi 8
Bronchial breath sound 47, 165
 high-pitched 166
Bronchial hyperreactivity 34
Bronchial secretions 17
Bronchiectasis 39, 43, 46, 169, 224, 227, 228*f*
 cylindrical 228*f*
 signs of 227
Bronchitis 34
 chronic 169
Bronchoalveolar lavage 45, 240
Bronchodilator response 202

Bronchogenic carcinoma 43, 46, 117
Broncholithiasis 35
Bronchophony 166
Bronchopleural fistula 208, 230*f*
Bronchopneumonia 217, 218*f*
Bronchoprovocation test 34
Bronchopulmonary lymph nodes 9
Bronchopulmonary segments 15
Bronchoscopy 45
 techniques 170
Bronchus
 left main 215*f*
 right main 8
Bucket handle movement 158
Bulla 121
Butterfly rash over cheeks 142*f*

C

Cachexia 128
Calcium deposition 138
Candidiasis 154
Capillary refill time 147
Carbon dioxide 21, 22, 25
 dissolved 25
 forms of 26*t*
 partial pressure of 23
 removal of 30
 values 24*t*
Carbon monoxide 22, 65
Cardiac activities 61
Cardiac notch 10
Cardiac percussion 164
Cardiac silhouette 177, 185
 enlarged 212
Cardiomyopathy 3
Cardiopulmonary exercise 64
Cardiothoracic ratio 177
Cardiovascular abnormalities, palpation of 162
Cardiovascular disorders 43
Cardiovascular system 5, 62, 148
Carotene 124
Carotid artery 114*f*
Carotid pulse 104*f*, 114, 114*t*
Cartridge design 233*f*
Cartridge-based nucleic acid amplification test 37, 171, 238, 240, 241
 indications of 233
Cataract 138
Cellular respiration 104
Central airway obstruction 202

Index

Central nervous system 72, 241
Central venous pressure 113
Centrilobular emphysema 225f, 226
Cerebellar gait 120
Cervical
 myelitis 14
 sympathetic chain 10
Charcot-Marie-tooth disease 150
Cheeks 117
Chemotherapy 4
Chest
 barrel 156, 156f
 drain 180
  insertion, indications of 60
 flail 107
 funnel 156
 injuries 7
 lobes, both sides of 184f
 movement of 160
 pigeon 156
 shape of 155
 tightness 33
Chest pain 2, 49, 53
 cardiac causes of 49
 causes of 53t, 56, 57b, 58
 etiology of 49, 52
 gastrointestinal causes of 55, 56b
 musculoskeletal causes of 56
 pleuritic 36
 psychiatric causes of 56
 pulmonary causes of 52
Chest wall 208, 230
 bulging 156
 cutaneous lesions over 157
 diseases of 62
 expansion 161
 lateral 181
 subcutaneous lesions over 157
Chest X-ray 2, 45, 174, 183, 207, 240
 abnormal 172
 interpreting 174
 role of 183
Cheyne–Stokes breathing 64, 106, 106f, 155
Chloral hydrate 138
Chloroquine hydrochloride 73
Cholestasis, extrahepatic 94
Cholestatic hyperbilirubinemia 94
Chondrosarcoma 230
Chorea 151
Choreiform gait 121

Chronic cough 31-33
 evaluation of 34
Chronic fibrotic hypersensitivity pneumonitis 220, 225f
 mediastinitis 117
Chronic kidney disease 78
Chronic obstructive pulmonary disease 1, 3, 32, 53, 61, 143, 172, 200, 204
 assessment score 66f
 assessment test 66
 diagnosis of 3
Chylothorax 59, 204
 with rib, right-sided 211f
Chylous pleural effusion 58
Ciliary dyskinesia, primary 9
Cirrhosis, alcoholic 145
Clarithromycin 36
Claw hand 146
Clofazimine 242
Clubbing 87, 90, 90f
 mechanics of 88
Cobalamin 133
Cognition, disorder of 81
Coin test 167
Cold extremities 144, 145f
Collapse 40, 160
Columnar ciliated epithelium 15
Commercial kits 232
Compensation, degree of 193
Computed tomography 208
 contrast-enhanced 206
 pulmonary angiography 45
Concomitant pericardial effusion 212
Conjugated hyperbilirubinemia 93f
Conjunctiva 70, 137
Connective tissue diseases 205
Consciousness 80
Consequent pneumothorax 12
Cornea 139
Corneal arcus 139, 140f
Corneal scar 139
Cortical cataract, peripheral 138
Costophrenic angle, right-sided 182f
Cough 31, 32, 35, 36
 acute 32
 causes of 32, 32t
 chronic 31-33
 onset of 38
 prevalence of 31
 subacute 32

 tic 35
 variant asthma 34
COVID-19 pandemic 238
Crazy-paving pattern 45
Crepitation 151, 167
Cretinism 142
Curb-65 criteria 36
Cyanosis 70, 73, 74, 76, 86, 148
 age of 87
 appearance of 71f
 causes of 71, 75
 central 71-73, 74t, 86, 87f
 detection of 74
 differential 73, 87
 mixed 87
 pathophysiology of 70
 peripheral 72, 73, 74t, 86, 87f
 types of 72, 75, 86, 86t
Cycloserine 242
Cyst 223, 224
 bronchogenic 15
 carinii 172
 duplication 228
 enterogenous 15
 mediastinal 15
 neuroenteric 15, 228
 parenchymal 225f
 pericardial 15
 thymic 228
Cystic bronchiectasis 228f
Cystic fibrosis 43, 224
Cystic lung disease 225b
Cystic metastasis 225
Cytomegalovirus 126

D

D'Espine sign 167
Dantrolene 212
Dasatinib 212
Dead space 11
Debakey classification 50
Deep vein thrombosis 72
Dentistry 171
Deoxyribonucleic acid 207
Depression 244
Diabetes mellitus 238
Diabetic ketoacidosis 78
Diaphragm 13, 26, 178
 anatomy of 9
 eventration of 14
 opening of 13
 paralysis of 13, 14
Diaphragmatic defects 204
Diaphragmatic pleura, part of 10

Index

Diminished vesicular breath sound 165
Dipalmitoylphosphatidylcholine 28
Direct amplification test 232
Dithiothreitol 34
Dorsal respiratory group 28
Dorsal spine, concavity of 158
Dorsalis pedis 104*f*
Down's syndrome 119, 140, 145
Doxycycline 36
D-penicillamine 43
Drug
　anticoagulant 43
　antiplatelet 43
　anti-tubercular 235
　antituberculosis 69, 93
　classification of 243*t*
　mycobacterial 232
　overdose 72
　sensitivity test 235, 240
　toxicity 221
Dupuytren's contracture 145, 145*f*, 147
Dyspepsia, history of 85
Dyspnea 2, 3, 61-64, 69, 108, 154
　analysis of 64
　cardiac 109
　　origin of 63
　cardiovascular 63
　causes of 62
　etiology of 61
　expiratory 109
　inspiratory 109
　paroxysmal-nocturnal 109
　psychological 63
　respiratory 63
　　origin of 63
　signs of 157
　worsening 53
Dystonia 150

E

Ear 70
　nose, and throat 33, 154
Echinococcus granulosus 171
Edema 90, 92*f*
　causes of 91
　periorbital 136
　postural 91
　pulmonary 32, 180, 220, 220*f*, 221
　signs of 91, 92*f*
　symptoms of 91, 92*f*

Effusion 62
　development of 37
Ehler-Danlos syndrome 146
Electrocardiography 50
Electrolytes 197
Elicit coin sound 67
Emphysema 26, 165, 223
Empyema 12, 208
　thoracis 59
Encephalitis 14, 111
Encysted pleural fluid 184
Endemic fungi 32
Endobronchial mass, enhancing 227*f*
Endocrine 126, 142
Endotracheal tubes 180
Enophthalmos 136
Ensure trachea 177
Enterogenous cyanosis 87
Eosinophilia 205
Epigastric vessels, superior 13
Episodic wheezes 33
Epitrochlear lymphadenopathy 127
Epstein-Barr virus 126
Erythema nodosum 122, 122*f*
Erythroderma 121
Escherichia coli 171
Esophageal carcinoma 117
Esophageal rupture 55, 56, 204
Esophagitis 56
Esophagus 6
Ethambutol 238
Ewing's sarcoma 230
Exacerbations 169
Exanthems 121
Exercise 28, 34
Exophthalmos 136, 136*f*
Expectoration 31
Extramedullary hematopoiesis 228
Extrapulmonary tuberculosis 245
　management of 245
　sample for 234
Extrathoracic airway, upper 28
Extravascular origin, transudates of 204
Extrinsic disorders 200
Exudative pleural effusion 204
Eye 136
　examination of 136
　movement of 137
　partial ptosis of 157

F

Face examination 140
Facial plethora 85
Facies 140
　acromegaly 143*f*
　aortic 141
　cardiovascular 141
　cretin 143*f*
　Cushing 142, 143*f*
　Down's 141*f*
　elfin 140, 141*f*
　frog 143
　Graves' 142, 142*f*
　hatchet 141, 141*f*
　hepatic 143, 143*f*
　leonine 143
　lions 143
　marfanoid 141, 142*f*
　Marshall Hall's 143
　masked 141*f*
　metabolic 142
　mitral 141
　myasthenic 141
　myotonic 141, 142*f*
　myxedematous 142
　neurologic 140
　Potter's 140
　renal 142
　rheumatologic 142
　snarling 141
　tabetic 143
　thalassemic 143, 144*f*
Falcon tube 233, 234
Fallacy 99
Fasciculation 119
Febrile illness 24
Fetor hepaticus 78
Fever 2, 110
　drug 112
　factitious 112
　hectic 111
　high 28, 36
　intermittent 110, 111*f*
　pattern of 110
　Pel-Ebstein 110
　quartan 111, 112*f*
　quotidian 111, 112*f*
　relapsing 111
　remittent 110, 111*f*
　saddle back 110
　tertian 111, 111*f*
　vontinuous 110, 111*f*
Fiberoptic bronchoscopy 35

Fibrosis 40, 160, 168
  interstitial thickening to 220
Fibrotic sarcoidosis 220
Fibrous dysplasia 230
Fine crackles 167
Fissure 19t, 226
  surface marking of 10
  transverse 10
Fixed drug combination, number of 241t
Fluid 180, 220
  abnormal accumulations of 12
  accumulation of 90
  level, horizontal 164
  movement of 91fc
Fluorescent in situ hybridization 206
Fluoroquinolone 36
Folic acid 133
Forced vital capacity 198
Foul smell 78
  belching 78
Fungal elements 44
Furrow 120

G

Gait 120
  different types of 120
Ganglia, sympathetic 15
Ganglioneuroma 15
Gas 179
  molecules 22
Gastric tubes 180
Gastroesophageal reflux 32, 35
  disease 33, 56, 172
Gastrointestinal etiology, chest pain of 56
Gastrointestinal investigations 35
Gastrointestinal reflux disease 78
Gastrointestinal system 147
Generalized lymphadenopathy 124
  causes of 126
GeneXpert 171
Germ cell tumor 117, 228
Giant bulla 55f
Gilbert's syndrome 93
Glossitis 119
Glucose-6-phosphate dehydrogenase 93
Gorham's syndrome 211f
Gram stain 44
Granulomatous inflammation 177

Gravitational pull 22
Ground-glass 219
  opacities 45, 214f, 221, 222, 223f
Growth hormone 88
Gum 42, 118
Gun pellets lodged 176f
Gynecomastia 244

H

Haemophilus influenzae 36
Hair 151
  growth, abnormal 151, 152f
  loss 151
Haldane effect 25
Halitosis 78
Hamman's sign 168
Hand 144
  examination 144, 147, 150
Handshake 77
Hard palate 117, 144
Harsh vesicular breath sound 165
Headache 244
Heart
  borders of 178
  disease, alcohol-related 101
  failure 5, 52, 72, 77, 101
  lies 5
  rate, irregular 97
  right displacement of 186f
Heat stroke 112
Heberden's node 146, 146f, 151
Hematemesis 43t, 47
Hematologic disorders 43
Hemidiaphragm, right 178
Hemiplegic gait 120
Hemithorax 38
  movement of 57
  right 230f
    lower 230f
    upper 230f
  symmetry of 64
Hemoglobin 44, 71
  concentration 71f
  deoxygenated 25
  hereditary 87
  reduced 25
  saturating 24
Hemoptysis 42, 43t, 45, 46fc, 48, 240
  causes of 47
  massive 47
  etiology of 43
  history of 211

  management of 45
  massive 47
  severe 42
Hemorrhage 138
  control 45
  intracranial 72
  pulmonary 180, 220, 221
  retinal 139, 140f
  splinter 148f
Hemorrhagic pleural effusion 58
Hemothorax 12, 59, 205
Hepatic flap 147
Hepatic hydrothorax 212
Hepatitis 48
Hering–Breuer reflex 29
Hernia, congenital 13
Hiatus hernia 187f
Hilar points
  left 180f
  right 180f
Hilum 179
Hippocampal damage, bilateral 82
Hirsutism 151
Histamine 34
Holt–Oram syndrome 146
Honeycombing 222f
Hoover's sign 159
Horner's syndrome 136
Human chorionic gonadotropin, beta 208f
Human erythrocytes, normal 24
Human immunodeficiency virus 126, 172
  infection 238
Hutchinson's pupil 138
Hydrogen
  ions 29
  peroxide 35
Hydropneumothorax 164
Hyperbilirubinemia
  mixed 93
  unconjugated 93
Hypercapnia 26
Hypercarotenemia 124
Hyperlucency, right-sided 182f
Hyperpigmentation 124f, 145
Hyperpnea 106, 109
Hypersensitivity pneumonitis 217
Hypertension 101
  pulmonary 53
Hyperthermia 112
  malignant 112
Hyperthyroidism 77

Index

Hypertonic saline 34
Hypertrophy 118
Hyperventilation 106
Hypoechoic thickening,
  ultrasound detects 207
Hypopnea 109
Hypoproteinemia 212
Hypotension, prolonged 53
Hypothalamus 110
Hypothermia 112
Hypothyroidism 119, 244
Hypovolemia 72

I

Idiopathic interstitial
  disease 38
Idiopathic pulmonary
  fibrosis 221
  diagnosis of 2
Image reconstruction techniques
  215
Immune thrombocytopenic
  purpura 44
Immunocompromised host 172
Immunologic tests 206
Indolent infections 32
Ineffective respiratory
  movements 7
Infection 43, 214
  recurrent childhood 43
Infiltration 220
Inflammation 12, 118, 177
Infrascapular areas 161
Intercostal nerve 7
  block 7
Intercostal spaces 6
Interlobular septal thickening
  219, 220t, 223f
Intermittent fever 110, 111f
  types of 111
Interstitial lung disease 3, 32, 33,
  172, 200
Interstitial septal thickening
  225f
Intrahepatic cholestasis 94
Intralobular septal thickening
  219
Intrapulmonary airways
  structure of 17f
  subdivisions of 17f
Iris 138
Iritis 138
Iron 124

J

J receptors 30
Janeway lesion 148, 148f
Jaundice 93, 138, 138f, 144, 244
Jugular vein 113f
  external 113
  internal 113, 114f
Jugular venous pressure 113,
  114, 114t
  waveform 114, 115f
Juxtacapillary receptors 30

K

Kartagener's syndrome 9
Kayser–Fleischer ring 139, 140f
Ketones 78
Klebsiella pneumoniae 36
Koilonychia 133, 149f
Kronig's isthmus 163, 163f
Kussmaul's breathing 64
Kussmaul's sign 116
Kyphoscoliosis 62, 200
Kyphosis 83, 155

L

Lamellar effusion 182f
Langerhans cell histiocytosis
  224
Laplace's law 28
Laryngeal dyskinesia 35
Laryngopharyngeal reflux 35
Larynx 30, 154
Legionella infection 37
Lens 138
  dislocation of 137
Lesion 184
  descriptors 179
  tubercular 235
Leukonychia 135, 149f
Leukoplakia 120, 120f
Levofloxacin 36, 242
Ligament, pulmonary 11
Line probe assay 236
  application of 237
Linezolid 242
Lingular collapse, left 181f
Lipoma, low-density 187f
Lips 70, 144
Liver
  dullness 164
  function abnormalities 244

Liver abscess 212
  accidental detection of 209f
  chronic 78
  discovers 207
Lobular air trapping 225f
Lovibond's angle 88, 88f
Lower chest wall movement,
  examination of 161f
Lower limb around ankle 122f
Lower lobe 226f
  distribution 226
  right 176f, 184
Lower palpebral conjunctiva
  84, 84f
Lower respiratory
  system, examination of 154
  tract 153
Lower ribs, movement of 20
Low-pitched bronchial breath
  sound 166
Low-pleural fluid glucose 205
Lung 9
  abscess 46, 78
  anatomy of 9
  apex of 19
    malignancy of 10
  attenuation 223f
    decreased 223
    increased 221, 222t
  border of 10
    collapsed 182f
  cancer 32, 172
  collapse of 38
  compliance of 27
  diffuse fibrosis of 38
  fibrosis of 38, 168
  fluke 172
  injury, acute 27
  left 211f
  lobar distribution of 11f
  mass, left lower 186f
  movement of apex of 161
  opposite 211f
  parenchyma 21, 23, 223
  parenchymal diseases 168
    dyspnea of 62
  posterior borders of 19
  receptors 29
  segmental distribution of 11f
  surface marking of 10, 19t
  tissue 180
  volumes 175
Lymph node 177, 228, 245
  aspirate 236
  examination of 125f

Index

Lymphadenitis
  different patterns of 125
  pattern of 125*t*
Lymphadenopathy 228
Lymphangioleiomyomatosis 224, 225
Lymphangiomas 15
Lymphangitic carcinomatosis 220
Lymphatic drainage 9
Lymphatic duct, right 9
Lymphatic obstruction 92*f*
Lymphocytes, small 205
Lymphocytic interstitial pneumonia 216, 225
Lymphocytic leukemia, acute 126
Lymphocytosis 205
Lymphoma 3, 126, 127, 205, 206, 228, 229*f*
Lytic vertebral obstruction 210*f*

M

Macrocytic anemia 85
Macroglossia 119
Macule 121
Malignancy 12, 53
  tests for 206
Malignant pleural
  disease 205, 211
  thickening 209*f*
Malnutrition 128
Mannitol 34
Marcus Gunn pupil 139
Marfan's syndrome 50, 144, 148, 148*f*
Mass 121, 214
  lesions 177
Mean arterial pressure 96
Median nerve damage 150
Mediastinal adenopathy, extensive 208
Mediastinal diseases 168
Mediastinal germ cell tumors 15
Mediastinal goiters 15
Mediastinal lymphomas 15
Mediastinal mass 228*t*
  anterior 15, 208, 208*f*, 229*f*
Mediastinal percussion 165
Mediastinal tumor 117
Mediastinitis 15, 177
Mediastinum 5, 14, 20, 214, 228
  anterior 228
  borders of 178
  tumor of posterior 15

Medical Research Council Scale for Dyspnea, modified 65*b*
Mees' line 135
Meigs's syndrome 204, 212
Melanin 123
Melanoptysis 171
Memory 82
Meningoceles 228
Metabolic acidosis 21, 191, 193, 197
Metabolic alkalosis 192, 193
Metabolic disorders 43
Methacholine 34
Methemoglobin 86
Methicillin-resistant Staphylococcus aureus 172
Microbiological tests 207
Microcytic anemia 85
Microglossia 119
Mid-arm circumference 131
  measurement 132*f*
Midclavicular line 163*f*
Middle lobe syndrome 39
Middle mediastinal mass 229*f*
Middle mediastinum, tumor of 15
Miliary metastasis 219*f*
Miliary tuberculosis 218*f*
Mini-mental state examination 78
  chart 79*f*
Minimum intensity projection 215*f*
Miosis 138
Mitral valve disease 52, 101
Molecular techniques 207
Mononucleosis, infectious 126
Monophonic wheezing 166
Morphine 138
Mosaic attenuation 224
Mosaic perfusion 223, 224*f*, 224*t*
Motor neuron disease 150
Motor skills 4
Mouth 118
  dryness of 118
Mphoric breath sound 166
Mucosal glands 7
Mucus 169
Müller's muscle 157
Multiloculated pleural effusion 230*f*
Muscles 6
Music wheezy sound heard 62
Myasthenia gravis 137
Mycobacterial tests, common 236*t*

Mycobacterium tuberculosis 171, 207, 232, 234, 236
Mycoplasma pneumoniae 36
Mydriasis 139
Myocardial infarction 101
Myocardial ischemia 49
Myogenic lesions 137
Myopathic gait 121
Myopericarditis 52
Myotonic dystrophy 77

N

Nail
  bed 70
  black 135
  blue 134
  blue-red discoloration of 135
  cherry-red discoloration of 136
  different type of 133
  half-and-half 149*f*
  Lindsay 134
  movement of 89*f*
  plummer 134
  rat-bitten 134
  red 134
  terry 136
  white 134
Naked ears 62
Nasal bridge, depression of 154
Nasopharynx 30
National Sample Survey 239
National Tuberculosis Control Program 170, 238, 246
  revised 172, 238
National Tuberculosis Elimination Program 238-241, 243*t*, 247
National Tuberculosis Prevalence Survey 239
Neck
  bent backward 83
  vein, engorgement of 64
Neologism 82
Neoplasms 43
Nephropathy 244
Nerve
  root irritation 59
  sheath tumors 15
Neuritis, peripheral 244
Neuroblastoma 228
Neurofibroma 15, 228
Neurogenic tumors 15
Neurological disorder 150
Neuromuscular disease 199

Neuropathic gait 120
Neurovascular bundle 6
Neutropenia, cyclic 110
Niacin 133
Night sweats 110
Nikshay Poshan Yojana 246
Nitric oxide, exhaled breath 35
Nitrofurantoin 205, 212
Nitrogen 23
Nodular interlobular septal
    thickening 220, 220*f*
Nodule 121, 216
    centrilobular 217
        distribution of 218*f*
    distribution of 217*t*
    miliary 215*f*
    perilymphatic 216, 217
        distribution of 218
    pleural 208*f*
    random 217
        distribution of 218*f*
    tree-in-bud branching pattern
        of 218*f*
Nonasthmatic eosinophilic
    bronchitis 32, 33
Non-Hodgkin's lymphoma 127
Nonpalpable purpura 122*f*
Nonpulmonary diseases 31
Nonsteroidal anti-inflammatory
    drugs 43
Noonan's syndrome 144
Normal lung 27, 185*f*
    parenchyma 223, 224*f*
Normocytic anemia 85
Nose 30, 42, 144, 154
Nucleic acid amplification 173
    techniques 207
    test 232, 236
Nutrition 130
Nutritional risk index 131
Nystagmus 137

O

Oblique fissure 10, 19
Obstructive airway diseases 32
Obstructive apnea 107
Ocular myopathy 137
Odors 78
Oliver's sign 160
Onycholysis 135
Onychomycosis 135
Ophthalmoplegic migraine 137
Opportunistic infection 172
Oral candidiasis 119, 119*f*
Oral cavity 154
Organophosphorus 138
    poisoning, acute 169
Orthopnea 83, 109
Osler's node 148, 148*f*
Osler-Weber-Rendu syndrome
    118
Osteoarthritis 151
Osteogenesis imperfecta 138,
    138*f*
Ovarian malignancy 212
Ovarian tumors 207
Oxygen 23
    adequate supply of 30
    cascade 23
    partial pressure of 22, 24*t*
    utilization of 25
Oxyhemoglobin dissociation
    curve 25*f*

P

Palate 144
    high-arched 144, 144*f*
Pallor 84, 137
Palmar erythema 145, 145*f*, 147
Palpable purpura 44, 122*f*
Palpation 159
    superficial 159
Pancoast syndrome 10
Pancreatic pleural effusion,
    chronic 212
Pancreaticopleural fistula 204
Papule 121
Paragonimus westermani 171
Paraphasia 82
Paraplegic gait 120
Parapneumonic effusion 208
Paraseptal emphysema 225*f*
Parasternal percussion, right
    164
Parathyroid hormone 88
Paratracheal nodes 9
Parenchyma, pulmonary 214
Parenchymal lung
    abscess 208
    diseases 33, 63
Parkinson's disease 140
Parkinsonism 150
    gait 120
Paronychia 135
Paroxysmal-nocturnal
    hemoglobinuria 93
Patches 119, 119*f*
Peak expiratory flow
    measurements 34
Pectus
    carinatum 156
    excavatum 156
Pediatric pulmonary
    tuberculosis 233
Pel-Ebstein fever 110
Pemberton's sign 117
Pericardial lipoma 187*f*
Pericarditis 52
Perinuclear antineutrophilic
    cytoplasmic antibody 45
Peripancreatic collections 207
Peripheral distribution 226
Peripheral vertical column,
    right-sided 182*f*
Peroneal arterial pulse 104
Peutz-Jeghers syndrome 118
Peyronie's disease 145
Pharyngeal wall, posterior 118
Pharynx 42
Phenol 138
Phenothiazines 73
Phenytoin 93, 126
    therapy 145
Phlegm 169
Phrenic nerve 10, 13
Pigmentation 123
    around mouth 118, 118*f*
Pigtail drainage catheter
    placements 207
Plaque 121
Plasmodium
    falciparum 111
    malariae 111
Platypnea 83, 109
Pleura 11, 214, 226, 229
    anatomy of 9
    inflammation of 12
    markings of 17
    needle biopsy of 211
    surface marking of 12, 18*t*
Pleural calcification, unilateral
    230
Pleural cavity 11
Pleural diseases 168
    investigations for 204
Pleural effusion 12, 58, 68, 69,
    168, 180, 204, 208*f*, 211*f*, 230,
    230*f*
    bilateral 58
    cause of 209*f*
    chronic 230
    drug-induced 58

Index

left 210f, 230
recurrent 230
ultrasound detects 207
undiagnosed 212
Pleural fibrosis 12, 161
Pleural fluid 12, 207
- abnormal collection of 180
- amylase 206
- antinuclear antibody 206
- cytology 206
- differential 205
- eosinophilia 205
- glucose 205
- lactate dehydrogenase 204, 205
- pH 205
- protein 204

Pleural metastasis 208f
Pleural rub 167
Pleural thickening, enhancing parietal 230f
Pleurisy 5, 12, 58
Pleuritis 12, 53
Pleurodesis, indications of 60
Pneumocystis jirovecii 171
Pneumomediastinum 14, 185, 186f
- secondary 14

Pneumonia 5, 32, 37, 53, 143, 172
- chlamydia 36
- community-acquired 36
- complications of 37
- eosinophilic 226
- healthcare-associated 36
- hospital-acquired 36
- interstitial 2, 168, 220, 221, 226f
- investigate 37
- lobar 110
- management of 37
- nonspecific interstitial 220
- organizing 226
- physical signs of 37
- severe 36
- types of 36
- viral 221

Pneumonitis, acute hypersensitivity 219f
Pneumotaxic center 28
Pneumothorax 12, 20, 54, 54f, 55f, 62, 67, 69, 168, 181, 205
- diagnose 185
- recurrent 67
- spontaneous

primary 55
secondary 55
types of 67
Polycythemia 85
Polydactyly 145
Postazygos 116
Postnasal drip syndrome 32
Praxia 82
Prealbumin 132
Preazygos 116
Prematurity, apnea of 108
Pressure, difference of 26
Private sector, strategies for 246
Protein 28
Proteinuria 212
Pseudohemoptysis 42
Pseudohypertension 96
Pseudomacroglossia 119
Pseudomonas aeruginosa 36
Psychogenic cough, diagnosis of 35
Psychotic symptoms 244
Ptosis 136, 136f
Puffy face 157
Pulmonary alveolar proteinosis 223f
Pulmonary artery 216f
- catheters 180
- narrow caliber of 224f
- spirals 8

Pulmonary circulation 9, 12
Pulmonary diseases 31
- diagnosis of 171

Pulmonary embolism 5, 32, 53, 53fc, 60, 205
- management of 54fc

Pulmonary hypertension, primary 62
Pulmonary infarction 14
Pulmonary lobule, secondary 216f
Pulmonary stretch receptors 29
Pulmonary thromboembolic diseases 62
Pulmonary thromboembolism 43, 64
Pulmonary tuberculosis 171
- clinical features of 39
- sample for 233

Pulmonary vasculature 23
Pulmonary vasculitis 62
Pulmonary veins 27
Pulsation 157
Pulse 99
- collapsing 101, 102f

deficit 101
dicrotic 102, 103f
femoral 104f
oximetry 73
popliteal 103f
radial 103f
volume, high 101
wave, flow of 99f
Pulsus alternans 101, 102f
Pulsus bisferiens 102f
Pulsus paradoxus 102
Pulsus parvus et tardus 101, 102f
Pupil 138
Pus 180
Pustule 121
Putrid smell 78
Pyrexia of unknown origin 112
Pyridoxine 133

Q

Quetelet's index 130

R

Raccoon eyes 143
Radial nerve damage 150
Radiofemoral delay 103
Radiograph viewing, technique for 176
Radiological signs, common 180
Rash 244
Raynaud's disease 144
Raynaud's phenomenon 77
Recoil, loss of 26
Red blood cells 42
Renal function tests 44
Renal system 149
Respiration 104, 155
- abnormal 107
- center activity, control of 29
- cycle of 105f
- movement of 19
- pattern of 106
- regulation of 28
- types of 155

Respiratory acidosis 192
Respiratory alkalosis 193
- primary 196

Respiratory alternans 107
Respiratory bronchiolitis interstitial lung disease 217
Respiratory center 28
Respiratory compensation 197
Respiratory depth 155

Index

Respiratory diseases 21, 63
Respiratory distress syndrome 28
Respiratory dysfunction 23
Respiratory failure 75, 76
  types of 75
Respiratory medicine 1
Respiratory rate 155
Respiratory symptoms, analysis of 31
Respiratory system 5, 21, 39, 44, 149, 183
  evaluation of 153
  examination of 168
Respiratory tract 169
Rest tremor 150
Restrictive abnormalities 200
Reticular opacities, pattern of 220t
Retina 139
Retrosternal goiter 14
Retrosternal thyroid 117
Reverse D'Espine sign 167
Reverse transcriptase 236
  polymerase chain reaction 233
Rheumatoid arthritis 3, 77, 151
Rheumatoid pleural effusion 3
Rheumatological disorder 151
Rhythm 101
Rib 5
  chrondrosarcoma of 231f
  crowding of 161
  fractures 20, 31
  osteolytic lesion of 231f
Riboflavin 133
Rifampin 171, 207
Right middle lobe 184
  atelectasis 185f
  collapse, collapse of 181f
Right upper lobe 184
  consolidation 181f
Ring around artery sign 186f
Rolling hernia 14
Röntgen rays 174
Rubella 126
Rusty sputum 171

S

Saddle nose 154
Salbutamol 100
Salicylate poisoning 196
Sandwich, bald tongue of 119
Sarcoidosis 32, 53, 126, 127, 218f, 220f, 226f
Sarcopenia 128
Scalene lymphadenopathy 127
Scapula
  inferior angle of 6
  winging of 158
Schamroth's window sign 88f, 89
Schwannoma 228
Scissors gait 120
Sclera 93, 138
Scleritis 138
Scleroderma 62, 142
Sclerosis, multiple 137
Scoliosis 83, 158
Scratch sign 168
Seizures 244
Serratia marcescens 42
Serum protein 204
Severity classification 201
Short arm span, abnormal 130
Short stature 130
  disproportionate 130
  proportionate 130
  short limb 130
  short trunk 130
Shorter film-focus distance 185
Shoulder, dropping of 156f, 158
Silhouette sign 178
Silver
  deposits 134
  iodide 73
  nitrate 73
Simian crease 145, 146f
Sinus 154
  rhythm 100
Sjögren's syndrome 118, 142
Skeletal muscles 110
Skin
  discoloration of 93
  lesions 121, 157
Skinfold thickness, triceps 131, 131f
Sleep apnea 108
Sleepiness, daytime 1
Slender fingers, long 145
Sliding hernia 14
Smooth interlobular septal thickening 220, 220f
Sodium
  chloride 233
  hydroxide 171
Soft palate 117, 144
Solid glass 219
Spherocytosis 93
Sphygmomanometers 94f
Spine, examination of 158
Spirometric tests 199
Spirometry 34
  interpretation of 198, 199
  results, reporting 199
Split pleura sign 210f
Spurious cyanosis 73
Sputolysin 34
Sputum 169, 172
  analysis 169, 172
  clinical application of 171
  examination of 169, 172
  microscopic features of 170
  production 33
  sample 170
    initiating test with 234
Squint 137
  nonparalytic 137
  paralytic 137
Stagnant hypoxia 70
Stanford classification 50
Sternomastoid sign 58, 159
Sternum 5
  body of 165
Stomping gait 121
Strabismus 137
Streptococcus pneumoniae 36
Stress cardiomyopathy 52
Stridor 167
Subcapsular cataract, posterior 138
Subcostal groove 7
Subcutaneous crepitation 168
Subcutaneous emphysema 67
Subcutaneous tissue 176f
Succinylcholine anesthesia 112
Succussion splash 69, 167
Superior vena cava 43, 113f
  formation of 113f
  obstruction 3, 116
  syndrome 15, 109, 157f
Surface tension 27
Surgery 9
Swan neck 146f
  deformity 146
Sweating 145
Swyer-James syndrome 224
Sympathetic trunk 13
Syphilis, secondary 127
Systemic lupus erythematosus 32, 53, 142

T

Tachycardia
  causes of 100
  supraventricular 100
Tachypnea 106, 109
Teeth 117
Telangiectasia 44, 121
  over gum 118
Temperature pulse dissociation 112
Tender joints 151
Tendonitis 244
Tension 22
  pneumothorax 182f
Thiamine 133
Third nerve palsy 136
Thoracentesis 204
  complications of 204
Thoracic anatomy 20
Thoracic cage 5, 20
  communicates 6
  landmarks 18t
Thoracic cavity 5, 6, 14
Thoracic diseases 214
Thoracic kyphoscoliosis 156, 156f
Thoracic kyphosis 158
Thoracic movement 158
Thoracic operation, signs of 156
Thoracic outlet syndrome 6, 14
Thoracic paradox 107
Thoracocentesis 207
  indications of 60
Thoracoscopic surgery, video-assisted 69
Thorax 5, 20, 208f
  basic anatomy of 5
  clinical anatomy of 5
  clinical examination of 18t
  computed tomography scan of 54f, 214
  contrast-enhanced computed tomography 45
  examination of 64
  movement of 64
  surface marking of 17
  transverse diameter of 162f
Thumb
  fingerization of 146
  sign 148
  Z-shaped 146
Thymolipoma 228
Thymoma 15, 117, 228
Thymus 228

Thyroid
  acropachy 89
  carcinoma 9
  function tests 243
  gland 9
    enlargement of 8
  lesions 228
Thyrotoxicosis 89, 101
Tidal percussion 69, 164
Tietze's syndrome 159
Tinel's sign 147
Tongue 117, 118
  beefy red 119, 119f
  black 119
  geographic 119
  strawberry 119
Tonic-clonic seizure, generalized 72
Tonsil 117
Total lung capacity 200
Toxic fumes exposure 224
Trachea 6, 7, 30, 57, 182f
  examination of 159, 159f
  part of 7
  posterior wall of 215f
  shifting of 160
Tracheal movement 160
Tracheal position 159
Tracheal tug 160
Tracheobronchial nodes 9
Tracheobronchopathia 35
Traction bronchiectasis 222f, 227
Trail sign 159
Tram-track appearance 228f
Transmit splanchnic nerves 13
Transradiancy, increased 175
Traube's space 17, 163f, 164
  obliteration of 3
  percussion of 164
Trauma 43, 120, 145, 150, 205
Tree-in-bud
  appearance 211f
  branching pattern 217
Trepopnea 83, 109
Triglyceride, level of 205
Tuberculosis 2, 14, 32, 33, 127, 218f, 225, 229f, 230f
  active 111
  certification of elimination of 246
  classification of 240
  diagnosis of 240
    regimens of 241fc
  drug-resistant 238, 240, 243t
  drug-sensitive 241

  management of 241, 242
    drug-resistant 242
  molecular diagnosis of 232
  multi-drug-resistant 240
  notification of 245
  patients 242
  prevention treatment 245
  treatment regimens of 241fc
  uncomplicated 153
Tuberculous infections 39
Tuberculous pleural effusion 207
  diagnosis of 207
Tubular bronchiectasis 228f
Tumor 177, 180
  markers, estimation of 206
Turner syndrome 144

U

Ulcer 118, 119
  aphthous 119
  painful 119
  single nonhealing 119
Ulnar deviation 146
Ulnar nerve damage 150
Ultrasound 207
Upper airway
  cough syndrome 32
  obstruction 199, 202
Upper lobe
  branch 8
  distribution 226
Upper respiratory
  infections 32
  tract 153
    secretions 170
Uremic fetor 78
Urinary tract 44
Urine
  analysis 197
  anion gap 197
Urticaria 121
Uvula 117

V

Vagal stimulation 88
Varicose bronchiectasis 228f
Vascular disorders 43
Vasculitis 44
Vasodilators 100
Ventilation
  chemical control of 29
  maximal voluntary 201

mechanical 14
minute 26
normal minute 28
Ventilator defects 200*f*
types of 199
Ventral respiratory group 28
Ventricular tachycardia 100
Vertebral column 5, 7
Vesicle 121
Vesicular breath sound 165
Vestibular toxicity 244
Viral hepatitis 93
Viral respiratory illness, acute 34
Visceral pleura 12
Visual constructional
inability 83
Vital capacity 198
Vitamin
A 133
B1 133
B12 133
B2 133
B3 133
B6 133
B7 133
B9 133
C 133
D 133
deficiency 118, 133
E 133
fat-soluble 133*t*
K 133
water-soluble 133*t*
Vitiligo 124*f*
Vocal fremitus 161
Vocal resonance 166

W

Waist circumference 129, 129*f*
Water 174
hammer pulse 101

Wegener's granulomatosis 44
Weight gain 128, 128*b*
Weight loss 128, 128*t*
Wernicke's aphasia 81, 83
Wheeze 2, 28, 64
White patch 154
Williams-Campbell syndrome 227
Wilson's disease 134, 139
Wrist
joint, hypermobility of 146
sign 148, 148*f*
subluxation 146

X

Xanthelasma 136, 136*f*
Xanthomata 148, 149*f*
Xiphisternal joint 6
Yellow nail syndrome 135
Z-shaped thumb 146